Mechanism of Drug Action

Academic Press Rapid Manuscript Reproduction

Proceedings of a Symposium on The Biochemical Basis of
Drug Action Held at Stanford University, Stanford, California,
June 20–23, 1983

MECHANISM OF DRUG ACTION

Edited by

Thomas P. Singer

Department of Pharmaceutical Chemistry, School of Pharmacy
Department of Biochemistry and Biophysics, School of Medicine
University of California, San Francisco
and
Molecular Biology Division
Veterans Administration Hospital
San Francisco, California

Tag E. Mansour

Department of Pharmacology
Stanford University
Stanford, California

Raul N. Ondarza

Center of Ecological Research of the Southeast
San Cristobal de las Casas
Chiapas, Mexico
and
Faculty of Medicine
National Autonomous University of Mexico
Mexico City, Mexico

1983

ACADEMIC PRESS, INC

(Harcourt Brace Jovanovich, Publishers)

ORLANDO   SAN DIEGO   SAN FRANCISCO   NEW YORK   LONDON
TORONTO   MONTREAL   SYDNEY   TOKYO   SÃO PAULO

ACADEMIC PRESS, INC.
Orlando, Florida 32887

United Kingdom Edition published by
ACADEMIC PRESS, INC. (LONDON) LTD.
24/28 Oval Road, London NW1   7DX

Library of Congress Cataloging in Publication Data

Symposium on the Biochemical Basis of Drug Action (1983 :
    Stanford University)
    Mechanism of drug action.

    Includes index.
    1. Pharmacology--Congresses. 2. Biological chemistry--
Congresses. I. Singer, Thomas Peter, Date.
II. Mansour, Tag. III. Ondarza, Raul N. IV. Title.
RM301.S9386   1983   615'.7   83–22362
ISBN 0–12–646680–7 (alk. paper)

PRINTED IN THE UNITED STATES OF AMERICA

83 84 85 86   9 8 7 6 5 4 3 2 1

CONTENTS

I RECEPTORS

II MOLECULAR AND GENETIC ANALYSIS OF DRUG ACTION

III ANTIPARASITIC AGENTS

IV PROSTAGLANDINS AND LEUKOTRIENES

V BIOCHEMICAL BASIS OF THE ACTION OF TOXIC SUBSTANCES

VI   CNS-DIRECTED AGENTS

CONTRIBUTORS

Numbers in parentheses indicate the pages on which the authors' contributions begin.

George K. Aghajanian (375), *Departments of Psychiatry and Pharmacology, Yale University School of Medicine, New Haven, Connecticut 06508*

James W. Apriletti (79), *The Metabolic Research Unit, and The Departments of Medicine and Biochemistry and Biophysics, University of California, San Francisco, California 94143*

Christian Auclair (305), *Laboratoire de Biochimie, Institut Gustave Roussy, Villejuif, France*

Cyrus J. Bacchi (159), *Haskins Laboratories, and Department of Biology, Pace University, New York, New York*

John D. Baxter (79), *The Metabolic Research Unit, and The Departments of Medicine and Biochemistry and Biophysics, University of California, San Francisco, California 94143*

James L. Bennett (187), *Department of Phamacology and Toxicology, Michigan State University, East Lansing, Michigan*

Stephen Beverley (107), *The Department of Biological Sciences, Stanford University, Stanford, California 94305*

Nigel J. M. Birdsall (27), *Division of Molecular Pharmacology, National Institute for Medical Research, Mill Hill, London, United Kingdom*

Morris J. Birnbaum (79), *The Metabolic Research Unit, and The Departments of Medicine and Biochemistry and Biophysics, University of California, San Francisco, California 94143*

Arthur J. Blume (341), *Department of Physiological Chemistry and Pharmacology, Roche Institute of Molecular Biology, Roche Research Center, Nutley, New Jersey 07110*

Peter Brown (107), *The Department of Biological Sciences, Stanford University, Stanford, California 94305*

Marc G. Caron (37), *Howard Hughes Medical Institute, Departments of Medicine (Cardiology), Biochemistry, and Physiology, Duke University Medical Center, Durham, North Carolina*

Richard Cassin (107), *The Department of Biological Sciences, Stanford University, Stanford, California 94305*

Anthony Cerami (175), *Laboratory of Medical Biochemistry, The Rockefeller University, New York, New York*

Alger Chapman (91), *Department of Pharmacology, Stanford University, Stanford, California*

Maureen Costello (91), *Department of Pharmacology, Stanford University, Stanford, California*

Paul Culver (9), *Division of Pharmacology, Department of Medicine, University of California, San Diego, La Jolla, California 92093*

John W. Daly (351), *Laboratory of Bioorganic Chemistry, National Institute of Arthritis, Diabetes, and Digestive and Kidney Diseases, National Institutes of Health, Bethesda, Maryland*

Deborah Dobson (91), *Department of Pharmacology, Stanford University, Stanford, California*

Norman L. Eberhardt (79), *The Metabolic Research Unit, and The Departments of Medicine and Biochemistry and Biophysics, University of California, San Francisco, California 94143*

Pedro A. Lehmann F. (61), *Departamento de Farmacología y Toxicología, Centro de Investigación y Estudios Avanzados, Instituto Politécnico Nacional, México D. F., México*

Nancy Federspiel (107), *The Department of Biological Sciences, Stanford University, Stanford, California 94305*

Peter H. Fishman (363), *Membrane Biochemistry Section, Developmental and Metabolic Neurology Branch, National Institute of Neurological and Communicative Disorders and Stroke, National Institutes of Health, Bethesda, Maryland*

Barbara Fox (317), *Departments of Biology and Chemistry, Massachusetts Institute of Technology, Cambridge, Massachusetts 02139*

F. Friedman (259), *Laboratory of Molecular Carcinogenesis, National Cancer Institute, National Institute of Health, Bethesda, Maryland 20205*

T. Fujino (259), *Laboratory of Molecular Carcinogenesis, National Cancer Institute, National Institute of Health, Bethesda, Maryland 20205*

Donna Galeazzi (327), *Department of Pharmacology, Stanford University School of Medicine, Stanford, California*

David G. Gardner (79), *The Metabolic Research Unit, and The Departments of Medicine and Biochemistry and Biophysics, University of California, San Francisco, California 94143*

Charles Gasser (107), *The Department of Biological Sciences, Stanford University, Stanford, California 94305*

H. V. Gelboin (259), *Laboratory of Molecular Carcinogenesis, National Cancer Institute, National Institutes of Health, Bethesda, Maryland 20205*

Edward J. Goetzl (221), *Howard Hughes Medical Institute Laboratories, and Division of Allergy and Immunology, University of California, San Francisco, California*

Daniel W. Goldman (221), *Howard Hughes Medical Institute Laboratories, and Division of Allergy and Immunology, University of California, San Francisco, California*

Avram Goldstein (49), *Addiction Research Foundation, and Stanford University, Palo Alto, California*

J. Russell Grove (91), *Department of Pharmacology, Stanford Unviersity, Stanford, California*

Carol Hall[1] (91), *Department of Pharmacology, Stanford University, Stanford, California*

Anna Hill (107), *The Department of Biological Sciences, Stanford University, Stanford, California 94305*

Edward C. Hulme (27), *Division of Molecular Pharmacology, National Institute for Medical Research, Mill Hill, London, United Kingdom*

Robert B. Innis (375), *Departments of Psychiatry and Pharmacology, Yale University School of Medicine, New Haven, Connecticut 06508*

David Israel (327), *Department of Pharmacology, Stanford University School of Medicine, Stanford, California*

Iain F. James (49), *Addiction Research Foundation, and Stanford University, Palo Alto, California*

Kenneth D. Jenkins (277), *Department of Biology, California State University, Long Beach, California*

David A. Johnson (9), *Division of Pharmacology, Department of Medicine, University of California, San Diego, La Jolla, California 92093*

Randal Johnston (107), *The Department of Biological Sciences, Stanford University, Stanford, California 94305*

Michael Karlin[2] (79), *The Metabolic Research Unit, and The Departments of Medicine and Biochemistry and Biophysics, University of California, San Francisco, California 94143*

Nancy C. Lan (79), *The Metabolic Research Unit, and The Departments of Medicine and Biochemistry and Biophysics, University of California, San Francisco, California 94143*

Frank Lee[3] (91), *Department of Pharmacology, Stanford University, Stanford, California*

Rober J. Lefkowitz (37), *Howard Hughes Medical Institute, Departments of Medicine (Cardiology), Biochemistry and Physiology, Duke University Medical Center, Durham, North Carolina*

Tag E. Mansour (197), *Department of Pharmacology, Stanford University, Stanford, California*

[1]*Present address: DNAX Research Institute, Palo Alto, California.*

[2]*Present address: Department of Microbiology, School of Medicine, University of Southern California, Los Angeles, California 90023.*

[3]*Present address: DNAX Research Institute, Palo Alto, California.*

Brian Mariani (107), *The Department of Biological Sciences, Stanford University, Stanford, California 94305*

J. Joseph Marr [4] (147), *Division of Infectious Diseases, Departments of Medicine and Microbiology, University of Colorado Health Sciences Center, Denver, Colorado*

Peter P. McCann (159), *Merrell Dow Research Center, Cincinnati, Ohio*

Synthia H. Mellon (79), *The Metabolic Research Unit, and The Departments of Medicine and Biochemistry and Biophysics, University of California, San Francisco, California 94143*

Bernard Meunier[5] (305), *Laboratoire de Pharmacologie et Toxicologie Fondamentales CNRS, Toulouse, France*

Arthur G. Miller[6] (327), *Department of Pharmacology, Stanford University School of Medicine, Stanford, California*

S. Moncada (209, 229), *Wellcome Research Laboratories, Langley Court, Beckenham, Kent BR3 3BS, United Kingdom*

Joel Moss (289), *National Heart, Lung, and Blood Institute, National Institutes of Health, Bethesda, Maryland*

Elise Mosse (107), *The Department of Biological Sciences, Stanford University, Stanford, California 94305*

K. M. Mullane (229), *Department of Prostaglandin Research, Wellcome Research Laboratories, Langley Court, Beckenham, Kent BR3 3BS, United Kingdom, and Department of Pharmacology, New York Medical College, Valhalla, New York*

Henry C. Nathan (159), *Haskins Laboratories, and Department of Biology, Pace University, New York, New York*

Fred R. Opperdoes (121), *Research Unit for Tropical Diseases, International Institute of Cellular and Molecular Pathology, Brussels, Belgium*

Claude Paoletti (305), *Laboratoire de Biochimie, Institut Gustave Roussy, Villejuif, France*

S. S. Park (259), *Laboratory of Molecular Carcinogenesis, National Cancer Institute, National Institutes of Health, Bethesda, Maryland 20205*

Ralph A. Pax (187), *Department of Zoology and Neuroscience Program, Michigan State University, East Lansing, Michigan*

Donald G. Payan (221), *Howard Hughes Medical Institute Laboratories, and Division of Allergy and Immunology, University of California, San Francisco, California*

Heidi Rath (107), *The Department of Biological Sciences, Stanford University, Stanford, California 94305*

Gordon Ringold (91), *Department of Pharmacology, Stanford University, Stanford California*

[4]*Present address: Division of Infectious Diseases B-168, University of Colorado Health Sciences Center, 4200 E. 9th Avenue, Denver, Colorado 80262.*

[5]*Present address: Laboratoire de Chimie de Coordination CNRS, Toulouse, France.*

[6]*Present address: The Salk Institute, San Diego, California.*

D. Robinson (259), *Laboratory of Molecular Carcinogenesis, National Cancer Institute, National Institutes of Health, Bethesda, Maryland 20205*

Brenda M. Sanders (277), *Duke University Marine Laboratory, Beaufort, North Carolina*

Robert T. Schimke (107), *The Department of Biological Sciences, Stanford University, Stanford, California 94305*

Steven M. Sine[7] (9), *Division of Pharmacology, Department of Medicine, University of California, San Diego, La Jolla, California 92093*

Albert Sjoerdsma (159), *Merrell Dow Research Center, Cincinnati, Ohio*

Emily P. Slater (79), *The Metabolic Research Unit, and The Departments of Medicine and Biochemistry and Biophysics, University of California, San Francisco, California 94143*

David Smouse (107), *The Department of Biological Sciences, Stanford University, Stanford, California 94305*

B. J. Song (259), *Laboratory of Molecular Carcinogenesis, National Cancer Institute, National Institutes of Health, Bethesda, Maryland 20205*

Gary L. Stiles (37), *Howard Hughes Medical Institute, Departments of Medicine (Cardiology), Biochemistry and Physiology, Duke University Medical Center, Durham, North Carolina*

Jane M. Stockton (27), *Division of Molecular Pharmacology, National Institute for Medical Research, Mill Hill, London, United Kingdom*

William G. Sunda (277), *National Marine Fisheries Service, NOAA, Southeast Fisheries Center, Beaufort Laboratory, Beaufort, North Carolina*

John F. Tallman (387), *Department of Psychiatry and Pharmacology, Connecticut Mental Health Center, Yale University School of Medicine, New Haven, Connecticut 06508*

Palmer Taylor (9), *Division of Pharmacology, Department of Medicine, University of California, San Diego, La Jolla, California 92093*

David P. Thompson (187), *Department of Zoology and Neuroscience Program, Michigan State University, East Lansing, Michigan*

Thea Tlsty (107), *The Department of Biological Sciences, Stanford University, Stanford, California 94305*

J. R. Vane (209), *Wellcome Research Laboratories, Langley Court, Beckenham, Kent BR3 3BS, United Kingdom*

James Vannice (91), *Department of Pharmacology, Stanford Unviersity, Stanford, California*

Martha Vaughan (289), *National Heart, Lung, and Blood Institute, National Institutes of Health, Bethesda, Maryland*

Christopher Walsh (317), *Departments of Biology and Chemistry, Massachusetts Institute of Technology, Cambridge, Massachusetts 02139*

Ching Chung Wang (133), *Department of Pharmaceutical Chemistry, University of California, School of Pharmacy, San Francisco, California*

---

[7]*Present address: Neurobiology Group, The Salk Institute, San Diego, California 92138.*

Allessandro Weisz (79), *The Metabolic Research Unit, and The Departments of Medicine and Biochemistry and Biophysics, University of California, San Francisco, California 94143*

Babette B. Weksler (243), *Division of Hematology-Oncology, Department of Medicine, Cornell University Medical College, New York, New York 10021*

James P. Whitlock, Jr. (327), *Department of Pharmacology, Stanford University School of Medicine, Stanford, California*

Erik H. F. Wong (27), *Department of Biochemistry, University of California, Riverside, California*

PREFACE

The discovery of therapeutically useful classes of drugs has been largely accidental. New pharmacological agents are developed through modification of already known drugs. This type of approach was forced on us by limitations in our knowledge of the pathophysiology of disease processes and lack of detail with regard to the chemistry of enzymes and receptor proteins. Recent conceptual advances in enzymology, protein chemistry, molecular biology, and medicine, as well as the discovery of new mediators of physiological functions, indicate that it is possible now to approach directly the problem of designing useful drugs. Fusing of ideas in the above disciplines indicates not only that drugs can be designed for specific purposes, but that such drugs will have fewer side effects and greater ratios of efficacy to toxicity than any now available. The knowledge required for rational design of therapeutic agents is at the frontier of every established discipline that relates to the life sciences. Only a few scientists, however, have seen the value for society in bringing these diciplines to bear on the common problem of designing drugs ''from the ground up.'' It is important, we believe, to bring together scientists interested in the development of drugs not only to discuss what has been learned but to see what can be accomplished. This will require interaction between disciplines that normally do not communicate with each other.

The First International Symposium on the Molecular Basis of Drug Action, which took place in Queretaro, Mexico, in 1980, was organized to achieve this purpose and to bring together scientists from a diversity of disciplines who have as common goals the elucidation of rational approaches to the development of therapeutic agents.

The reaction of the participants to that meeting was most gratifying. In fact, two of us (Raul N. Ondarza and Thomas P. Singer), who organized the symposium, were urged by many of the participants to hold a second symposium on the subject in 1983. Although the prospects of obtaining adequate funding for the meeting in the economic climate of 1981–1982 did not seem bright, the rapid advances in the area covered in the first sympsoium and the plethora of important subjects on the cutting edge of biochemical pharmacology that were not covered prompted us to go ahead with it. When Tag E. Mansour agreed to join the original team of joint chairmen, the splendid facilities of the Stanford Campus became available. An organizing committee was selected consisting of Jere E. Goyan, Christopher Walsh,

C. C. Wang (who acted as Secretary–Treasurer), David Zakim, and the three Joint Chairmen, T. E. Mansour, R. N. Ondarza, and T. P. Singer. One of the first actions of the committee was the decision to include a session on biochemical toxicology, which seemed conceptually closely interrelated with the biochemical basis of drug action, in fact, often an integral part of it.

Sponsorship and initial funding for the meeting were provided by the symposium committee of the International Union of Biochemistry, for which the organizers are grateful. Without the generous support of industry, however, the symposium could not have taken place. We wish to express our special thanks to the following industrial sponsors: Abbott Laboratories, Allergan Pharmaceuticals, Barnes-Hind Pharmaceuticals, Inc., Ciba-Geigy Corporation, E. I. Dupont de Nemours & Company, Inc., Hoffman-La Roche, Inc., ICI Americas, Inc., Instrumentation Specialties Company, Merck & Company, Inc., Merrell Dow Pharmaceuticals, Inc., Smith-Kline Beckman Corporation, Sterling-Winthrop Research Institute, Syntex USA, Inc.

We also wish to convey our warm gratidute to Mrs. Nancy Schonher, who was responsible for all the local arrangements and the smooth running of the symposium. In the final analysis, however, the success of every scientific meeting hinges primarily on the quality of the presentations. And these, as we trust the readers will agree, were almost uniformly excellent.

THE EDITORS

LISTS OF SPONSORS

International Union of Biochemistry
Stanford University School of Medicine
School of Pharmacy, University of California, San Francisco
Abbott Laboratories
Allergan Pharmaceuticals
Barnes-Hind Pharmaceuticals, Inc.
Ciba-Geigy Corporation
E. I. Dupont de Nemours & Company, Inc.
Hoffman-La Roche, Inc.
ICI Americas, Inc.
Instrumentation Specialties Company
Merck & Company, Inc.
Merrell Dow Pharmaceuticals, Inc.
Smith-Kline Beckman Corporation
Sterling-Winthrop Research Institute
Syntex USA, Inc.

ORGANIZING COMMITTEE

Jere E. Goyan
T. E. Mansour, *Joint Chairman*
R. N. Ondarza, *Joint Chairman*
T. P. Singer, *Joint Chairman*
Christopher Walsh
C. C. Wang, *Secretary-Treasurer*
David Zakim

Mechanism of Drug Action

THE SCIENTIST'S BURDEN

Jere E. Goyan[*]

In the past several weeks grave concern about the state of
education in the United States has been expressed in many
quarters. In particular, the National Committee on Excellence
in Education, in its report entitled "A Nation at Risk,"
reports "...that while we can take justifiable pride in what
our schools and colleges have historically accomplished and
contributed to the United States and the well-being of its
people, the educational foundations of our society are presently being eroded by a rising tide of mediocrity that
threatens our very future as a Nation and a people." It went
on to note, "If an unfriendly foreign power had attempted to
impose on America the mediocre educational performance that
exists today, we might well have viewed it as an act of war."

I certainly agree with all of this concern and "gnashing
of teeth" and believe that if the situation is bad in the
humanities, it is disastrous in the sciences. Dr. David
Saxon, immediate past president of the University of California, put it well in a recent speech in which he noted: "Simply
stated, the problem is that we are unable, as a society, to
distinguish between sense and nonsense when it comes to
science. The problem is that educated, intelligent, inquisi-
tive people are unable consistently to bring informed judgment
to bear on questions connected in almost any way to science
and technology, questions often vital to the welfare of each
of us and indeed to the future of the world.... A liberal
education should provide just that critical sense which makes
it possible to winnow out the meretricious from the meritori-
ous. Yet, many liberally educated people are unable to do
anything of the sort when it comes to science and technology."

---

[*]Keynote address delivered by Dean Goyan, School of Pharmacy,
University of California, San Francisco, and former
Commissioner of the Food and Drug Administration.

The reasons for this lack of scientific understanding by
the public are undoubtedly complex, but certainly related to
our educational system. One reason was recently elucidated in
an article in Science by Dr. Lauren Resnick who noted that
"...all students, the weak as well as the strong learners,
come to their first science classes with surprisingly
extensive theories about how the natural world works. They
use these 'naive' theories to explain real world events before
they have had any science instruction. Then, even after
instruction in new concepts in scientifically supported
theories, they still resort to their prior theories to solve
any problems that vary from their textbook examples."

It is argued by some that such "naive" theories and
beliefs are a matter of only individual concern and should not
concern society. I do not believe that, because many value
decisions profoundly affecting our society as a whole depend
on at least some understanding of scientific principles.

For example, the Merrell Dow Corporation recently found it
necessary to remove the anti-nauseant drug Bendectin from the
market, apparently because of its concern that insurance and
court costs in the coming year would be greater than any
potential profit. Thus, a decision about the safety of the
drug has been made not by the scientific community nor even
the regulatory community represented by the FDA, but rather by
a series of lay people sitting as members of juries across our
land. There is nothing inherently wrong in that process,
except that few individuals sitting on such juries have any
understanding of the niceties of epidemiologic research which
would be necessary to make informed decisions about the probability that the drug was responsible for the birth defect that
led to the lawsuit. The outcome is thus to remove from the
market the only anti-nauseant drug available for use in severe
"morning sickness," to a large degree based on the "naive"
theories of the lay public.

Before we go too far in damning education for the scientific illiteracy of our population, it would be well to consider the role of some other parts of our society. First, let
us consider the role of industry. When the FDA proposed to
ban saccharin, based on the Delaney Clause which indicates
that no food additive can be approved that has been found to
cause cancer in man or animal, the furor heard around the land
was quite incredible. In particular, the Calorie Council, a
creature of the soft drink industry, saw fit to take out full
page ads in newspapers throughout the Nation, showing literally hundreds of soda pop cans and indicating that an individual would have to drink that many in order to receive the
same dose that laboratory rats had received in the Canadian
studies which demonstrated that saccharin is an animal carcinogen. Entirely lost in the rhetoric was the scientific

validity of high-dose testing for carcinogens.

The proprietary drug industry has also mounted a number of "educational" efforts, primarily on TV. The outcome of which is that there are millions of people who do not know that the active ingredient in Anacin is aspirin, a simple fact not mentioned once in the $27.5 million its makers spent on advertisements in 1981. There are as many who still believe that mouth washes cure or prevent colds, who resort to ineffective topical anesthetics for relief of sunburn, who are convinced that alkalinizers mixed with aspirin are good for upset stomach, and who believe that the best cold products are the ones that contain the most ingredients. They are naive on a grand scale but not by accident and certainly not cheaply. It cost millions to misinform them for which they, in turn, pay billions and in so doing expose themselves to the hazards of drugs, for many of which there is little if any benefit, only potential adverse effects.

Much has been said and written about proprietary drug hucksterism over the years, but re-education of the misinformed is a slow process because deep-seated beliefs yield slowly to truth, and because slick advertisements have greater access to the population than do the critics or educators, one need only twist the knob to obtain a fresh supply. (I am able to contain my enthusiasm for prescription drug advertising directly to the public by the same people!)

Advertising is an effective educational "tool" even with those who are supposedly scientifically trained. For example, in a recent article, Avorn et al. found that 71 percent of physicians in a random survey in the Boston area believed that senile dementia is related to inadequate cerebral blood flow, and 80 percent believed that Darvon was equal to or greater than aspirin in its analgesic potency. Both such beliefs are congruent with commercial information but totally at odds with the scientific literature.

While talking about advertising, perhaps we should spend a little time considering the role of the media in general. I recently was on a television program and the host asked me why the FDA had approved the drug Cimetadine with its unfortunate anti-androgenic side effects? I hope that I was able to persuade him and at least a few of the viewers that the FDA's decision was a proper one, based on the benefit to risk ratio, for this the first truly effective drug for use in ulcer therapy. One could, of course, go on for some time with other examples such as the 60-Minute segment on dimethylsulfoxide which resulted in a veritable frenzy of people attempting to get the drug to "cure" their arthritis, a hope foreordained to disappointment.

Unfortunately, I must also note the role of government in encouraging scientific illiteracy. Recently, the FTC modified

its 1974 consent order with the manufacturer of Lysol brand
disinfectant to allow claims that environmental surfaces play
a significant role in the transmission of colds. In a separate statement, Commissioner Michael Pertschuk noted: "The
primary piece of evidence which Sterling cites is a study,
partly funded by Sterling, conducted by two eminent scientists
at the University of Virginia. They directed volunteers with
colds to blow their noses on their hands and wipe them on some
plastic tiles. Ten minutes later, some tiles were given a
three-second shot of Lysol; other were not. After fifteen
minutes, healthy volunteers were directed to rub their fingers
on the tiles and then pick their noses and rub their eyes. Lo
and behold, about half of the healthy volunteers touching the
tiles got colds; fewer got colds from touching the tiles that
had been sprayed with Lysol, although the results were not
statistically significant." Imagine, serious government
regulatory decisions are being made on the basis of such
results!

With all of the misinformation and poor, if not wretched
science being promulgated on our citizenry, how do we prevent
the American people from becoming a bunch of present-day
scientific Luddites? In 1884, Lord Raleigh said, "Men who
devote their lives to investigation cultivate a love of truth
for its own sake, and endeavor instinctively to clear up, and
not, as is too often the object in business and politics, to
obscure a difficult question." Thus, I believe that those of
us who have had the privilege of a scientific education must,
and I emphasize must, accept the attendant responsibility of
public commitment. That is, we must each be willing to "stand
up" and be counted relative to the many debates whose outcomes
are influenced by scientific or pseudo-scientific arguments.
This responsibility is often a burden but is, I believe, our
best hope of avoiding total disillusionment of the public with
science.

As an illustration, I have been concerned for some time
about the use of subtherapeutic doses of antibiotics in animal
feeds because of the potential for compromise of human drug
therapy. It is my belief that industrial sponsors have not
met their statutory burden to show the relevant uses to be
safe. Unfortunately, industrial sponsors have been able to
convince Congress that the lack of direct evidence -- that
specific resistant bacteria selected by antibiotic feeding
were transferred from specific animals to specific humans
where they were the cause of untreatable disease -- makes
discontinuance of this use unnecessary and undesirable.
Almost all of the evidence is epidemiological and thus, in a
sense, circumstantial. I might add that Thoreau, referring to
the practice of watering milk, once observed that "some circumstantial evidence is very strong, as when you find a trout

in the milk." Thus, I am at present serving as chairman of a committee of the Natural Resources Defense Council, which is attempting to bring this potential problem to the attention of the Congress and the American people.

My purpose today is not to ask you to join with me in this effort but rather to suggest that each of you should play some pro bono publico role in matters of public debate, especially those which have some scientific basis. Of course, some of you will be concerned about all of the potential risks such as being seen as a "popularizer" by your peers, being misquoted in newspapers, etc. I would like to try to allay such fears by noting that most of your peers will not read the popular articles anyway, and anyone who has had any experience with the press knows that being misquoted is only a minor hazard. I would also note that many of my friends who have left the halls of academe to take part in high technology industrial enterprises seem to have lost their former reticence when it comes to speaking out on scientific matters, especially those that affect the performance of their stock! On the other hand, I would like to underscore the single most rewarding benefit, the good feeling that comes from doing something which you know is in the best interest not only of yourself but of your fellowman. It is my fond hope that if you do not choose to accept my challenge, you at least will accept a slight feeling of guilt for not doing so!

I   RECEPTORS

THE COUPLING BETWEEN LIGAND OCCUPATION AND RESPONSE

OF THE NICOTINIC ACETYLCHOLINE RECEPTOR:

CORRELATIONS WITH RECEPTOR STRUCTURE[1]

Palmer Taylor
Paul Culver
Steven M. Sine[2]
David A. Johnson

Division of Pharmacology
Department of Medicine
University of California, San Diego
La Jolla, California 92093

Simultaneous measurements in intact cells of receptor
occupation and the change in ion permeability elicited by
the ligands enable one to define the linkage between
agonist association and activation of the ion channel of
the nicotinic acetylcholine receptor. The irreversible
antagonists, cobra α-toxin and lophotoxin, have been
employed to inactivate a specified number of sites on the
receptor and the residual responses to agonist compared
with those of native receptor. The receptor behaves
effectively as a cooperative dimer. Two agonist molecules
are required for activation while a single bound antagonist is sufficient to block the response of the receptor
oligomer. The two agonist binding sites on the oligomer
do not show precise equivalence in the binding of reversible ligands and lophotoxin. Such an inequivalence would
be expected from the arrangement of the five subunits of
this protein in the membrane.

[1]Supported by grants GM 24307 and GM 18360 from the
National Institutes of Health.
[2]Present address: Neurobiology Group, The Salk Institute,
San Diego, CA 92138

I. INTRODUCTION

Studies of the acetylcholine receptor from the neuromuscular junction have been directed primarily to the permeability changes resulting from activation by agonists and to the structure of the receptor in relation to properties of ligand association. The excellent temporal resolution of electrophysiologic studies has permitted definition of primary events of channel opening and closing associated with receptor activation (1), while the abundant quantities of receptor that can be isolated from the electric fish have facilitated the characterization of the molecular structure of the receptor (2-4). With our knowledge of the structure and the electrophysiology of the receptor developing to an advanced stage, it becomes important to understand the precise relationship between ligand association with the receptor and the attendant activation or antagonism of the functional event. To approach this fundamental question, we have employed a mammalian muscle cell line, BC3H-1 (5). Being a clonal cell line which grows to a confluent monolayer and subsequently elaborates diffusely distributed receptors on the cell surface, the system provides a homogeneous population of cells to which equivalent exposure of ligand can be achieved. Thus, ligand occupation of the receptor and the resulting change in permeability can be simultaneously monitored. Quantitation of permeability relationships requires that the measured ion flux be proportional to the number of receptors activated and constant over the interval of measurement. Under conditions which limit desensitization of the receptor response, it may be possible to approach these criteria in the intact cell.

Experiments directed to occupation-response relationships in intact cells possess a number of potential advantages: First, receptor densities in BC3H-1 cells are comparatively low and the internal volume of the cell is large, hence measurements of initial rates of influx can be achieved over periods of several seconds rather than being restricted to a millisecond time frame. Second, since the cell line is derived from a single precursor cell and a relatively uniform cell shape is achieved at confluence, the variance in rate of approach to equilibrium that could result from structures with a wide distribution of internal volumes relative to the membrane surface area is minimized. Third, permeability is measured by an inward directional flux of external Na^+ and it is this permeability change that is primarily responsible for the conductance seen <u>in situ</u>. Lastly, although the receptors on BC3H-1 cells desensitize rapidly, the allosteric constant which governs the fraction of receptors in the desensitized state is heavily weighted towards the activatable state

(10,000 to 1) (6). Hence, even with prolonged exposure to agonists desensitization does not result in complete inactivation of the receptor nor can an initial burst of influx be detected when measurements are monitored over 20-60 second intervals.

II. MEASUREMENTS OF LIGAND OCCUPATION AND RECEPTOR ACTIVATION IN INTACT CELLS

Ligand occupation can be ascertained from its capacity to inhibit the initial rate of cobra α-toxin association with surface receptors on the intact cell. The low receptor densities in the BC3H-1 cells preclude direct measurements of agonist binding and hence require a competition assay with a high affinity ligand. By relying on competition with an initial rate rather than equilibration of competing ligands, such measurements may be completed within a 15-30 second time frame. There is substantial evidence in the Torpedo receptor, where receptor concentrations are high and ligand association can be measured directly, that competition with the initial rate of α-toxin binding provides a satisfactory means for quantitating ligand occupation (7,8). Initial rates of $^{22}Na^+$ influx can also be monitored over the same time interval. To ensure that permeability is not affected by changes in membrane potential associated with channel opening, measurements are conducted with a depolarizing medium containing 140 mM K^+ and 18 mM Na^+. Hence, membrane potentials should approach zero and net movements of the prevailing current carrying ions are small. Under such circumstances unidirectional fluxes are ascertained with tracer quantities of $^{22}Na^+$. When initial rates of influx are measured at 3°C and over short time intervals (15-30 s), a significant portion of the dose-response relationship can be generated without appreciable interference from receptor desensitization.

III. MEASUREMENT OF RECEPTOR ACTIVATION AND OCCUPATION

Figure 1a shows the kinetics of $^{22}Na^+$ influx into the cell under conditions of immediate exposure to agonist and where desensitization has been achieved by prior exposure to agonist. A slow desensitization step is illustrated here since, following instantaneous exposure to agonist, the rate constant for $^{22}Na^+$ influx shows a gradual decrement until it approaches the influx rate constant seen with 30 min prior exposure to

agonist. Previous studies have demonstrated that a slow
conversion from the ligand-associated activatable (and active)

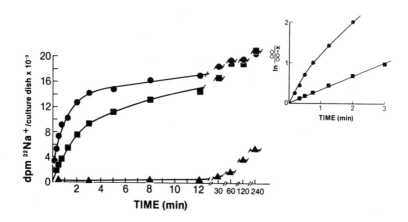

FIGURE 1A. $^{22}Na^{+}$ influx elicited by 100 µM carbamylcholine at
3.5°C. Cells were cooled slowly to 3.5°C and incubated for
30 min in the presence or absence of 100 µM carbamylcholine.
Influx of tracer $^{22}Na^{+}$ elicited by 100 µM carbamylcholine was
monitored for the durations indicated: ● , influx in the presence of carbamylcholine when cells were previously incubated
in buffer for 30 min; ■ , influx in the presence of carbamylcholine when cells were previously exposed to 100 µM carbamylcholine for 30 min; ▲ , influx in the presence of carbamylcholine monitored in cells initially incubated with α-toxin
(0.5 µM) for 20 min. <u>Inset</u>, first-order plot of specific
influx where the contribution of the slow phase of uptake has
been eliminated, providing kinetics of $^{22}Na^{+}$ exchange between
extracellular and freely exchangeable intracellular volumes, x
is the influx determined in the interval, t, and ∞ is the
equilibrium influx value corresponding to the capacity of the
freely exchangeable internal volume (61% of uptake achieved in
4 h) (10).

states which are characterized by low agonist affinities to a
non-responsive, high affinity state is responsible for
desensitization (7-9).

Initial studies established that association of the
essentially irreversible antagonist, cobra α-toxin, with
surface receptors behaved as a bimolecular reaction in intact
BC3H-1 cells (Fig. 1b). Agonists and reversible antagonists

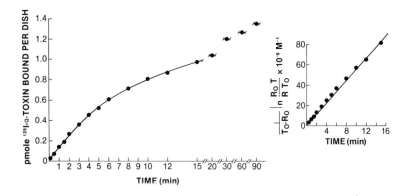

FIGURE 1B. Kinetics of association between ^{125}I-labelled α-toxin and surface receptors on BC3H-1 cells. Cells were rinsed and equilibrated in assay buffer at 21°C and incubated with ^{125}I-labelled α-toxin (17.5 nM) for the specified intervals. Non-specific binding determined in the presence of 3 mM carbamylcholine has been subtracted. Inset, second-order plot of specific binding to surface receptors according to the bimolecular rate equation. Linear regression of these data reveals a bimolecular rate constant, k_T, of $1.04 \times 10^5 M^{-1} s^{-1}$. Cells in this experiment were also examined for functional capacity and actually correspond to the data in Fig. 2(c).

competitively inhibit the binding reaction and the bimolecular kinetics demonstrate that each site associates equivalently with α-toxin and access to the sites is not limited by diffusional barriers (9,10). Thus, agonist and antagonist occupation can be measured by their capacities to inhibit the initial rate of [125I]α-toxin binding to the intact cells.

IV. IRREVERSIBLE INACTIVATION OF AGONIST-ANTAGONIST SITES ON THE RECEPTOR

It has long been known that the peptide α-toxins isolated from snake venoms bind with high affinity to the nicotinic acetylcholine receptor and that their dissociation rates are sufficiently slow that α-toxin association can be treated as an irreversible process. More recently, a toxin from coral, lophotoxin, has been shown to inactivate the receptor irreversibly (11). Unlike the peptide α-toxins of molecular weight between 7,000-8,000, lophotoxin has a small cyclic terpinoid

structure. Hence its overlap with multiple sites on the
receptor surface would be unlikely. The binding rates of
both α-toxins (2-4) and lophotoxin (11) are competitive with
agonists and antagonists, yet compounds such as local anesthe-
tics or histrionicotoxin which non-competitively influence
agonist-elicited channel opening do not impede association of
either of the toxins (6,11).

V. FRACTIONAL α-TOXIN OCCUPANCY AND THE PERMEABILITY RESPONSE

The equivalent reactivity of the individual binding sites
to α-toxin association (Fig. 1) enables one to analyze how
prior occlusion of α-toxin sites influences the functional
response to agonists. There is a considerable body of electrophysiologic data demonstrating positive cooperativity in the
conductance response (1). Similarly, positive cooperativity
in the concentration dependencies of both the permeability
response and ligand occupation is evident when analyzed in
BC3H-1 cells (9,10). Thus, the receptor behaves as an oligomeric protein, and minimally a two-site model can be considered to describe the activation data. With α-toxin showing
equivalent association with its sites, fractional α-toxin
association will yield a binomial distribution of unoccupied,
singly occupied and doubly occupied receptor species. If we
let y be the fraction of the total sites occupied by α-toxin
and k_G/k_{Go} reflect the fractional permeability response, a
simple linear relationship between α-toxin occupation and the
reduction in permeability, i.e. $k_G/k_{Go} = 1 - y$, would require
hybrid species of the dimer to exhibit one-half of the conductance of the dimer totally unoccupied by α-toxin. Hybrids
of the dimer would be defined as receptor molecules with only
one of their two sites occupied by α-toxin. If the hybrid
species cannot respond to agonist then the relationship is
described by $k_G/k_{Go} = (1 - y)^2$. When the hybrid species is
equally responsive, then $k_G/k_{Go} = 1 - y^2$. These relationships
can be distinguished through experiment by measuring fractional α-toxin occupation and $^{22}Na^+$ influx on the same culture
dish. Measurements of the residual response and the sites inactivated are best described by the equation $k_G/k_{Go} = (1 - y)^2$
(Fig. 2). Thus, at least two bound agonist molecules are
required for receptor activation and hybrid species carrying a
bound α-toxin molecule and the agonist (i.e. carbamylcholine)
remain mute with respect to ion permeability.

VI. LOPHOTOXIN OCCUPATION AND THE PERMEABILITY RESPONSE

When lophotoxin instead of cobra α-toxin is employed to inactivate the receptor irreversibly and the residual response is correlated with the available sites, a greater curvature is found than would be predicted from the parabolic $k_G/k_{GO} = (1-y)^2$ relationship. If we assume that lophotoxin can occupy the same sites as cobra α-toxin then the simplest interpretation for the enhanced lophotoxin inactivation indicates a selectivity of this toxin for one of the two available sites. Thus, if the sites y are designated as y_A and y_B and $y = (y_A + y_B)/2$, then $(1 - y_A)(1 - y_B) < (1 - y)^2$. Under these circumstances, with the inactivation of an equivalent number of sites, k/k_{GO} for lophotoxin inactivation would always be smaller than the values obtained when the two sites exhibit equal propensities for inactivation (Fig. 3).

VII. REVERSIBLE ANTAGONIST OCCUPATION AND BLOCKADE
OF THE PERMEABILITY

The binding profiles of reversible antagonists, which obviously lack the capacity to initiate the concerted transition associated with opening of the channel, exhibit Hill coefficients considerably smaller than 1.0. Theoretically, this could be a consequence of (a) negative cooperativity where the individual subunits are similar and occupation of one site reduces the affinity of the neighboring site in the oligomer, or (b) as we have seen for lophotoxin, an intrinsic non-equivalence in binding sites. Negative cooperativity mechanisms can be ruled out since prior fractional occupation by α-toxin causing hybrid species to predominate does not influence the concentration dependence of antagonist binding at the remaining sites (10). If a negative cooperativity mechanism were tenable, then Hill coefficients would approach 1.0 as more hybrid species are formed. Hence, the non-equivalence in binding sites for antagonists is not a consequence of conformationally linked binding of a neighboring site. The other possibility for the low Hill coefficient involves the nonequivalence of binding sites and here we can develop two limiting cases; either the two nonequivalent sites, A and B, are confined to a single oligomer (i.e. AB oligomers), or two types of receptors which contain identically paired subunits are present (AA and BB oligomers). In the event that the two types of receptors (AA and BB) were present in near-equal

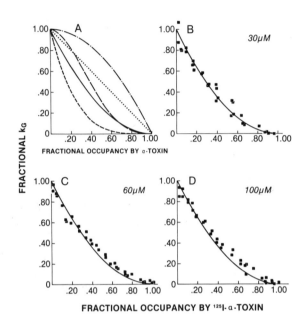

FRACTIONAL OCCUPANCY BY ^{125}I-α-TOXIN

FIGURE 2. Reduction of the permeability increase, k_G, elicited by carbamylcholine resulting from progressive occupancy of receptors by ^{125}I-labelled α-toxin. (a) Theoretical relationships for the fractional permeability response versus fractional occupancy of receptors by α-toxin.

.—., Model 1: Functional receptor contains two binding sites and full activation results when one or two binding sites are occupied by agonist under saturating agonist concentrations. Occupation of both sites by toxin is required to block function. Therefore $k_G/k_{Go} = 1 - y^2$.

..., Model 2: Functional receptor contains two binding sites and activation results when one or two binding sites are occupied by agonist. Occupation of each site by α-toxin reduces the response capacity of that receptor by one-half. $k_G/k_{Go} = (1 - y)$.

——, Model 3: Functional receptor contains two binding sites and activation requires occupation of both binding sites by agonist. Occupation of either site by α-toxin will completely block function. $k_G/k_{Go} = (1 - y)^2$.

---, Model 4: Functional receptor contains four binding sites and activation requires occupation of both binding sites by agonist. Occupation of either site by α-toxin will completely block function. $k_G/k_{Go} = (1 - y)^4$.

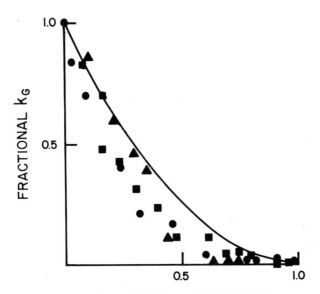

FRACTIONAL OCCUPATION

FIGURE 3. Reduction in agonist-elicited permeability
following progressive occupation by lophotoxin. Cells were
exposed to lophotoxin (0.06-100 μM) for 120 min and washed
with four 3 ml changes of buffer. Plates were divided into
two groups and assayed in parallel for $^{22}Na^{+}$ permeability
elicited by 60 μM carbamylcholine at 4° or the initial rate of
[^{125}I]cobra α-toxin binding. Fractional permeability values
(k_G/k_{Go}) were calculated relative to controls which were
treated in an identical manner but in the absence of lophotoxin. The individual symbols denote separate experiments and
the solid line describes the equation $k_G/k_{Go} = (1 - y)^2$ where
y is the number of sites inhibited by lophotoxin.

— —, Model 5: Functional receptor contains four binding
sites and activation requires occupation of three or four
binding sites by agonist. Occupation of more than one site by
α-toxin will completely block function. Occupation of only
one site has no inhibitory effect. $k_G/k_{Go} = (1 - y)^3(3y + 1)$.
     In each panel, the solid line corresponds to the function
$k_G = k_{Go}(1 - y)^2$ resulting from Model 3. In each experiment,
fractional occupancy of receptors by ^{125}I-labelled α-toxin was
achieved as detailed in the legend to Fig. 1b, and the cells
were cooled to 3.5°C for 30 min prior to measuring the initial
rate of sodium influx upon addition of the specified concentration of carbamylcholine and tracer $^{22}Na^{+}$.

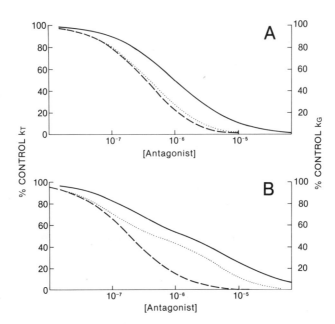

FIGURE 4. Concentration dependencies for occupation and functional antagonism using a two-site description of antagonist binding where the sites are present in equal populations. The solid lines in each panel depict the occupation curves. The corresponding dashed lines represent inhibition of the agonist-elicited permeability, k_G, for AB oligomers where non-equivalent sites are confined to a single oligomer (equation 4). The dotted lines represent inhibition of agonist-elicited permeability where the sites exist on two distinct oligomers and the sites are identically paired on each oligomer (AA and BB oligomers) (equation 6). In panel A antagonist affinities for the A and B sites differ by a factor of 4 ($K_A = 5 \times 10^{-7}$, $K_B = 2 \times 10^{-6}$M) while in panel B they differ by 50-fold ($K_A = 2 \times 10^{-7}$M, $K_B = 1 \times 10^{-5}$M).

populations, binding experiments alone would not distinguish between these two possibilities. In both cases

$$\text{fractional occupation} = 0.5(X_A) + 0.5(X_B) \qquad (1)$$

$$= 0.5(\frac{L}{L + K_A}) + 0.5(\frac{L}{L + K_B}) \qquad (2)$$

where L is the ligand concentration, X_A and X_B are the fractional occupations of the A and B sites, respectively, and K_A and K_B are the respective dissociation constants.

It is to be expected that reversible antagonists, like α-toxin, will block an agonist-elicited response by binding to

a single site. Then, if the binding sites are confined to a
single oligomer

$$k_G / k_{G_0} = (1 - X_A)(1 - X_B) \tag{3}$$

$$= (\frac{K_A}{L + K_A})(\frac{K_B}{L + K_B}) \tag{4}$$

If the non-equivalent sites exist on separate oligomers each
containing identically paired subunits, then

$$k_G/k_{Go} = 0.5(1 - X_A)^2 + 0.5(1 - X_B)^2 \tag{5}$$

$$= 0.5(\frac{K_A}{L + K_A})^2 + 0.5(\frac{K_B}{L + K_B})^2 \tag{6}$$

When $K_A \rightarrow K_B$, equations 4 and 6 converge, whereas when K_A and K_B
differ, the overall functions differ substantially. Shown in
Fig. 4 are the corresponding functions for binding and functional antagonism when $K_B = 4K_A$ and $K_B = 50K_A$. In the latter
case we should be able to distinguish between mechanisms. Data
for the association of five classical nicotinic antagonists
reveal Hill coefficients of less than one (Table 1) and the
binding curves can all be fitted to a two-site model in which
there are equal populations of sites with differing dissociation constants. Within this series of antagonists K_B/K_A ranges
between 4 and 89. Thus, by obtaining dissociation constants
from the occupation curves (equation 3) one can compare the
concentration dependence for functional antagonism with the
predictions of equations 4 and 6. Our experimental observations in the mammalian cells clearly show a close correspondence with equation 4 or the limiting case where the two sites
are confined to a single oligomer [12] (see Fig. 5).

VIII. RELATIONSHIP BETWEEN THE SITE SELECTIVITY OF
LOPHOTOXIN AND REVERSIBLE ANTAGONISTS

Since independent evidence has been developed for both
lophotoxin and the reversible alkaloid antagonists showing
selectivity for one of the two sites binding cobra α-toxin, it
should be possible to determine if the order of selectivity is
identical for the reversible and irreversible antagonists. By
irreversibly inhibiting a substantial fraction of sites by

Table 1. Parameters for antagonist occupation of receptors on BC3H-1 cells: inhibition of the permeability change elicited by carbamylcholine.

Antagonist	K_p,M [a]	n_{Hp} [a]	K_A,M [b]	K_B,M [b]	K_B/K_A	K_{ant},M [c]	n_{Ha} [c]	$\dfrac{K_p}{K_{ant}}$
Alcuronium	4.18×10^{-8}	0.87 ± 0.03	2.14×10^{-8}	1.68×10^{-8}	4.1	1.28×10^{-8}	0.99 ± 0.02	3.3
Pancuronium	2.33×10^{-8}	0.86 ± 0.02	9.11×10^{-9}	6.83×10^{-8}	7.6	7.38×10^{-9}	1.16 ± 0.07	3.2
AH8165	6.01×10^{-7}	0.78 ± 0.01	1.83×10^{-7}	1.84×10^{-6}	10.3	2.08×10^{-7}	1.08 ± 0.03	2.9
Gallamine	1.46×10^{-5}	0.70 ± 0.03	3.70×10^{-6}	5.50×10^{-5}	14.8	3.68×10^{-6}	1.00 ± 0.06	4.0
Dimethyld-tubocurarine	3.07×10^{-6}	0.51 ± 0.03	3.09×10^{-7}	2.75×10^{-5}	89.0	4.69×10^{-7}	0.85 ± 0.05	6.9

[a] K_p is the concentration of antagonist at 50% occupation and n_{Hp} is the associated Hill coefficient. Occupation was ascertained by the antagonists' capacity to inhibit the initial rate of α-toxin association.

[b] K_A and K_B are the high and low affinity intrinsic dissociation constants resulting form the fit of experimental data to equation 3.

[c] K_{ant} is the concentration of antagonist which decreases the permeability increase elicited by 30 μM carbamylcholine by 50% and n_{Ha} is the associated Hill coefficient (cf. ref. 10).

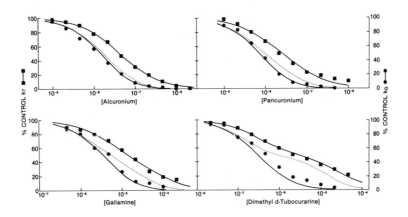

FIGURE 5. Concentration dependence for antagonist inhibition of the initial rate of ^{125}I-labelled α-toxin binding and inhibition of the carbamylcholine-mediated permeability increase to ^{22}Na$^+$. Cells were cooled slowly to 3.5°C, and incubated for 20 min in the presence of the specified concentrations of antagonist. Antagonist occupation was then measured by its competition with the initial rate of α-toxin binding (squares) and is expressed relative to the control rate, k_T, in the absence of antagonist. Functional antagonism was measured by replacing the prior incubation solution with an identical solution supplemented with 30 μM carbamylcholine and tracer ^{22}Na$^+$, and the initial rate of sodium uptake monitored (circles). The resulting permeability change, k_G, is expressed relative to k_{GO} measured in the absence of antagonist. The solid curve associated with the squares is the best fit for antagonist binding to two sites of equal populations with values of K_A and K_B: alcuronium, 0.021 μM and 0.087 μM; pancuronium, 0.0091 μM and 0.069 μM; gallamine, 3.7 μM and 55 μM; and dimethyl-d-tubocurarine 0.31 μM and 28 μM. The remaining solid and dotted curves are the predicted concentration dependencies for functional antagonism by equations 4 and 6, respectively.

lophotoxin, reversible antagonist binding to the remaining sites should reveal lophotoxin's preference. As shown in Fig. 6, after lophotoxin inactivation binding to the residual sites, the sites of higher affinity for the antagonist predominate. Thus, lophotoxin exhibits a preference for inactivation of sites with lower affinity for the reversible antagonist.

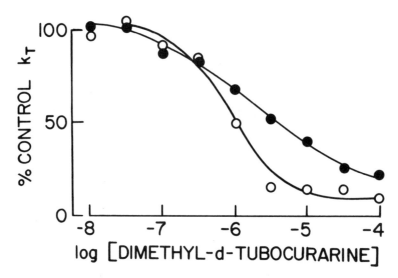

FIGURE 6.   Influence of partial inactivation of receptor
sites by lophotoxin on antagonist competition with $[^{125}I]\alpha$-
toxin binding. Cells were exposed to buffer containing either
1% DMSO (●) or 2 μM lophotoxin in 1% DMSO (o) for 120 min,
washed with four 3 ml changes of buffer, incubated with
dimethyl-d-tubocurarine for 30 min, and then replaced with an
identical solution containing $[^{125}I]\alpha$-toxin. Initial rates of
$[^{125}I]\alpha$-toxin binding are given on the ordinate as a percen-
tage of the rate observed in the absence of dimethyl-d-tubocurarine for the control and lophotoxin-treated cells.

IX. RELATIONSHIP TO RECEPTOR STRUCTURE

The arguments suggesting that the receptor functions as a
cooperative dimer in which the two individual sites are not
equivalent are based entirely on occupation-response relationships of a mammalian receptor in cell culture and we have not
required a priori assumptions regarding receptor structure.
Nevertheless, it is instructive to consider these findings in
the light of our knowledge of receptor structure. Four distinct subunits have been identified in the pentameric Torpedo
receptor in the apparent ratio of $2\alpha{:}\beta{:}^{\gamma}{:}^{\delta}$ and there is one
mutually exclusive site for agonist and α-toxin association on
each α-subunit (2-4). Based on fluorescence energy transfer
the respective sites on the two α-subunits are a substantial
distance apart (13) and hence a concerted event among the
subunits is required to open the channel. Since considerable

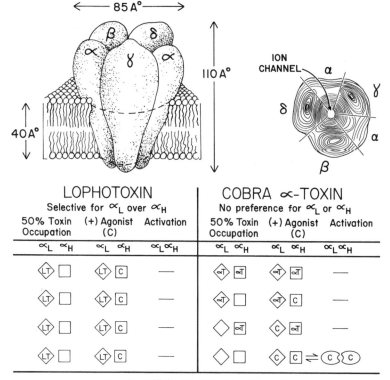

LOPHOTOXIN				COBRA α-TOXIN			
Selective for α_L over α_H				No preference for α_L or α_H			
50% Toxin Occupation	(+) Agonist (C)	Activation		50% Toxin Occupation	(+) Agonist (C)	Activation	
α_L α_H	α_L α_H	$\alpha_L \alpha_H$		α_L α_H	α_L α_H	$\alpha_L \alpha_H$	
⟨LT⟩ ☐	⟨LT⟩ ⊏C⊐	—		⟨αT⟩ ⊏αT⊐	⟨αT⟩ ⊏αT⊐	—	
⟨LT⟩ ☐	⟨LT⟩ ⊏C⊐	—		⟨αT⟩ ☐	⟨αT⟩ ⊏C⊐	—	
⟨LT⟩ ☐	⟨LT⟩ ⊏C⊐	—		◇ ⊏αT⊐	⟨C⟩ ⊏αT⊐	—	
⟨LT⟩ ☐	⟨LT⟩ ⊏C⊐	—		◇ ☐	⟨C⟩ ⊏C⊐ ⇌ ⊂C⊃⟨C⟩		

α_L - low affinity for reversible antagonists
α_L - preferred site of lophotoxin

FIGURE 7. Structure of the receptor and a description of the species of receptor capable of antagonist inactivation and agonist occupation and activation. The receptor is depicted with two binding sites. A concerted transition is required for activation and the two sites do not show precise equivalence. A plausible structural organization of subunits, α, β, γ, δ, is shown and summarized from x-ray and electron microscopic studies (15,16). This structure allows for non-equivalence of both agonist and antagonist binding on each oligomer, the positive cooperativity and presumed concerted interaction required for activation. Ligand binding sites are found on the α-subunits and all five subunits form the perimeter of the ion channel. In the lower portion cobra α-toxin (αT) is shown to lack selectivity for one of the two α-subunits and thus will yield binomial distribution of α-toxin-occupied species. Lophotoxin (LT) shows selectivity for one of the two subunits. This selectivity increases the proportion of hybrid species. Since hybrid species are inactive lophotoxin yields a greater loss of response than α-toxin at similar levels of occupation.

sequence homology exists among the four subunits (14), it is likely that all of the subunits span the membrane (cf. Fig. 7). This disposition of subunits would preclude a twofold axis of symmetry existing within the molecule and the two α-subunits could differ simply by virtue of non-equivalent intersubunit contacts. Thus, the structure of the receptor is consistent with a dimeric arrangement of ligand sites suitable for cooperative activation and this arrangement also provides a plausible structural basis for the observed functional non-equivalence of the subunits. Cobra α-toxin can associate to either of the two sites on the two α-subunits and, in fact, displays no selectivity in its binding. Fractional occupation by cobra α-toxin yields a parabolic relationship between the residual response and the sites occupied (Fig. 2). Moreover, prior occupation with this toxin does not change the ratio of high- and low-affinity sites for antagonist occupation (10). By contrast, a relationship possessing greater curvature than the parabolic $k_G/k_{GO} = (1 - y)^2$ is found for lophotoxin inactivation of sites. Moreover, lophotoxin inactivation will alter the ratio of low- and high-affinity sites for antagonist occupation (Fig. 6). Interestingly, lophotoxin is selective for the site or α-subunit of lower affinity for antagonists. These considerations are summarized in Fig. 7. By carrying out α-toxin inactivation in the presence of a reversible antagonist, α-toxin can also be directed to the low affinity subunit (10). Under these circumstances, inactivation by cobra α-toxin would yield a distribution of inactivated sites similar to that found for lophotoxin.

REFERENCES

1. Steinbach, J.H., in "The Cell Surface and Neuronal Function" (G. Poste, G.L. Nicolson and C.W. Cotman, eds.), p. 119. Elsevier North Holland, New York, (1980).
2. Karlin, A., in "The Cell Surface and Neuronal Function" (G. Poste, G.L. Nicolson and C.W. Cotman, eds.), p. 191. Elsevier North Holland, New York (1980).
3. Changeux, J.-P., Harvey Lect. 75:85-254 (1981).
4. Taylor, P., Brown, R.D. and Johnson, D.A., in Current Topics of Membranes and Transport, Vol. 18 (A. Kleinzeller and B.R. Martin, eds.) Academic Press, N.Y., pp. 407-444.
5. Schubert, D., Harris, A.J., Devine, C.E. and Heinemann, S., J. Cell Biol. 61:398-413 (1974).
6. Sine, S. and Taylor, P., J. Biol. Chem. 257:8106-8114 (1982).

7. Weber, M., David-Pfeuty, T. and Changeux, J.-P., Proc. Natl. Acad. Sci. USA 72:3443-3447 (1975).
8. Weiland, G., Georgia, B., Lappi, S., Chignell, C.F. and Taylor, P., J. Biol. Chem. 252:7648-7656 (1977).
9. Sine, S. and Taylor, P. (1979) J. Biol. Chem. 254:3315-3325.
10. Sine, S. and Taylor, P., J. Biol. Chem. 255:10144-10156 (1980).
11. Culver, P., Fenical, W. and Taylor, P., submitted for publication (1983).
12. Sine, S. and Taylor, P., J. Biol. Chem. 256:6692-6699 (1981).
13. Johnson, D.A., Voet, J.A. and Taylor, P., submitted for publication (1983).
14. Raftery, M.A., Hunkapiller, M.W., Strader, C.D. and Hood, L.E., Science, N.Y. 208:1454-1457 (1980).
15. Kistler, J., Stroud, R.M., Klymkowsky, M.W., Lalaneette, R.A. and Fairclough, R.H., Biophys. J. 37:371-383 (1982).
16. Wise, D.S., Wall, J. and Karlin, A., J. Biol. Chem. 256:12624-12677 (1981).

PROSPECTS FOR THE DESIGN OF NOVEL
MUSCARINIC DRUGS

Nigel J.M. Birdsall
Edward C. Hulme
Jane   M. Stockton

Division of Molecular Pharmacology
National Institute for Medical Research
Mill Hill, London, U.K.

Erik H.F. Wong

Department of Biochemistry
University of California
Riverside, California

I.   INTRODUCTION

In order to develop drugs which have a selective action
on a subclass of a receptor, it is necessary in the first
instance to demonstrate the existence of such subclasses.
In many cases this requires the observation of a selective
effect of an agonist or antagonist. Hence a prototype
selective drug must have been synthesised or isolated.
However, now that the binding assay technique can be used to
give information about the <u>direct</u> interaction of drugs with
their receptors, it is sometimes possible to obtain evidence
of receptor heterogeneity even in the absence of a selective
agonist or antagonist. This may be accomplished by demonstrating that a receptor binding site is capable of being
coupled directly to two different effector systems or that
an allosteric modification of the receptor binding site can
amplify or express undetected differences between the receptor
subtypes. In both instances one is obtaining information not
just from the immediate locale of the binding site but from
any site which may be allosterically coupled to the binding
site. This considerably extends the scope of binding studies.

Clearly binding studies can never supplant whole tissue
and whole animal pharmacological studies in the investigation

Copyright © 1983 by Academic Press, Inc.
All rights of reproduction in any form reserved.
ISBN 0-12-646680-7

of drug selectivity. Nevertheless they can be used to confirm
whether or not the selectivity of a drug resides in its
binding to the receptor and to pinpoint novel approaches to
the design of drugs. In this chapter, we consider how these
approaches have provided evidence for the existence of
muscarinic receptor subclasses. In particular, studies of
allosteric interactions at these receptors will be considered.

II. MUSCARINIC RECEPTORS - HETEROGENEOUS OR HOMOGENEOUS?

     Muscarinic receptors have a widespread distribution in
both the central and peripheral nervous systems where they are
linked to a wide variety of biochemical and physiological
responses (both excitatory and inhibitory)(1). The question
as to whether there are muscarinic subclasses has been
debated for at least twenty years without, until recently,
coming to a firm conclusion. The initial studies of Barlow
and co-workers (2) suggested that, as far as the action of
competitive antagonists in smooth muscle was concerned, there
appeared to be only one type of receptor. Binding studies in
the rat cerebral cortex agreed with this suggestion: antagonists bound to an apparently uniform population of muscarinic receptor sites with affinities which were very close to
those estimated by antagonism of contraction of smooth muscle
(3). However, Barlow and co-workers (4) reported that a
number of competitive antagonists had lower affinities for
heart muscarinic receptors than for the smooth muscle
receptors. This is summarised in Figure 1 which depicts the
structure-activity relationships for a number of competitive
antagonists acting on myocardial and smooth muscle receptors.
The affinity constants for an antagonist in the two tissues
are joined by a tie-line. The gradients of the lines are
related to the differences in affinity and any changes in the
structure-activity relationships are depicted by a crossover
of lines. It is clear from the tie-lines for the competitive
antagonists (solid lines) that the structure-activity relationships of the receptors in the two tissues are very similar
but not identical. There is one antagonist which is very much
weaker in the heart than in smooth muscle (4-diphenylacetoxy-
N-methylpiperidine methiodide) and one (pirenzepine) which
has essentially equal affinity in the two tissues. [The
cardioselective drugs shown by dashed tie-lines will be
discussed in section III].

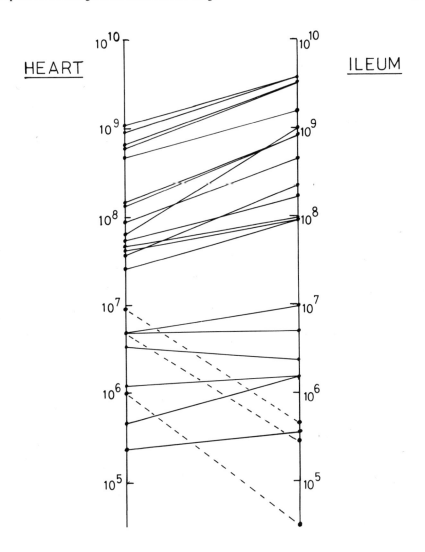

FIGURE 1.   Structure-activity relationships for 23 muscarinic
    antagonists in their action on the heart and smooth muscle.
    The affinities for a drug in these two tissues are joined
    by a line. Solid lines represent the data of Barlow and
    co-workers (4), the dashed lines, the data of Mitchelson
    and co-workers (8,9).

Pirenzepine is a novel muscarinic antagonist which is used
clinically in the treatment of ulcers. It differs from classical muscarinic antagonists in inhibiting vagally stimulated
acid secretion at much lower doses than those which are required to affect other muscarinic responses e.g. regulation of
heart rate, smooth muscle contraction and salivation. It is
also quite hydrophilic and only crosses the blood-brain
barrier to a very limited extent and hence, when administered
peripherally, does not inhibit central muscarinic responses.
Pirenzepine binds with differing affinities to muscarinic
receptors in different tissues (5). It has a low affinity for
myocardial and smooth muscle receptors but has a higher
potency and furthermore does not give simple mass action
binding curves in some other tissues, e.g. cerebral cortex,
hippocampus, sympathetic ganglia and the sublingual gland.
In general, the pattern of selectivity found in the binding
studies agrees with the pharmacological and clinical picture.
Interestingly, benzhexol exhibits a similar but lower binding
selectivity to that found for pirenzepine (Stockton et al., in
preparation). Therefore there seem to be at least two classes
of selective antagonist exemplified by 4-diphenylacetoxy-N-
methylpiperidine methiodide (high affinity in smooth muscle,
salivary glands and cerebral cortex, low affinity in heart(6)),
and pirenzepine (low affinity in heart and smooth muscle, high
affinity plus heterogeneous binding in the cerebral cortex and
other neuronal tissues). A further candidate for an antagonist
with a different selectivity is secoverine which is a potent
inhibitor of smooth muscle contraction but exhibits little
effect on cholinergically induced secretions(7). The selectivity of this drug has not yet been confirmed in a binding
assay. It therefore appears clear that there are subclasses
of muscarinic receptors with a discrete tissue distribution.
At the present time there seem to be at least three receptor
subtypes, being the predominant species in heart, smooth muscle
and neuronal tissue respectively (1).

III. A SECOND DRUG BINDING SITE
ON MUSCARINIC RECEPTORS

In Figure 1, there are also three drugs, which are ca 20
times more potent on heart muscarinic receptors (dashed lines).
These are data of Mitchelson and co-workers (8,9) and the drugs
are the neuromuscular blocking agents gallamine, pancuronium

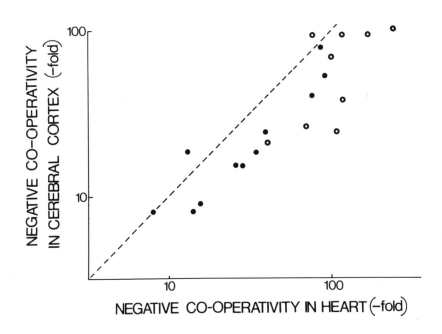

FIGURE 2. Comparison of the negative heterotropic cooperativity between gallamine and a series of agonists (O) and
antagonists (●) for the binding to myocardial and cortical
muscarinic receptors. The dashed line is the line of
identity.

and stercuronium. We have investigated the interaction of
gallamine with muscarinic receptors in different tissues and
have confirmed the cardioselective nature of its interaction
(10). However gallamine does not act as a competitive antagonist. It binds to a novel binding site, distinct from the
site to which acetylcholine and atropine bind, and allosterically decreases the binding of agonists and antagonists to
the conventional site. The extent of negative heterotropic
cooperative varies with the different drugs (Figure 2) and
therefore the conformational change induced by gallamine
changes the structure-binding relationships.

It is apparent from Figure 2 that the negative cooperativity in the heart and cortex are not identical as the points
deviate from the line of equivalence. Furthermore, the rank
order of negative cooperativity is different in the two

tissues. There is also a tendency for the cooperativity of agonists (open circles, Figure 2) to be greater than that of antagonists (closed circles, Figure 2) However the values of negative cooperativity for agonists are an average as the binding of agonists to the receptors in these tissues is complex (11,12). A detailed investigation of ligands, such as agonists and pirenzepine, which can distinguish between subclasses of muscarinic receptor binding sites, revealed differences in the interactions of gallamine with the subclasses of these sites (10). A number of other drugs besides gallamine will bind to this second site and some bind to both the conventional and the allosteric site.

The finding that responses to muscarinic drugs can be altered by the binding of drugs to an allosteric site provides the possibility of developing drugs with novel structures. Such drugs would have a maximum effect on acetylcholine binding and hence the possibility of overdosing is minimised. Secondly, drugs which have varying degrees of cooperativity would have different maximum effects and hence there is the possibility of developing a series of drugs with defined graded actions. Thirdly, there is the possibility that drugs might be found which have a positively cooperative interaction with acetylcholine, enhancing rather than inhibiting muscarinic responses. A selective drug of this type could be useful in enhancing muscarinic neurotransmission in diseases where there are low acetylcholine levels, for example in Alzheimers disease. Finally, since muscarinic receptors in different tissues are not identical and the pattern of selectivity of competitive and allosteric drugs is not identical, the development of a drug which has a selective action on different tissues is also a possibility.

We have also found that, in contrast to conventional agonists, McN-A-343 (13), binds non-competitively with muscarinic antagonists in the heart but apparently competitively in the cerebral cortex (14). It is not certain whether it binds to the same allosteric site as gallamine in the heart but its binding (like other muscarinic agonists) is inhibited by guanine nucleotides. As McN-A-343 is an agonist on myocardial muscarinic receptors (15) it would appear that it is possible to activate muscarinic receptors in two ways, via the acetylcholine binding site and the allosteric McN-A-343 site. If this proposition is confirmed pharmacologically, it would represent a novel mechanism of receptor activation.

IV. MODIFICATION OF THE SULFHYDRYL
GROUPS ON MUSCARINIC RECEPTORS

There have been numerous reports in the literature that
chemical modification of sulfhydryl groups on muscarinic
receptors will change the binding of ligands to the receptors.
We have examined these phenomena closely and have been able
to delineate at least four different classes of sulfhydryl
groups on muscarinic receptors based on the selective action
and effects of a number of sulfhydryl reagents (16). The
subclasses of muscarinic receptors exhibit both a different
reactivity to these reagents and are affected differently
by chemical modification. In this paper we consider two of
the effects of p-chloromercuribenzoate (PCMB) (16-18).

At low concentrations (10^{-5} - 10^{-4}M) PCMB produces a
selective change in the binding of agonists to muscarinic
receptors in the cerebral cortex. In the cerebral cortex,
there are two predominant classes of agonist binding site (11),
termed H and L, which in the absence of divalent cations,
correspond to the receptor sites which have a low and high
affinity for pirenzepine respectively (1). These two sites
are affected quite differently by low concentrations of PCMB,
both structure-binding relationships being affected. For
example oxotremorine binding to the H site is reduced by a
factor of 15 whereas the affinity for the L site is unaffected.
On the other hand, acetylcholine binding to the H site is
unaffected whereas it binds with a six-fold higher affinity
to the L site. This is an example of how subtypes of receptor
site are affected differently by this modification, and a
subtle but significant conformation change has been produced
in the active states (but not ground states) of the receptors.
This selective action of PCMB on agonist binding could not be
observed in myocardial membranes, providing an example of the
different reactivity of the muscarinic binding sites in these
two tissues.

At higher concentrations of PCMB (10^{-4} - 10^{-3}M), a
profound effect on antagonist and agonist binding is observed.
The structure-binding profile of antagonists is changed
(Figure 3). For example in the cerebral cortex, the affinity
of N-methylscopolamine is decreased over 100-fold whereas the
affinity of the structurally related N-methyl atropine
(lacking only the epoxide group) binds only 3-fold weaker.
On the other hand the affinity of the benzilate esters,
lachesine and propylbenzilylcholine, are increased.

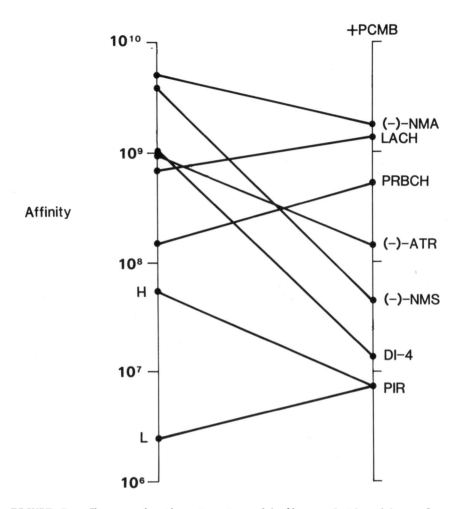

FIGURE 3.   Changes in the structure-binding relationships of
    antagonists for muscarinic receptors in the cerebral cortex
    after treatment with p-chloromercuribenzoate (-)-NMA; N-
    methylatropine, LACH;   lachesine, PrBCh;   propylbenzilyl-
    choline, (-)-ATR;   atropine, (-)-NMS;   N-methylscopola-
    mine, Di-4;   4-diphenylacetoxy-N-methyl-piperidine
    methiodide, PIR;   pirenzepine

Furthermore, pirenzepine binding heterogeneity has been
abolished. The dramatic extent of the change in the structure-
binding relationships and hence the conformation of the binding
site can be readily seen from the extent of crossover of the
tie-lines. Associated with the large changes in antagonist

binding are equally dramatic changes in agonist binding. The binding heterogeneity for potent agonists (11) is eliminated and affinity constants are decreased up to 10^5-fold. Interestingly, under these conditions PCMB seems to have created a binding site in which heterogeneity in agonist and antagonist binding both within and between tissues has been eliminated (16,17). However there is one drug out of $\sim$ 40 examined that actually exhibits an increased heterogeneity of binding and this is pilocarpine (16,18), which is the only putative selective agonist (19) that we have examined. It remains to be ascertained whether this PCMB treatment has amplified the selective binding characteristics of such drugs.

In summary, there appear to be subclasses of muscarinic receptors which can be distinguished by selective agonists and antagonists and the reactivity and effects of sulfhydryl group modification. Besides the conventional binding site to which acetylcholine and atropine bind, there is a second drug binding site to which antagonists and at least one agonist can bind, and allosterically modulate the binding of ligands to the conventional site. These findings offer the prospect of development of novel and selective muscarinic drugs.

REFERENCES

1. Birdsall, N.J.M., and Hulme, E.C. (1983) Trends Pharmac. Sci. submitted
2. Barlow, R.B., Franks, F.M., and Pearson, J.D.M. (1972) Brit. J. Pharmacol. 46, 300
3. Hulme, E.C., Birdsall, N.J.M., Burgen, A.S.V., and Mehta, P. (1978) Mol. Pharmacol. 14, 737
4. Barlow, R.B., Berry, K.J., Glenton, P.A.M., Nikolaou, N.M., and Soh, K.S. (1976) Brit. J. Pharmacol. 58, 613
5. Hammer, R., Berrie, C.P., Birdsall, N.J.M., Burgen, A.S.V., and Hulme, E.C. (1976) Nature (London) 283, 90
6. Birdsall, N.J.M., Hulme, E.C., Hammer, R., and Stockton, J. (1980) in Psychopharmacology and Biochemistry of Neurotransmitter Receptors. Eds. Yamamura, H.I., Olsen, R.S., and Usdin, E. Elsevier, N.Y. p97
7. Zwagemakers, J.M.A., and Claasen, V. (1981) Eur.J. Pharmacol. 71, 165

8. Li, C.K., and Mitchelson, R. (1980) Brit.J. Pharmacol. 70 313

9. Clark, A., and Mitchelson, F. (1976) Brit. J. Pharmacol. 58, 523

10. Stockton, J.M., Birdsall, N.J.M., Burgen, A.S.V., and Hulme, E.C. (1983) Mol. Pharmacol. 23, in press

11. Birdsall, N.J.M., Burgen, A.S.V., and Hulme, E.C. (1976) Mol. Pharmacol. 14, 725

12. Berrie, C.P., Birdsall, N.J.M. Burgen, A.S.V., and Hulme E.C. (1979) Biochem. Biophys. Res. Commun. 87, 1000

13. Roszkowski, A.P. (1961) J. Pharmac. Pharmacol. 132, 156

14. Birdsall, N.J.M., Burgen, A.S.V., Hulme, E.C., Stockton J.M., and Zigmond, M.J. (1983) Brit. J. Pharmacol. 78, 257

15. Fozard, J.R., and Muscholl, E. (1972) Brit. J. Pharmacol. 45, 616

16. Wong, E.H.F. (1981) Ph.D. Thesis C.N.A.A./N.I.M.R.

17. Birdsall, N.J.M., Burgen, A.S.V., Hulme, E.C., and Wong, E.H.F. (1983) Brit. J. Pharmacol. in press

18. Birdsall, N.J.M., Burgen, A.S.V., Hulme, E and Wong, E.H.F. (1983) Brit. J. Pharmacol. in press

19. Caulfield, M., and Straughan, D.W. (1983) Trends Neurosci, 6, 73

THE β-ADRENERGIC RECEPTOR:
STRUCTURE, FUNCTION AND REGULATION

Gary L. Stiles*
Marc G. Caron
Robert J. Lefkowitz

Howard Hughes Medical Institute
Departments of Medicine (Cardiology),
Biochemistry and Physiology
Duke University Medical Center
Durham, North Carolina

I. INTRODUCTION

Catecholamines such as epinephrine and norepinephrine initiate physiologic alterations by first interacting with specific membrane-bound adrenergic receptors. Ahlquist was the first to subdivide these receptors into two subtypes termed alpha and β-adrenergic receptors based on the relative potency order of various sympathetic amines for producing physiologic responses (1). Lands later provided physiologic evidence for the existence of two subtypes of β-adrenergic receptors (β-AR) which he termed β_1 and β_2 (2). A feature common to both subtypes of β-ARs is that they are coupled to the membrane-bound enzyme adenylate cyclase. Activation of either subtype by catecholamines is associated with stimulation of adenylate cyclase and an increased accumulation of intracellular cyclic AMP (3). Cyclic AMP appears to be the second messenger of β-adrenergic agonists in all tissues examined.

Although both subtypes appear to have a similar mechanism of action, they can be differentiated by their relative responsiveness to a series of catecholamine agonists. For

---

*GLS is supported by a Clinical Investigator Award from the National Heart, Lung and Blood Institute #HL01027.

37

example, β_1 receptors demonstrate a potency series of
isoproterenol > epinephrine ≅ norepinephrine for the
production of cyclic AMP. In contrast, β_2-adrenergic
receptors demonstrate a potency series of isoproterenol >
epinephrine >> norepinephrine (2).

Our understanding of the structure and function of β-
adrenergic receptors has evolved through three technological
stages. The first was the use of physiologic studies which
demonstrated that there were two types of β receptors which
were nonhomogeneously distributed throughout the tissues of
the body and that these receptors demonstrated marked
pharmacologic specificity and high affinity. The second was
the development of radioligand binding techniques which
brought about the first direct quantification of β-ARs in
tissues and has provided a tool for characterizing the
distribution of the subtypes of β-adrenergic receptors in
various tissues. In addition, radioligand binding has
provided insight into how agonists interact with the
β-AR-adenylate cyclase system to initiate the transmembrane
signal which results in increased cellular levels of cyclic
AMP (3). The most recent advances consisting of purification
and photoaffinity labeling techniques for the β-AR have
provided new insight into the protein structure of β-ARs in
both mammalian and nonmammalian systems (3). This paper
shall present recent information from the authors' laboratory
on the structure and function of the β-AR.

II. RADIOLIGAND BINDING

The first successful direct radioligand binding methods
for studying β-adrenergic receptors were first developed in
1974 (4-6). A variety of radiolabeled agonists and
antagonists have been developed since then and all
demonstrate the appropriate characteristics, namely
specificity, stereospecificity and saturability (3).
Radioligand binding techniques have now been successfully
utilized to: 1) characterize the pharmacologic binding
properties of receptors in intact cells, isolated membranes
and solubilized receptors; 2) study the regulation of
receptor number in tissues under pathophysiologic conditions;
3) study the mechanisms of receptor-effector coupling under
pathophysiologic conditions; and 4) characterize the
distribution of β_1 and β_2 receptor subtypes in various
tissues (3). The most frequently used method for
characterizing this heterogeneous distribution of receptor
subtypes involves the construction of competition binding

curves in which the binding of a nonsubtype selective
radioligand antagonist is competed for by a subtype selective
antagonist (7). The data derived from these curves can be
analyzed by a nonlinear least squares curve fitting technique
based on the law of mass action to quantitate the number of
β_1- and β_2-ARs as well as their affinity for a competing
antagonist. Such studies reveal that β_1- and β_2-adrenergic
receptors exist in the same tissue and that their relative
proportions vary markedly depending on the tissue studied.
These distributions have recently been reviewed (3).

III. STRUCTURE OF THE β-ADRENERGIC RECEPTOR

Until very recently the goal of identifying and
characterizing the structure and molecular properties of the
β-AR has remained elusive. However, the elucidation of the
structure of the β-AR is critical if one is to attempt to
understand at a biochemical level how hormones and drugs
interact with membrane receptors. The identification of the
two subtypes of β-ARs has intensified the interest in
understanding the sturcture of the β-AR as it relates to the
possible structural differences which could explain the
pharmacologic specificity characteristic of each receptor
subtype. Two approaches have led to our current
understanding of the structure of β-adrenergic
receptors--purification of the receptor binding subunit and
photoaffinity labeling of these receptor subunits.

A. Purification

In order to characterize the membrane-bound β-ARs
solubilization of the receptors must first take place under
conditions which do not alter their ability to interact with
appropriate ligands. The plant glycoside, digitonin, has
been found to be an effective detergent for solubilizing β-
adrenergic receptors (3,8). The initial approach to
purification was through the use of affinity chromatography
which utilizes the immobilization of the antagonist
alprenolol on an affinity support system such as Sepharose
(8). Chromatography of solubilized receptor preparations on
these affinity columns yields an extensive purification
(100-1,000 fold) of the receptor. This procedure was
originally coupled to sequential ion exchange chromatographic
steps to yield the first purification of the β_2-adrenergic
receptor from frog erythrocyte membranes (9). This technique

demonstrated that the binding subunit is composed of a single peptide of M$_r$ 58,000 (9). This purified peptide had all the characteristics expected of a β$_2$-adrenergic receptor. Figure 1 demonstrates an autoradiograph of a sodium dodecyl sulfate-polyacrylamide gel electrophoresis (SDS-PAGE) of the purified radioiodinated peptide as well as photoaffinity labeled frog erythrocyte β$_2$-adrenergic receptors (described below). It is apparent that the purified radioiodinated receptor migrates as a single peptide (right panel).

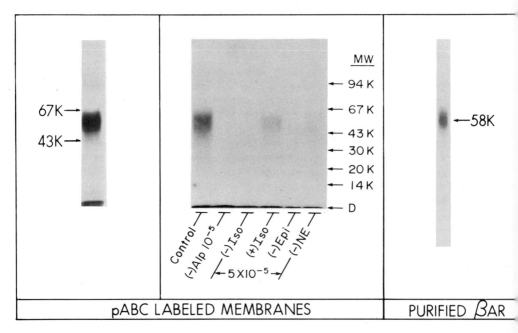

FIGURE 1. Identification of the β$_2$-adrenergic receptor binding subunit of frog erythrocytes by photoaffinity labeling and purification. Left and center panels represent membranes photolabeled with [^{125}I]p-azidobenzylcarazolol (13) alone (left panel and control lane of center panel) or in the presence of (-)alprenolol, 10^{-5} M (Alp), or 10^{-5} M of the following drugs: (-)isoproterenol ((-)Iso), (+)isoproterenol ((+)Iso), (-)epinephrine ((-)Epi), (-)norepinephrine ((-)NE). The membranes were then processed as recently described and subjected to SDS-PAGE (13) followed by autoradiography. Right panel: For comparison a purified β$_2$-adrenergic receptor preparation from frog erythrocyte membranes obtained by affinity chromatography and high performance liquid chromatography on steric exclusion columns (10) was iodinated by chloramine-T and Na[^{125}I] and electrophoresed on SDS-PAGE.

Recently the affinity chromatographic technique has been coupled to a molecular sieving process on high pressure liquid chromatography (HPLC) columns to produce a purified receptor preparation with all the appropriate characteristics but with a much higher overall yield than the previous methods (10).

These same procedures have now been applied to the β_1-adrenergic receptor from turkey erythrocytes and the receptor has been purified to a specific activity of > 15,000 pmol binding activity/mg protein (10). Purified receptor preparations display the appropriate β_1 pharmacologic specificity characteristic of this model system (10). In contrast to the single polypeptide seen in the β_2-adrenergic receptor from frog erythrocytes, two peptides of M_r 40, 000 and 45,000 have been identified. Figure 2 demonstrates iodinated purified turkey β_1-adrenergic receptor on SDS-PAGE and autoradiography as well as photoaffinity labeled turkey erythrocyte β_1-adrenergic receptors. As assessed by biochemical and pharmacologic techniques, each of these peptides possess a ligand binding site typical of this β_1 system suggesting that these two peptides represent different forms of the receptor. The biologic or physiologic significance of these two forms remains unknown at this time. It should be noted, however, that these same two peptides have been seen by photoaffinity labeling techniques as demonstrated in Figure 2 and these results are similar to those published by others (10,11).

The ultimate proof that these purified polypeptides are the complete functional unit of the β-AR rather than just the binding subunit will require reconstitution-fusion studies in which the purified receptor protein can confer β-adrenergic responsiveness to a previously unresponsive adenylate cyclase system. Early results suggest that the binding subunit is in fact the complete functional unit (12).

B. Photoaffinity Labeling

Photoaffinity labeling is a relatively new technique in terms of the characterization of hormone and drug receptors. For a photoaffinity probe to be useful in characterizing the β-AR, the compound must fulfill certain criteria including: 1) possess high affinity for the β-adrenergic receptor; 2) possess a high degree of specificity; 3) be labeled to high specific radioactivity; and 4) contain a light sensitive group that can be covalently incorporated into the structure of the binding site. One such compound, para-azido-m-[^{125}I]-iodobenzylcarazolol ([^{125}I]pABC), has recently been

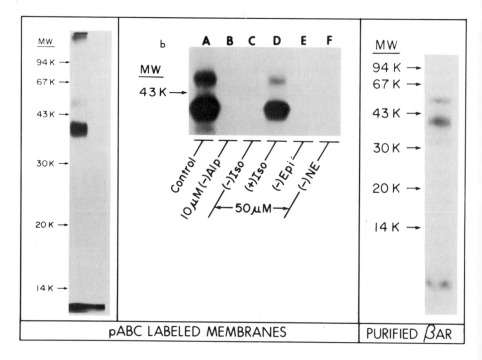

FIGURE 2.   Identification of the β_1-adrenergic receptor
binding subunit of turkey erythrocytes by photoaffinity
labeling and purification.   Left and center panels: Aliquots
of turkey erythrocyte membranes photolabeled with [^{125}I]ABC
alone or in the presence of the indicated concentrations of
the various adrenergic drugs indicated.   Abbreviations are as
in Figure 1.   All procedures are as stated in Figure 1 and as
recently described (10).   Right panel: A purified β_1-
adrenergic receptor preparation from turkey erythrocyte
membrane obtained by affinity chromatography and high
performance liquid chromatography as recently described (10)
was iodinated and electrophoresed on a 10% SDS–polyacrylamide
slab gel and an autoradiograph developed.

synthesized and characterized (13).   The compound's basic
structure is built around carazolol, a high affinity,
nonsubtype selective β antagonist to which has been added an
aryl azide, the light sensitive group which can covalently
incorporate into proteins, and ^{125}iodine to radiolabel it.
Upon exposure to ultraviolet light the azide will covalently
incorporate into proteins.   To validate that the
photoaffinity labeling approach is useful it first must be
demonstrated that incorporation of the ligand into the

macromolecule is specifically blocked by a variety of ligands that specifically occupy the receptor. A validation for [^{125}I]pABC is demonstrated in Figure 1 for the β_2-AR of frog erythrocyte membranes and in Figure 2 for the β_1-AR of turkey erythrocyte membranes. Photoincorporation of [^{125}I]pABC can be blocked by β-adrenergic ligands with a specificity consistent with the notion that incorporation is occurring into the receptor binding subunit. For example, in Figure 1 the antagonist alprenolol (10 μM) and (-)isoproterenol (50 μM) completely blocked incorporation into the binding subunit while (+)isoproterenol (50 μM) was less effective. This is consistent with the stereospecificity characteristic of the β-AR. Moreover, (-)epinephrine and (-)norepinephrine are equipotent in preventing photoincorporation in turkey erythrocyte β_1-AR (Figure 2) whereas (-)epinephrine is more potent than (-)norepinephrine in the β_2-AR of the frog erythrocyte membranes as seen in Figure 1. This is to expected from the known pharmacologic characteristics of these receptors. In addition, it is apparent that the peptides labeled with the photoaffinity probe are exactly the same peptides purified by affinity chromatography and high performance liquid chromatogrpahy and then radioiodinated. This further supports the contention that [^{125}I]pABC does photoincorporate into the receptor binding subunit.

The observation that the β_2-adrenergic receptor binding subunit from frog erythrocytes resides on a M_r 58,000 peptide while the β_1 subunit resides on two peptides immediately raised the question whether this difference was responsible for the different characteristics of β_1- and β_2-adrenergic receptors and whether these same peptides would be seen in mammalian tissues. When photoaffinity labeling techniques were applied to a variety of mammalian tissues containing β_1- and β_2-adrenergic receptors, either two or three peptides have been found in varying ratios (13-15). All of these peptides displayed the appropriate pharmacologic characteristics of either a β_1-AR or a β_2-AR as determined by inhibition of photoincorporation. These peptides were usually of $M_r \cong 62,000$, 55,000 and 40,000 (13-15). Recent evidence suggests that proteolysis may be responsible for the generation of the smaller peptides. Thus when membranes are prepared in the presence of proteinase inhibitors particularly those effective in inhibiting metalloproteinases there is an enhancement of the $M_r = 62,000$ peptide. For example when these techniques are applied to the canine heart β_1-adrenergic receptor, two peptides of $M_r = 62,000$ and 55,000 are specifically labeled as demonstrated in Figure 3.

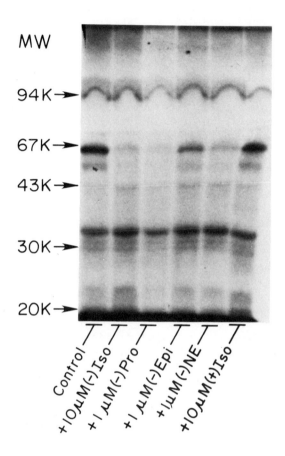

FIGURE 3.   Photoaffinity labeling and pharmacological
specificity of incorporation of [^{125}I]pABC in canine
myocardial membranes.   Aliquots of highly purified myocardial
membranes (16) were incubated with [^{125}I]pABC alone (control)
or in the presence of the indicated concentration of
competing ligand and photolabeled as recently described (15).
The samples were solubilized and electrophoresed on an 8%
SDS-polyacrylamide gel which was then subjected to
autoradiography (15).   The small arrows indicate the M_r
62,000 and 55,000 proteins.   The molecular weights (MW) shown
x 1,000 (K) as recently described (15).   Abbreviations are:
(-)Pro, (-)propranolol; (-)Iso, (-)isoproterenol; (-)Epi,
(-)epinephrine; (-)NE, (-)norepinephrine; (+)Iso,
(+)isoproterenol.   Data are from reference 15.

Both peptides display the appropriate characteristics of a β_1-adrenergic receptor, i.e. stereospecificity with the (-)isomer being more potent than the (+)isomer of isoproterenol in preventing photoincorporation while norepinephrine is slightly more potent than epinephrine also consistent with a β_1 pharmacologic specificity. As noted above the minor component, the M_r 55,000 peptide is thought to represent a degradation product of the M_r 62,000 peptide and its relative abundance can be decreased with proteinase inhibitors (15). Thus the β_1-adrenergic receptor binding subunit appears to reside on the M_r 62,000 peptide. To assess if this peptide is unique to the canine heart, we have photolabeled the β_1-adrenergic receptor binding subunit from canine, porcine and human heart as well as the β_2-adrenergic receptor from frog heart and then subjected these to electrophoresis on SDS-PAGE. An autoradiograph of just such an experiment is demonstrated in Figure 4. In this experiment membranes were photolabeled either in the absence (control) or in the presence of 10^{-5} M (-)isoproterenol. It can be appreciated that the binding subunit from each of these tissues resides on a peptide of M_r 62,000 regardless of whether it is of the β_1 or β_2 subtype (15). Although it is not demonstrated here we have shown that the 62,000 M_r peptide from frog heart has the appropriate characteristics of a β_2-adrenergic receptor (15). The M_r 55,000 peptide breakdown product is readily apparent as a minor contaminant in each system.

Benovic et al. (14) have recently demonstrated that the β_2-AR from rat and hamster lung membranes also resides on a M_r = 62-64,000 peptide which is also subject to in situ proteolysis. All these data taken together suggest that the β-AR from mammalian tissues resides on a M_r 62-64,000 peptide regardless of whether it is of a β_1 or β_2 subtype. Thus the avian species appears to be the exception rather than the rule. To date there has been no evidence to suggest that the M_r 40,000 and 45,000 peptides are breakdown products or that any higher molecular weight peptides exist which have the characteristics of the avian erythrocyte β_1-adrenergic receptor.

It is clear that further work will be required to determine what structural characteristics of the β-ARs from mammalian tissues confer the β_1 or β_2 pharmacologic specificity. The possibilities would include alterations in the primary structure of these subunits, i.e. the amino acid sequence or the secondary or tertiary structure of the proteins or their position in the membranes themselves. This work is currently under investigation in the laboratory at this time.

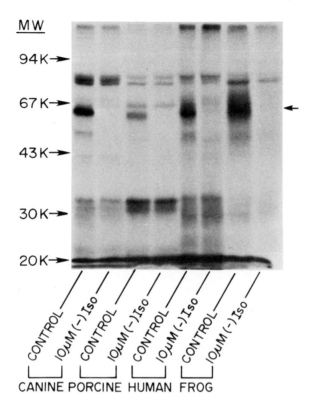

FIGURE 4. Photoaffinity labeling and simultaneous gel electrophoresis of frog, human, canine and porcine myocardial membranes. Aliquots of each type of membrane were prepared (15,16) and photolabeled (15) as recently described either with [^{125}I]pABC alone or in the presence of 10^{-5} M isoproterenol ((-)Iso). The samples were then subjected to SDS-PAGE and autoradiography. The small arrow represents the M_r 62,000 peptide. The molecular weight standards (MW) are shown x 1,000 (K). This gel was provided by Dr. R. Strasser.

IV.   CONCLUSION

In this brief chapter we have attempted to highlight recent advances in the purification and photoaffinity labeling of β-adrenergic receptors. These techniques have provided evidence that in mammalian systems the β-adrenergic receptor binding subunit resides on a peptide of M_r 62-64,000 regardless of whether it is of the β_1 or β_2 subtype. A similar peptide has been found in the frog erythrocyte model system by both purification and photoaffinity labeling techniques. In contrast, the β_1-adrenergic receptor from the turkey erythrocyte appears to reside on two separate peptides of M_r 40,000 and 45,000 by both the photoaffinity labeling and purification techniques. Further work is underway in the laboratory to determine what structural characteristics confer β_1 or β_2 subtype specificity on these peptides.

REFERENCES

1. Ahlquist, R.P., Am. J. Physiol. 153:586-600 (1948).
2. Lands, A.M., Arnold, A., McAuliff, J.P., Cuduena, F.P., and Brown, T.G., Nature 214:597-598 (1967).
3. Stiles, G.L., Caron, M.G., and Lefkowitz, R.J., Physiol. Rev., in press (1983).
4. Lefkowitz, R.J., Mukherjee, C., Coverstone, M., and Caron, M.G., Biochem. Biophys. Res. Commun. 60:703-709 (1971).
5. Levitzki, A., Atlas, D., and Steer, M.L., Proc. Natl. Acad. Sci. USA 71:2773-2776 (1974).
6. Aurbach, G.D., Fudak, S.A., Woodard, C.J., Palmer, J.S., Hauser, D., and Troxler, T., Science 186:1223-1224 (1974).
7. De Lean, A., Hancock, A.A., and Lefkowitz, R.J., Mol. Pharmacol. 21:5-16 (1982).
8. Caron, M.G., Srinivasan, Y., Pitha, J., Kociolek, K., and Lefkowitz, R.J., J. Biol. Chem. 254:2923-2977 (1979).
9. Shorr, R.G., Lefkowitz, R.J., and Caron, M.G., J. Biol. Chem. 256:5820-5826 (1981).
10. Shorr, R.G., Strohsacker, M.W., Lavin, T.N., Lefkowitz, R.J., and Caron, M.G., J. Biol. Chem. 257:12341-12350 (1982).
11. Burgermeister, W., Hekman, M., and Helmreich, E.J.M., J. Biol. Chem. 257:5306-5311 (1982).
12. Cerione, R.A., Strulovici, B., Benovic, J.L., Strader, C.D., Caron, M.G., and Lefkowitz, R.J., Proc. Natl. Acad. Sci. USA, in press (1983).
13. Lavin, T.N., Nambi, P., Heald, S.L., Jeffs, P.W., Lefkowitz, R.J., and Caron, M.G., J. Biol. Chem. 257:12332-12340 (1982).
14. Benovic, J.L., Stiles, G.L., Lefkowitz, R.J., and Caron, M.G., Biochem. Biophys. Res. Commun. 110:504-511 (1983).

15. Stiles, G.L., Strasser, R.H., Lavin, T.N., Jones, L.R., Caron, M.G., and Lefkowitz, R.J., J. Biol. Chem. 258:8443-8449 (1983).
16. Jones, L.R., Maddock, S.W., and Besch, H.R., J. Biol. Chem. 255:9971-9980 (1980).

THE DYNORPHIN OPIOID PEPTIDES AND THE KAPPA OPIOID RECEPTOR[1]

Avram Goldstein
Iain F. James

Addiction Research Foundation and
Stanford University
Palo Alto, California

I. INTRODUCTION

In 1975 the discovery of two opioid peptides in pituitary was reported from this laboratory. These were of higher molecular weight than the enkephalins, the structures of which were at that time still unknown. One of the pituitary peptides (1) (we can see in retrospect) was β-endorphin. The other (2) had quite different properties, enough to encourage us to persist in the long and difficult task of its isolation. Finally, a few micrograms were obtained in a pure enough state to obtain a partial sequence -- the first 13 residues of a longer peptide, which proved to be an extended form of [Leu]enkephalin (3). It was evident from the behavior of the natural peptide -- and this was confirmed with the synthetic tridecapeptide -- that this novel endogenous opioid was extraordinarily potent. The natural peptide was named "dynorphin" in recognition of this high potency. Eventually, the remaining four amino acids were determined (4). Later, another novel opioid peptide was found to be

[1] The investigations conducted in our laboratory were supported by grant DA-1199 from the National Institute on Drug Abuse, grant NS18098-01 from the National Institutes of Health, and grant BNS-8107237 from the National Science Foundation.

part of the same precursor; it was named dynorphin B (5) [(also "rimorphin" by another group (6)], and the original dynorphin was accordingly re-named dynorphin A. Most recently, it was found that a third extended [Leu]enkephalin-containing peptide, α- (or β-)neo-endorphin, is also contained in pre-pro-dynorphin (7). Structures are shown in Fig. 1.

(H)Tyr-Gly-Gly-Phe-Leu^5(OH)
[Leu]enkephalin

(H)Tyr-Gly-Gly-Phe-Leu-Arg-Lys-Tyr-Pro-Lys^{10}(OH)
α-neo-endorphin

(H)Tyr-Gly-Gly-Phe-Leu-Arg-Lys-Tyr-Pro^9(OH)
β-neo-endorphin

(H)Tyr-Gly-Gly-Phe-Leu-Arg-Arg-Ile-Arg-Pro-Lys-Leu-Lys^{13}-
-Trp-Asp-Asn-Gln^{17}(OH)
dynorphin A

(H)Tyr-Gly-Gly-Phe-Leu-Arg-Arg-Ile^8(OH)
dynorphin A-(1-8)

(H)Tyr-Gly-Gly-Phe-Leu-Arg-Arg-Gln-Phe-Lys-Val-Val-Thr^{13}(OH)
dynorphin B

FIGURE 1. Opioid peptides contained in the deduced pro-dynorphin sequence (7) and identified in tissues.

The GPI bioassay served as guide to the initial purification of dynorphin A, the remarkable potency of which was first demonstrated in this tissue. The guinea pig ileum myenteric plexus-longitudinal muscle preparation (GPI) produces a measurable force of contraction when stimulated electrically under isometric conditions. This muscle twitch is due to the stimulated release of acetylcholine from cholinergic terminals onto muscarinic acetylcholine receptors on the smooth muscle. Opioids (e.g. morphine) diminish acetylcholine release and thereby inhibit the twitch. The potency of an agonist is expressed as EC_{50}, the concentration that produces half-maximal inhibition of the twitch amplitude. Other substances, such as atropine or catecholamines, also inhibit, but only the inhibition caused by opioids is blocked and reversed by the specific opioid receptor antagonist naloxone. The specificity of the antagonism is attested to by the fact that the enantiomer (+)-naloxone is without antagonist effect, just as (+) opiate agonists are much less potent than their (−) enantiomers.

In the GPI assay, the 13−residue synthetic peptide has the same potency as natural dynorphin A, i.e., the additional four residues at the COOH−terminus seem to contribute nothing to the potency. Dynorphin A−(1−13) proved to be some 700 times more potent than [Leu]enkephalin. The obvious question was: Which residues in the eight−residue extension of [Leu]enkephalin account for the enhanced potency? Besides, it was important to ascertain if the increased potency of the longer peptide was manifested through the same receptor as the one acted upon by [Leu]enkephalin, or through a different opioid receptor type.

Early evidence concerning structure−activity relationships in dynorphin A was obtained through successive truncations of the peptide from its COOH−terminus (8), it being the rule for opioid peptides that tyrosine−1 must be intact with its amino group free. Although potency in the GPI dropped off somewhat with each shortening of the chain by one residue, very great losses of potency occurred when lysine−11 and arginine−7 were removed. These findings have since been confirmed by others (9,10). Two "register-shift" peptides[5a] were also synthesized and tested. These were the endo−Gly derivative, in which a glycine residue is added as a spacer, immediately after the [Leu]enkephalin sequence, thus shifting the entire COOH−terminal extension to the right; and the des−Arg[6] derivative, in which the extension is shifted to the left. Both these rather small changes resulted in a potency drop of about 10−fold, showing the need for a precise critical placement of the key residues that contribute to potency.

II. MULTIPLE OPIOID RECEPTORS

Evidence for the existence of multiple types of opioid receptor (e.g., μ, δ, κ, ϵ, σ) began to accumulate in 1976, and since then several lines of evidence have converged to support the concept:

(a) Distinctive patterns of biologic effects are found in whole animals administered different opiate alkaloids, all of the effects, however, being antagonized by naloxone (11).

(b) Grossly different rank orders of potency can be observed with a series of opioids tested in different tissues (12).

(c) Different sensitivities to antagonism by naloxone are found for effects of various agonists in a single tissue (12). This important criterion is discussed further below.

(d) Different rank orders of effectiveness are obtained for competition displacement in binding assays, depending upon which of several opioid radioligands is used (13).

(e) Selective tolerance can be produced to one family of opioids when a member of that family is administered chronically, without crosstolerance to opioids of other families (14,15).

(f) Single receptor types can be inactivated selectively or protected selectively againist inactivation by the technique of site-directed alkylation, as described below. This indicates that the multiple receptor types are physically distinct and not interconvertible.

In the GPI there appear to be but two functional opioid receptor types, μ and κ, distinguished not only by their selective interactions with various classes of agonist, but also by their very different affinities for the antagonist naloxone. The naloxone affinity can be expressed as an apparent dissociation constant (K_e), estimated from the "dose ratio", i.e., the ratio of EC_{50} of an agonist in the presence of a given concentration of naloxone to the EC_{50} in the absence of the antagonist (16). The equation is $K_e = C/(DR-1)$ (where DR is dose ratio and C is concentration of antagonist). The potency of the agonist is irrelevant; what is measured is the parallel shift of the agonist log-concentration response curve, regardless of its initial position on the log-concentration axis. In GPI, when normorphine or morphine is the agonist, naloxone K_e is about 2 nM; but when ethylketazocine (EKC, a benzomorphan opiate considered to act principally upon κ opioid receptors) is the agonist, naloxone K_e is greater than 20 nM. Several other opiate alkaloids related closely to morphine yield naloxone K_e values in the 2 nM range, while several other benzomorphans yield high K_e values. Thus, in GPI, low K_e signifies action through μ receptors, high K_e signifies action through κ receptors. It is understandable that naloxone, with structure very closely related to that of morphine, should have highest affinity for μ receptors.

The enkephalins not only have low potency in GPI (EC_{50} about 200 nM), they also yield low naloxone K_e values, i.e., they are antagonized as readily as morphine. This behavior contrasts sharply with that in another bioassay preparation, the mouse vas deferens (MVD), in which the enkephalins display both higher potency (EC_{50} about 10 nM) and a high naloxone K_e. These widely replicated observations are interpreted to mean that in GPI, which contains predominantly μ and κ receptors, enkephalins act through μ receptors; but that MVD contains, in addition, δ receptors, which are especially sensitive to enkephalins as agonists and relatively insensitive to naloxone as antagonist. The evidence reviewed here, as well as evidence from binding studies, strongly supports the existence of three types of opioid receptor -- μ, δ, and κ -- in mammalian nervous system. Less firmly established are the ε and σ types, selective for β-endorphin and (possibly) phencyclidine, respectively.

The selectivity of dynorphin A for κ receptors was first suggested by our original investigations on the synthetic tridecapeptide and its truncated fragments in GPI (3,8), later confirmed by others (9,17,18). Naloxone K_e was 25-30 nM for the intact dynorphin A-(1-13), but it dropped abruptly to about 15 nM upon removal of lysine-11. This intermediate value of K_e persisted until removal of arginine-7, when it dropped abruptly into the μ-receptor range. We interpret intermediate K_e values to mean that a biologic response is mediated to some extent by both receptor types, μ and κ. We concluded that lysine-11 and arginine-7 were critically important, not only for potency but also for κ-selectivity. We see now that the high potency of dynorphin A is entirely attributable to its interaction with the κ receptors; this accounts for the correlation of potency change and selectivity change when the structure is modified. Thus, the original question -- what features of the structure are responsible for enhancing the potency of [Leu]enkephalin? -- was incorrectly phrased. The COOH-terminal extension of dynorphin A does not enhance the potency of [Leu]enkephalin at the same receptor (here the μ receptor) at all; rather, it acts as an "address" to direct the peptide to a different receptor type.

Evidence of selectivity based on naloxone K_e is indirect. More direct evidence for specific dynorphin receptors identifiable with the κ type came from studies on selective tolerance (14). In MVD from mice treated chronically with the μ agonist sufentanil and a δ agonist, [D-Ala^2,D-Leu^5]enkephalin (DADLE), the potencies of μ and δ agonists on the MVD were greatly diminished, but the potency of dynorphin A-(1-13) was unchanged, as was that of the κ-selective benzomorphan EKC (15,19).

The availability of an opioid site-directed alkylating agent, β-chlornaltrexamine (CNA) (20) gave us the opportunity to obtain an even more direct proof of the κ-selectivity of dynorphin peptides (21). The well-established method of selective protection was used, in which a ligand selective for one receptor type is present, at high concentration, during exposure to the alkylating agent. The relative specificity of CNA (itself an opiate derivative) for opioid receptors is a distinct advantage; indiscriminate alkylation would destroy the function of a tissue bioassay preparation. We showed, by the CNA technique (Table I), that dynorphin A-(1-13) selectively protected GPI responses to dynorphin, while responses to [Leu]enkephalin were attenuated, thus confirming that dynorphin A acts through different receptors (22). The quantitative measure of selective protection is the degree to which a potency shift (i.e., the ratio of EC_{50} after CNA treatment to EC_{50} before treatment) is prevented. It is noteworthy (not shown) that protection by any one of dynorphin A, dynorphin B, or α-neo-endorphin provided complete crossprotection of the other two; thus, we could obtain no indication of the existence of κ receptor subtypes in GPI.

There is a widespread misconception that MVD is some sort of special "δ-receptor tissue". However, the CNA technique has shown that dynorphin peptides act through κ receptors in MVD as well as in GPI (23), and that their high potency in this tissue, as in GPI, is due to their κ-receptor interaction. MVD contains μ, δ , and κ receptors, and apparently also ε receptors (specific for β-endorphin). It is not MVD that is unique, but rather GPI, which apparently lacks δ receptors. Thus, it is only for selective δ agonists that a very high ratio of potency in MVD to potency in GPI has any special significance. In general, potency comparisons of agonists in a single tissue or across tissues can not yield valid information about agonist selectivity.

TABLE I. Potency Shifts After CNA Treatment[a]

	Protector	
	None	Dynorphin A-(1-13)
[Leu]enkephalin	14 ± 1.5 (23)	12 ± 1.8 (4)
Normorphine	15 ± 4.4 (14)	19 ± 4.4 (10)
Dynorphin A-(1-13)	17 ± 2.4 (33)	2.9 ± 0.6 (6)
EKC	18 ± 3.9 (12)	2.7 ± 0.6 (6)

[a]For each ligand, EC_{50} was estimated before and after incuation with CNA in presence of a protector. Potency shift is the ratio of these EC_{50} values. Data are mean shifts ± SEM, with number of experiments in parentheses. Unchanged potency would correspond to a potency shift of 1.0. [From Chavkin et al (21), Table II.]

III. PHARMACOLOGIC SELECTIVITY AND BINDING SELECTIVITY

   Pharmacologic selectivity concerns the preferential
(i.e., at the lowest concentration) activation of a particular receptor type to produce a biologic response. Potency
is measured, not affinity for a receptor. And potency
depends on receptor affinity, intrinsic activity (24,25), and
receptor reserve (25-27), all three of which can vary independently between agonists and between tissues. An agonist
that shows pharmacologic selectivity for one receptor type
in a given tissue could be selective for a different type in
another tissue; the well-known example of enkephalins in MVD
and GPI was noted above. Moreover, an agonist need not display pharmacologic selectivity for the same receptor type for
which it has highest affinity, since increased receptor
reserve will cause increased potency, regardless of the
affinity. It follows that conclusions about pharmacologic
selectivity are limited to a single tissue. From the standpoint of molecular pharmacology, each of the three determinants of potency must be studied separately. The first step
in understanding the selectivity of various opioids for the
several types of opioid receptor is to analyze structure-activity relationships for receptor affinities in direct binding studies. Ideally, a highly selective radioligand would
be used for each receptor type, so that classical competition
experiments could yield K_i values for every competing ligand
at each type of binding site. Unfortunately, the opioid
radioligands most widely used are not sufficiently selective
for the purpose.
   How selective is "sufficiently selective"? Many investigators do not realize that an apparently linear Scatchard
plot offers no assurance of site homogeneity. As an example,
Fig. 2 presents a theoretical Scatchard plot, constructed on
the assumption of a 5% error in binding data (a very conser-
vative assumption). The almost perfect straight line, with
its impressive correlation coefficient, actually represents
the binding of a ligand at two sites present in equal numbers
and with a 5-fold difference in ligand affinity for those
sites. Linear Scatchard plots obtained with DADLE, which
have been assumed to represent binding to δ sites, actually
depict the composite binding of this poorly selective ligand
(see below) to both δ and μ sites.
   Another measure of "sufficiently selective" is obtained
from mass-law calculations on what fraction of bound ligand
occupies a non-preferred site. Assuming an equal number of
preferred (high-affinity) and non-preferred (low-affinity)
sites, and a concentration of free ligand equal to the

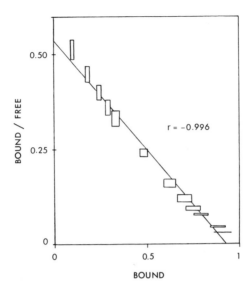

FIGURE 2. Theoretical Scatchard plot. Constructed for
the case of a ligand binding at two sites present in equal
numbers, with ligand dissociation constants for the two sites
differing by a factor of 5. Rectangles represent an error of
± 5% in each value of bound ligand. The line of best fit by
the method of least squares is shown, where r is the correlation coefficient.

dissociation constant at the high-affinity site, one finds
that with an affinity twice as great at the preferred as at
the non-preferred site (as with DADLE, see below), 40% of
bound ligand will be associated with the latter. With an
affinity ratio of 10, this fraction is still 15%. Only at
affinity ratios greater than 50 does the fraction fall below
5%. We conclude that "sufficiently selective" means that for
binding studies the affinity of a radioligand for its preferred site ought to be at least 50 times that for its next-
preferred site. Even greater selectivity is required in autoradiography or other cytochemical technique for mapping receptors; here the selectivity problem is similar to the crossre-
activity problem in immunocytochemistry, namely, that a high
local density of non-preferred sites can mimic a low density
of preferred sites.
     With the CNA technique we can obtain unambiguous measure-
ments of selectivity for opioid binding sites even with the
partially-selective radioligands currently available.
Furthermore, the same technique can be used to search for

ligands with better selectivity. By selectively inactivating
and protecting binding sites on guinea pig brain membranes,
we were able to obtain preparations that are, from a practi-
cal standpoint, homogeneous with respect to opioid receptor
type. Then competition experiments employing such μ, δ,
and κ membranes, with the appropriate partially selective
radioligands, permitted us to assign three K_i values to each
competing ligand studied.

We define the binding selectivity of a ligand as a ratio
of the equilibrium association constant at the preferred
(highest-affinity) site to that at a specified non-preferred
site. For multiple opioid receptor types we express the
overall selectivity pattern of a ligand as its binding
selectivity profile, namely, the set of binding selectivities
defined above, stated in a uniform sequence -- μ, δ, κ.
Instead of writing the tautologic ratio 1.0 for the preferred
site, we write, instead, the pK_i at that site, i.e., $-\log_{10}$
of the dissociation constant. Thus, three numbers provide
all the relevant information about a ligand's affinities and
selectivity. Examples are given in Table II. Some striking
facts emerge. DADLE, which has been used widely as a radioligand to label δ receptors, discriminates only by a factor
of 2 against μ receptors (although by a factor of 6,400
against κ). EKC has often been used to label κ receptors,
but its selectivity for κ over μ is only 8-fold. The remarkable κ-selectivity of the compound U50,488H (and to a

TABLE II. Some Binding Selectivity Profiles[a]

| | Binding Site Type | | |
	μ	δ	κ
DADLE	2.1	[8.82]	6,400
U50,488H	1,300	12,000	[9.14]
tifluadom	97	1,400	[10.1]
dynorphin A-(1-13) amide	30	78	[10.7]
EKC	7.5	78	[9.96]
morphiceptin	[6.97]	280	88
sufentanil	[10.3]	70	220
naloxone	[9.14]	18	4.0

[a] See text for explanation. Number in brackets is $-\log_{10}$
K_i at preferred site. Other numbers are binding selectivities for preferred site over each non-preferred site.

lesser degree, tifluadom) is noteworthy; these synthetic
compounds are substantially more κ-selective than the endogenous κ ligands, the dynorphin peptides. The "prototypic" μ
radioligands have been dihydromorphine (DHM) and naloxone,
but sufentanil has vastly superior selectivity.

Of theoretical interest is the finding, apparent in Table
II, that affinity and selectivity can vary quite independently. Sufentanil and morphiceptin, for example, have rather
similar selectivities for μ sites, but their affinities
differ by three orders of magnitude. Thus, high selectivity
can presumably result not only from a very close fit and
tight binding at a preferred site, but also from strong rejection (e.g., by steric hindrance or unfavorably placed
charges) at non-preferred sites. Examination of a large set
of opioid selectivity profiles reveals that no two types of
binding site are especially closely related; rather, all
three types have their own characteristic ligand preference
patterns. When multiple opioid receptors were first recognized it was generally supposed that the differences between
them were rather minor. Now, with increasing numbers of
highly selective ligands becoming available, we see that the
types of opioid binding sites are really quite different from
each other.

IV.   THE BASIS OF κ SELECTIVITY IN THE DYNORPHIN PEPTIDES

What molecular features of the dynorphin peptides account
for their κ-selectivity? The enkephalin sequence at the
NH_2-terminus is the common element required by all opioid
receptors. The flexibility of this sequence permits a
β-bend at Gly^2-Gly^3, which in turn allows a close approximation of the benzene ring of phenylalanine-4 to the benzene
ring of tyrosine-1. Thus, a three-dimensional structure can
be favored, in the binding site, that is remarkably like that
of some rigid opiate alkaloids of the morphine type. The
extension of [Leu]enkephalin at its COOH-terminus causes a
change in receptor selectivity, from δ-selective to κ-selective, if there is a positive charge at residue 7 (arginine-7
in dynorphin A and B, lysine-7 in the neo-endorphins).
Striking further enhancement of κ-selectivity is seen if
there is another positive charge at residue 10 or 11 (lysine-
10 in α-neo-endorphin and dynorphin B, lysine-11 in dynorphin A). The κ binding site could have complementary negative charges, so that two additional electrostatic bonds
would add to the binding energy and also serve to stabilize
a certain conformation of the enkephalin sequence, perhaps by
amphiphilic effects in the membrane (28). This conformation

of the dynorphin peptides would be preferred by the κ site
and quite different from that of [Leu]enkephalin itself, preferred by the δ site. In this connection, fluorescence energy transfer experiments recently showed (29) that the distance of tryptophan-4 from tyrosine-1 was substantially
greater in [Trp^4]dynorphin A than in [Trp^4,Leu^5]enkephalin.
In other words, free enkephalin in solution is compact,
whereas the enkephalin sequence in dynorphin is more open and
extended.

V. SUMMARY

The dynorphin peptides offer interesting possibilities
for studying some fundamental aspects of the molecular mechanisms of action of drugs, hormones, and neurotransmitters,
as well as for understanding the evolutionary significance of
multiple neuropeptide ligands encoded by the same gene and
interacting with one of the multiple types of related receptors. The principal question at the level of molecular
interaction is: What features account for the high affinity
and high selectivity of the dynorphin peptides for κ opioid
receptors? The ultimate question about post-receptor events
is: What is the physiological significance of the multiple
opioid receptors, and what is the special functional significance of the apparently redundant κ-selective dynorphin gene
products? A modest beginning has been made in answering
these and related questions.

REFERENCES

1. Teschemacher, H., Opheim, K.E., Cox, B.M.,and Goldstein,
      A. (1975). Life Sci. 16, 1771.
2. Cox, B.M., Opheim, K.E., Teschemacher, H.,and Goldstein,
      A. (1975). Life Sci. 16, 1777.
3. Goldstein, A., Tachibana, S., Lowney, L.I., Hunkapiller,
      M., and Hood, L. (1979). Proc. Natl. Acad. Sci. USA
      76, 6666.
4. Goldstein, A., Fischli, W., Lowney, L.I., Hunkapiller,
      M., and Hood, L. (1981). Proc. Natl. Acad. Sci. USA,
      78, 7219.
5. Fischli, W., Goldstein, A., Hunkapiller, M.W., and Hood,
      L.E. (1982). Proc. Natl. Acad. Sci. USA, 79, 5435.
6. Kilpatrick, D.L., Wahlstrom, A., Lahm, H.W., Blacher,R.,
      and Udenfriend, S. (1982). Proc. Natl. Acad. Sci.
      USA, 79, 6480.

7. Kakidani, H., Furutani, Y., Takahashi, H., Noda, M., Morimoto, Y., Hirose, T., Asai, M., Inayama, S., Nakanishi, S., and Numa, S. (1982). Nature, 298, 245.
8. Chavkin, C., and Goldstein, A. (1981). Proc. Natl. Acad. Sci. USA 78, 6543.
9. Yoshimura, K., Huidobro-Toro, J.P., Lee, N.M., Loh, H.H., and Way, E.L. (1982). J. Pharmacol. Exp. Ther. 222, 71.
10. Corbett, A.D., Paterson, S.J., McKnight, A.T., Magnan, J., and Kosterlitz, H.W. (1982). Nature 299, 79.
11. Martin, W.R., Eades, C.G., Thompson, J.A., Huppler, R.E., and Gilbert, P.E. (1976). J. Pharmacol. Exp. Ther. 197, 517.
12. Lord, J.A.H., Waterfield, A.A., Hughes, J., and Kosterlitz, H.W. (1977). Nature 267, 495.
13. Chang, K.J., and Cuatrecasas, P. (1979). J. Biol. Chem. 254, 2610.
14. Schulz, R., Wuster, M., Krenss, H., and Herz, A. (1980). Mol. Pharmacol. 18, 395.
15. Wuster, M., Schulz, R., and Herz, A. (1980). Neurosci. Lett. 20, 79.
16. Kosterlitz, H.W., and Watt, A.J. (1968). Br. J. Pharmac. Chemother. 33, 266.
17. Schulz, R., Wuster, M., and Herz, A. (1982). Peptides 3, 973.
18. Oka, T., Negishi, K., Suda, M., Sawa, A., Fujino, M., and Wakimasu, M. (1982). Eur. J. Pharmacol. 77, 137.
19. Wuster, M., Rubini, P., and Schulz, R. (1981). Life Sci. 29, 1219.
20. Portoghese, P.S., Larson, D.L., Jiang, J.B., Caruso, T.P., and Takemori, A.E. (1979). J. Med. Chem. 22, 168.
21. Chavkin, C., James, I.F., and Goldstein, A. (1982). Science 215, 413.
22. Chavkin, C., and Goldstein, A. (1981). Nature 291, 591.
23. Cox, B.M., and Chavkin, C. (1983). Mol. Pharmacol. 23, 36.
24. Ariens, E.J., van Rossum, J.M., and Koopman, P.C. (1960). Arch. Int. Pharmacodyn. 127, 459.
25. Stephenson, R.P. (1956). Br. J. Pharmacol. 11, 379.
26. Nickerson, M. (1957). Pharmacol. Rev. 9, 246.
27. Furchgott, R.F. (1978). Federation Proc. 37, 115.
28. Kaiser, E.T., and Kezdy, F.J. (1983). Proc. Natl. Acad. Sci. USA 80, 1137.
29. Schiller, P.W. (1983). Int. J. Pept. Prot. Res. 21, 307.

THE QUANTITATIVE ANALYSIS
OF
RECEPTOR STEREOSELECTIVITY[1]

Pedro A. Lehmann F.[2]

Departamento de Farmacología y Toxicología
Centro de Investigación y Estudios Avanzados
Instituto Politécnico Nacional
México D.F., México

SUMMARY

The stereoselective interaction of living beings with bioactive compounds takes on a great variety of forms. These can be classified on the basis of the molecular recognition between the chiral selector biomacromolecule and the stereo-isomeric selectands it interacts or reacts with. One type, that in which the isomers have the same kind of activity, is singled out for detailed examination. The notion that stereoselectivity increases with affinity is substantiated by a number of examples. For them, a quantitative analysis of receptor stereoselectivity can be made, which in turn sheds light on the pharmacon-receptor interaction at the submolecular level.

[1]Stereoselectivity and Affinity in Molecular Pharmacology, Part 10; for earlier parts see Ref. 19.

[2] A.P. 14-740, México 07000 D.F., MEXICO.

MECHANISM OF DRUG ACTION

I. INTRODUCTION

Over 125 years ago Pasteur discovered the existence of chiral compounds in nature **and** the selective character of living systems towards them. Since then countless further observations have been reported on such interactions and descriptions of them at the molecular level are beginning to appear. The purpose of this paper is to contribute to our understanding of this phenomenon by proposing a simple classification scheme of its various subtypes and showing that the stereoselectivity of receptors can be quantified. Both of these should aid our comprehension of the mechanism of drug action, and hopefully, in the rational design of new drugs.

The general aspects of stereoselective molecular recognition in biology have recently been reviewed extensively (1,2 and general references cited therein) and the reader is referred to them for a description of the underlying concepts (chirality, stereoisomerism, measurement of affinity, thermodynamics of association, etc.), which space limitations preclude repeating here.

Receptors and enzymes have not taken courses in organic stereochemistry and so are not impeded in their tasks by the chemist's complicated and sometimes overlapping classification into functional, positional, configurational and conformational isomers. To them they are all "stereo-isomers" which they recognize and/or react with on the basis of their overall shape, or stereostructure (3). It is in this general sense that we will employ the term stereoselectivity.

It should be emphasized once again that only these biomacromolecules can be said to be stereoselective since only they exist in chiral form and can select to interact or not with both (or all) isomers of a pharmacon. Statements such as "the methyl derivates are more stereoselective" are wrong and should not be made. Or, to use Gil-Av's terms (4), in this case only the selector can be stereoselective towards the selectands. The use of the term stereospecific should also be discouraged since countless cases are known in which both isomers interact with the biomacromolecule, and the process is really stereoselective although it may just not be possible to measure the weaker interaction.

The organic chemist's chiral molecules live mostly in an achiral world, but for the biologist, both chiral and achiral molecules inhabit a chiral jungle. In view of this, the organic chemist's stricture that only enantiomers possess identical physical and chemical properties may have less import in this setting and comparisons of interactions with isomers other than enantiomers, for example epimers, can furnish valuable information.

In Table I is given a list of the different types of stereoselective interactions that have been discerned in living systems. It is an arbitrary and incomplete classification, but serves to point out the complexity of the problem at hand. The recent literature on this subject is extremely lengthy and diffuse (for example an extensive treatise (5) has just been completed on the different effects of stereoisomers in psychopharmacology). Rather than attempt to review it, emphasis will be placed on an analysis of receptor stereoselectivity (subtypes I.A, I.F and II. H) which can be expected to shed light on the pharmacon-receptor interaction at the molecular and sub-molecular levels.

II. RECEPTOR STEREOSELECTIVITY

In receptor-preparation binding studies or in isolated tissue experiments with potent compounds conditions can be achieved in which it is certain that the pharmacon-receptor interactions that are measured reflect processes at the molecular level. In fact precise determinations of affinity constants (pA_2 or pD_2 values) provide excellent measures of the binding energies involved. It would be most desirable if the overall energy could be broken down into the separate contributions made to it by each molecular fragment which actively participates in the "molecular embrace". This would be similar to the molecular fragment approach of Rekker (6) in the calculation of partition coefficients. One of a few successful endeavors of this type was described by the late Professor Jorgensen in the first Symposium of this series (7). He showed that for a large series of thyromimetic compounds the overall binding energy to various receptors could be successfully accounted for by the sum of the individual contributions made by the substituents on the diphenyl ether core. This considerable advance in receptor understanding was possible because of the large number of analogues available and because the binding is such that the ligand is completely (or at least mostly) engulfed by the macromolecules so that all the substituents interact (positively or negatively) with groups lining the receptor cavity.

For the classical pharmacological receptors this has not been possible yet because a) their stereostructure is unknown, b) insufficient analogues have been examined, and c) because the thinking of molecular pharmacologists has long been dominated by the Easson-Stedman (8) formulation of the binding locus as lying on a plane. Perhaps the following analysis can help change this and eventually lead to quantitative **stereo**-structure-activity relationships for these receptors.

TABLE I. A classification of the different types of stereoselective processes found in living systems

I. In vitro stereoselectivity such as that displayed by receptors toward a series of stereo-
   isomers which can be interpreted at the molecular level due to the absence of interfering
   factors. Subclasses include:
   A. Stereoselectivity depends on affinity and/or efficacy
   B. Absence of stereoselectivity: both (or all isomers) have the same potency
   C. High stereoselectivity since for one isomer no effect is detectable
   D. Isomers have opposite effects on the same receptor (agonism/antagonism)
   E. The receptor interacts prochirally with an achiral pharmacon
   F. The stereoselectivities displayed by various receptors towards one chiral pair are
      different

II. Other types of stereoselectivity are those observed at the organ or whole-body level.
    The differences in final biological activity may be due to:
    G. Stereoselective pharmacokinetics (absorption, distribution and elimination)
    H. Stereoselective biotransformation
    I. Stereoselective chemical reactivity
    J. Interaction of isomers with different targets

   Alone or combined they can result in any of the following situations:
   1. Selective bioactivation or destruction
   2. Conversion of one enantiomer into the other
   3. Isomer interference
   4. Synergism
   5. Different or opposite final effects

A. The Dependence of Stereoselectivity on Affinity

1. Eudismic Analysis

Many years ago Pfeiffer (9) made the acute observation that for several common chiral drugs an increase in their potency was associated with an increase in their enantiomeric potency ratio. Although further series were found to behave similarly (10) little use was made of it until, after an exhaustive literature search, we (11) established that in general **stereoselectivity increases with affinity.** This will be the Leitmotiv of this paper, one which will reappear in various guises throughout. To reach this conclusion we (12) developed a method of analyzing quantitatively the interaction of a series of isomeric pairs with a given receptor. Since then it has been applied successfully to auxins (13), angiotensins (14), sweet-bitter compounds (15), cis, trans- antihistamines (16), proteolytic enzymes (17), enkephalins (18) and to the in vivo activities of oxotremorine analogues (19).

This method, which we call **eudismic analysis,** is applied to homologous series of isomeric pairs in which both isomers display measurable affinities (potencies, etc.). The more and less active member of each pair is called the **eutomer (Eu)** and **distomer (Dis),** respectively. These terms refer (20) to the good or bad "fit" between them and the receptor, and are independent of their absolute configuration, which may be irrelevant.

To illustrate our method it will be applied to recently published data of Ringdahl and Jenden (21) on the results of their elegant and painstaking studies on muscarinic receptor agonists and antagonists related to oxotremorine, and extending their own eudismic analysis somewhat.

2. The muscarinic receptor

In Fig. 1 is shown a plot of the affinities of both the eutomers and distomers against the affinity of the eutomers. Of course the eutomers lie on a line of unit slope but the distomers may form any pattern. The enantiomeric potency ratio is represented by the vertical separation between the members of any pair. On a logarithmic scale affinities are directly proportional to binding energies so that this separation corresponds to the difference in the binding energies of the eutomer and distomer (or to the logarithm of the enantiomeric potency ratio) which we term the **eudismic index (E.I.).** In the Easson-Stedman model of enantioselectivity (8) the distomers would all show similar low potencies since the third

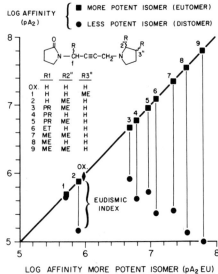

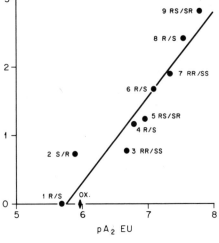

Figure 1. Structures of oxotremorine (OX.) and nine enantiomeric or diastereomeric pairs of analogues which are antagonists to it. Their affinities for muscarinic receptors in the isolated g.p.i. are plotted against the affinity of the more potent isomer which in all cases is the R-form. The s.d. of the pA₂ values are all less than 0.1. Data of Ringdahl and Jenden (21).

Figure 2. E.A.C. plot for the data in Fig. 1 of the enantioselectivity of the muscarinic receptor. The configurational descriptions are for C1 and C2″, Eu/Dis. The regression equation is E.I. = 7.1 + 1.2 pA₂ Eu, (n = 10, r² = 0.91).

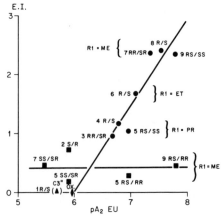

Figure 3. E.A.C. plot for the data in Fig. 1 of the epimeric stereoselectivity of the muscarinic receptor. The regression equation for the points marked with circles is E.I. = –8.6 + 1.4 pA₂ Eu, (n = 8, r² =0.92). The average E.I. for the square points is 0.42.

variable substituent would be oriented away from the binding
site, and the distomers would all lie on a horizontal line.
This is certainly not the case as can been seen from Fig. 1
where the distomers of **3** to **9** clearly fall on a descending
line.

The same data have been plotted in Fig. 2 in a slightly
different form which we call a **eudismic-affinity correlation
(E.A.C.) plot.** Here the eudismic index for each pair has been
plotted against the logarithm of the eutomer affinity. When
the regression between these two variables is analyzed, a
significant correlation is often found (11-19) as in this
case. The slope of the regression line **(E.A.Q., eudismic
affinity quotient)** represents the eudismic difference in
binding energy per unit increase in binding energy of the
eutomer. As such it can be considered a **quantitative measure
of stereoselectivity.** For the Easson-Stedman model it would be
unitary, as considered by Ringdahl and Jenden (21). Positive
slopes less than one have generally been found (12) and
interpreted at the molecular level in terms of alternate
binding modes. Slopes greater than one are found occasionally
and can be understood in terms of negative contributions to
the binding energy by steric hindrance.

Two further interesting details are to be found in Fig. 2.
Oxotremorine, which is the lowest achiral member of this
homologous series is also on the regression line and has been
included in its analysis. Similar observations have been made
in the case of some auxins (13), angiotensins (14) and
sweet-bitter compounds (15). The second notable point is that
in the compounds with a chiral center at C1 (**3** through **9** in
Fig. 1) the eutomer always has the same configuration, R̄.

The identical physical and chemical properties of enantiomers in achiral environments are very important in assuring
equal concentrations in the biophase. However, "chiral noise"
in the form of the stereoselective interactions with "silent"
chiral molecules in living systems (binding and carrier
proteins, phospholipids, etc.) may interfere, making difficult
the detection of enantiomeric eudismic-affinity correlations.
Diastereomers of course do not have identical properties but
they are often similar enough so that they can be included in
these correlations. Once the pharmacon-receptor complex has
formed, for compounds with two or more chiral centers, a
comparison between enantiomers may in fact be less informative
than one between epimers. The epimeric E.A.C. for these
compounds is shown in Fig. 3, from which some very interesting
new features emerge. It is immediately apparent that the
points fall into two groups: one comprises those which lie
along the regression line (circles) and the other shows 5
points (squares) that group themselves along a horizontal line

near the bottom of the figure. These groupings correspond without exceptions to the chiral center which was epimerized: the first to C1 and the second to C2" (see Fig. 1). Also shown (triangle) is a pair epimeric at C3" which will not be discussed   further. Note that oxotremorine itself once again falls squarely on the regression line (included in the analysis). These observations can be explained as follows: the chiral center at C1 is **critical** (10,11) to stereoselectivity whereas that at C2" is not; for the latter, epimerization results in small eudismic differences which are not correlated with affinity.

For the epimers at C1, once again and with no exceptions The R-isomers are the eutomers. The E.A.Q. here is 1.4, which clearly indicates the existence of steric hindrance, a point reinforced by the orderly progression from propyl through ethyl to methyl. To an unwary medicinal chemist this order would strongly suggest synthesizing the hydrogen analogue and he would be most disagreeably surprised to find that it (oxotremorine) would not only have a very low affinity but that it would be an agonist where the rest are antagonists at this receptor!

The seven epimeric antagonists **(3-9)** considered in Fig. 3 really belong to two different families. When these are considered separately as in Fig. 4, correlations are obtained with such high determination coefficients ($\geqslant$0.997) that they should dispel any doubts concerning the validity and importance of eudismic analyses.

The plots in Fig. 4 in turn suggested that further information could be extracted from these very precise data. The high E.A.Q. of these correlations (1.64 and 1.82, respectively) together with the orderly progression of the C1-substituent (propyl, ethyl, methyl) indicate clearly that this same substituent is contributing positively to binding in the distomeric series and negatively in the eutomeric series. This is schematically indicated in Fig. 5 from which can be extracted the average contribution per methylene group to the overall binding energy as -0.39 kcal/mole (attraction) in the distomeric series, and +0.53 kcal/mole (repulsion) due to steric hindrance in the eutomeric series. The former value falls within the range (-0.2 to -1 kcal/mole per methylene group) found for the binding of homologous series of compounds to various enzymes (22).

The above interpretation is incompatible with the Easson-Stedman model: the pharmacon's three substituents (excluding hydrogen) must be interacting with four subsites on the receptor disposed in space in a roughly tetrahedral arrangement such as can only obtain if the receptor's active site is a cleft or pouch.

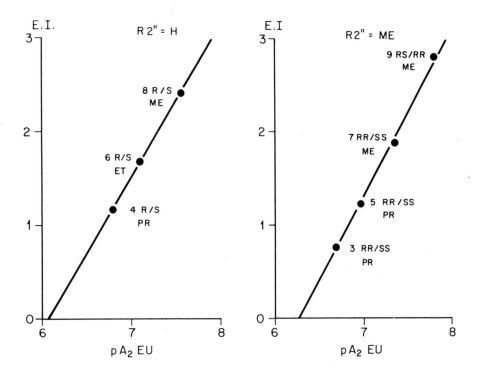

Figure 4. Separate E.A.C. for the 2''-hydrogen and 2''-methyl analogues. The regression equations are, respectively, E.I. = -10.0 + 1.64 pA₂ Eu, (n = 3, r² = 0.9998), and E.I. = -11.5 = 1.82 pA₂ Eu, (n = 4, r² = 0.997).

DISTOMERS   EUTOMERS

Figure 5. A schematic representation of the attractive and repulsive contributions to the overall binding energy per methylene group of the C1-substituent in the distomeric and eutomeric series, respectively.

5	6	pA₂ 7	8

6 CH₂ 4   4 CH₂ 6

8 CH₂ 6   6 CH₂ 8

7 (CH₂)₂ 3   3 (CH₂)₂ 7

9 (CH₂)₂ 5   5 (CH₂)₂ 9

+0.28   Av. Δ pA₂/CH₂   − 0.38
−0.39   Av. ΔF(kcal/mol)/CH₂   + 0.53
(ATTRACTION)   (REPULSION)

3. Other systems

During the ten years gone by since we concluded our survey
(11) of existing data bearing on this point, several hundred
new sets have become available. Although only a few dozen
fulfill the requirements for meaningful eudismic analysis
(three or more chiral pairs having measurable activities
covering a large potency span), the clear emergence of good
correlations such as those just described has been disappoint-
ing.
    Some of the better ones, each for a different type of
isomerism, are discussed below.
    a. Three enantiomeric pairs of methadone analogues were
examined for their ability to inhibit the binding of naloxone
to opiate receptors (23). In the absence of sodium (Fig. 6)
the increase of stereoselectivity with affinity is only hinted
at, but emerges clearly when the binding experiments were
carried out in the presence of 100 mM sodium ion.
    b. Some time ago (24) four pairs of E/Z isomers of
dibenzoxepins were evaluated for their chlorpromazine-like
behavioral activity (CPI). In spite of the complex measure of
activity employed, the correlation is excellent and has unit
slope (Fig. 7).
    c. Three pairs of diastereoisomeric tricyclic catecholamines
(25) show dopamine agonist activity. From Fig. 8 it would seem
that the dopamine receptor displays increasing stereoselectivity with increasing activity. Note that the E.A.Q. is
again close to 1, but that the variable substituent does not
affect the results in the expected progression.

4. Is receptor activation also stereoselective?

It is now well accepted in molecular pharmacology that the
pharmacon-receptor interaction takes place in at least two
stages: binding and activation (26). It is thus pertinent to
ask if stereoselectivity is also expressed during the
activation. Isolated data have been published, e.g. for
compound 2 in Fig. 1 the efficacy relative to oxotremorine is
0.073 for R-2 and 0.050 for S-2 (21), showing that the
efficacy of partial agonists is dependent on their stereochemistry. However, sufficient data for a eudismic analysis
seem not to have been reported. It is well known though, that
the enzyme-substrate complex resembles the receptor-pharmacon
complex in many ways, and for this interaction there is much
information available. Space allows citing only one example.
In a study of the carboxypeptidase-A catalyzed hydrolysis of
alanine peptides, Abramowitz et al. (27) reached the qualitative conclusion that kcat (the second step) is very sensitive

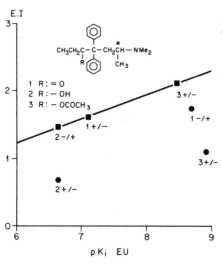

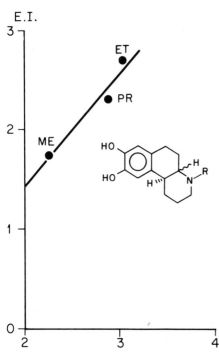

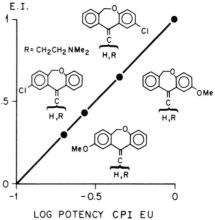

Figure 6. E.A.C. for the ability of methadone and two analogues to inhibit the binding of naloxone to opiate receptors in the absence (circles) and presence (squares) of 100 mM sodium. The regression equation for the latter is E.J. = -0.91 + 0.36 pK. Eu, (n = 3, r²∿1). Data from Ref. 23.

Figure 7. E.A.C. of the chlorpromazine-like potency in the conditioned avoidance response test of E,Z,-isomeric dibenzoxepins. In all cases the Z-isomer (ring substituent and amino side chain cis to each other) was the eutomer. Regression equation is E.J. = 1.00 + 1.00 log CPJ Eu, (n = 4,r²∿1). Data from Ref. 24.

Figure 8. E.A.C. of the cis,trans-stereoselectivity of the dopamine receptor for tricyclic catecholamines. Regression equation is E.J. = -0.84 + 1.13 log inhibitory potency Eu, (n = 3, r² = 0.94). Data from Ref. 25.

to epimerization whereas the first (binding, Km) is not. This
could be established quantitatively by a eudismic-affinity
analysis (1,17) in which the E.A.Q. for binding was zero and
that for reaction was 0.8.

B. Differences in Receptor Stereoselectivity Towards One or More Chiral Pairs

Some years ago we pointed out (11) that when the E.A.Q. is
taken as the measure of a receptor's stereoselectivity,
different receptors (e.g. histaminic and cholinergic) showed
different stereoselectivities (E.A.Q.) for the same set of
chiral diphenhydramine derivatives.

Recently Schunack and coworkers (28) reported on the
histaminergic activity of three pairs of chiral histamine
analogues (Fig.9). Although relatively high affinities are
involved, they found no stereoselectivity displayed by H1
receptors and a modest one by H2 receptors.

Very recently Robert et al.(29) pointed out that Pfeiffer's
Rule (9) has a corollary: for a given chiral pair interacting
with several different receptors the observed enantioselectivity shoud depend on affinity. To test this idea they examined
both enantiomers of methotrimeprazine, an analgesic/ neuroleptic, for their ability to interfere with the binding of
appropriate radioligands to three different (dopamine, opiate
and serotonin) CNS receptors. As Fig. 10 shows, a good
correlation was found: for this compound the opiate receptor
displays low affinity and stereoselectivity whereas the
dopamine and serotonin receptors display high affinities and
correspondingly high stereoselectivities.

C. Stereoselective metabolism

In a most interesting study Küpfer and Bircher (30)
studied the metabolic fate of both mephenytoin enantiomers in
the dog. The production of hydroxylated metabolites was
stereoselective (S/R = 1.4) while that of demethylated
metabolites was not. This difference is attributed to
differences in the apparent Km values of the transforming
enzymes: the high Km for hydroxylation leads to stereoselective transformation, while the low one for demethylation
does not.

CONCLUSION

In a few studies of stereoselective interactions of living
beings with bioactive compounds, the complexity of the system

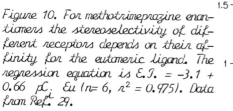

	HISTAMINERGIC		ACTIVITY	
	H1 RECEPTORS (G.P. ILEUM)		H2 RECEPTORS (G.P. ATRIA)	
	pD₂	I.A.	pD₂	I.A.
1	6.85	1.0	5.95	1.0
2R	4.31	0.57	3.42	0.48
2S	4.31	0.74	4.27	0.87
3R	4.35	0.7	5.58	1.0
3S	4.33	0.3	5.19	1.0
4R	4.33	0.6	5.66	1.0
4S	4.31	0.6	4.80	1.0

Figure 9. Structures and histaminergic activities of some chiral histamine analogues. Data from Ref. 28.

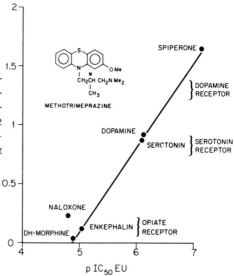

Figure 10. For methotrimeprazine enantiomers the stereoselectivity of different receptors depends on their affinity for the eutomeric ligand. The regression equation is E.I. = -3.1 + 0.66 pC. Eu (n= 6, r² = 0.975). Data from Ref. 29.

recedes into the background, allowing the pharmacon-receptor complex to be pictured at the molecular and submolecular levels. For such cases it has been verified that the receptor's stereoselectivity increases with the affinity it displays for the most potent isomer and that this stereo-selectivity can be analyzed quantitatively leading to a detailed description of their interaction.

REFERENCES

1. Lehmann F., P.A. (1978). In "Receptors and Recognition" (P. Cuatrecasas and M.F. Greaves, eds.), Series A, Vol. 5, p. 1, Chapman and Hall, London.
2. Lehmann F., P.A. (1980). Rev. Latinoam. Quím. 11, 82.
3. Fries, D.S., Dodge, R.P., Hope, H., and Portoghese, P.S. (1982). J. Med. Chem. 25, 9.
4. Mikeš, F., Boshart, G., and Gil-Av, E. (1976). J. Chromat. 122, 205.
5. Smith, D.F., ed. (1983). "Handbook of Stereoisomers. Drugs in Psychopharmacology", CRC Press, Boca Ratón, FL.
6. Rekker, R.F. (1977). "The Hydrophobic Fragmental Constant" Pharmacochemistry Library Vol. 1, Elsevier, Amsterdam.
7. Jorgensen, E.C. (1981). In "Molecular Basis of Drug Action" (T.P. Singer and Raúl N. Ondarza, eds.), p. 223, Elsevier, Amsterdam.
8. Easson, L.H., and Stedman, E. (1933). Biochem. J. 27, 1257.
9. Pfeiffer, C.C. (1956). Science 124, 29.
10. Ariëns, E.J., and Simonis, A.M. (1967). Ann. N.Y. Acad. Sci. 144, 842.
11. Lehmann F., P.A., Rodrigues de Miranda, J.F. and Ariëns, E.J. (1976). In "Progress in Drug Research" (E. Jucker, ed.), Vol. 20, p. 101, Birkhäuser Verlag, Basel.
12. Rodrigues de Miranda, J.F., Lehmann F., P.A. and Ariëns, E.J. (1976). In "Progress in Drug Research" (E. Jucker, ed.), Vol. 20, p. 126, Birkhäuser Verlag, Basel.
13. Lehmann F., P.A. (1978). Chem.-Biol. Interact. 20, 239.
14. Lehmann F., P.A. (1978). Chem.-Biol. Interact. 20, 251.
15. Lehmann F., P.A. (1978). Life Sci. 22, 1631.
16. Lehmann F., P.A. (1979). Rev. Latinoam. Quím. 10, 75.
17. Lehmann F., P.A. presented at the XIII Congreso Latino-americano de Ciencias Fisiológicas, México, D.F., 10-14 VII 1977.
18. Lehmann F., P.A. (1980). Proc. Third European Symposium on Chemical Structure-Biological Activity: Quantitative Approaches. Third Congress of the Hungarian Pharmacological Society, Budapest, Vol. 3, p. 285.

19. Lehmann F., P.A. (1982). TIPS 3, 103.
20. Derived analogously to those in Zeller, E.A. (1963). Ann. N.Y. Acad. Sci. 107, 811.
21. Ringdahl, B., and Jenden, D.J. (1983). Molec. Pharmacol. 23, 17.
22. Santi, D.V., and Kenyon, G.L. in "Burger's Medicinal Chemistry" (M.E. Wolff, ed.), 4th Ed., Part 1, p. 367 and 371, John Wiley, New York (1980).
23. Lattin, D.L., Caviness, B., Hudson, R.G., Greene, D.L., Raible, P.K., and Richardson, J.B. (1981). J. Med. Chem. 24, 903.
24. Tretter, J.F., Muren, J.F., Bloom, B.M., and Weissman A. (1966). Cited by Kaiser, C. and Setler, P.E. in "Burger's Medicinal Chemistry" (M.E. Wolff, ed.), 4th Ed., Part III, p. 901, John Wiley, New York, 1981.
25. Verimer, T., Long, J.P., Rusterholz, D.R., Flynn, J.R., Cannon, J.G. and Lee, T. (1980). Eur. J. Pharmacol. 64, 271.
26. van Ginneken, C.A.M. (1977). In "Kinetics of Drug Action" (J.M. van Rossum., ed.), Handbook of Experimental Pharmacology, Vol. 47, p. 357, Springer, Berlin.
27. Abramowitz, N., Schechter, I., and Berger, A. (1976). Biochem. Biophys. Res. Comm. 29, 862.
28. Gerhard, G., and Schunack, W. (1981). Arch. d. Pharm. 314, 1040; ibid., 312, 933 (1979).
29. Robert, T.A., Hagardor, A.N., and Daigneault, E.A. (1982). Mol. Pharmacol. 21, 315.
30. Küpfer, A., and Bircher, J. (1978). J. Pharmacol. Exp. Therap. 209, 190.

I would like to thank Susana Zamudio and Alfredo Padilla for their painstaking efforts in the preparation of this contribution.

II MOLECULAR AND GENETIC ANALYSIS OF DRUG ACTION

MECHANISM OF THYROID AND GLUCOCORTICOID HORMONE ACTION[1]

Morris J. Birnbaum,[2] Emily P. Slater, Michael Karin,[3]
Nancy C. Lan, James W. Apriletti, Synthia H. Mellon,
David G. Gardner, Alessandro Weisz, Norman L. Eberhardt,
and John D. Baxter

The Metabolic Research Unit
and
The Departments of Medicine
and Biochemistry and Biophysics
University of California
San Francisco, California 94143

I. INTRODUCTION

Glucocorticoid and thyroid hormones are ubiquitous as physiologic regulators. They affect not only important metabolic processes and homeostasis, but also differentiation and development of many higher species (for review, see 1-4). Determining the mechanisms of action of these hormones is critical to the understanding of their diverse functions. Also, the hormones have provided important models to understand more generally the regulation of gene expression.

---

[1]Supported by Grants AM-31347 and AM-19997 from the NIH and by a grant from California Biotechnology, Inc.
[2]A Fellow of The Helen Hay Whitney Foundation
[3]Present address: Department of Microbiology
University of Southern California
School of Medicine
Los Angeles, California 90023

In the current report, we have summarized some of our
studies of the actions of thyroid and glucocorticoid hormones. These investigations have involved analyses of the
receptors for both classes of hormones, the utilization of
model cell culture systems, and the transfer of hormone-
responsive genes to cells in which they ordinarily are not
expressed.

II. THYROID HORMONE RECEPTORS

Thyroid hormone receptors have been studied in a number of target tissues, and their predominant location is
within the nucleus (5). Occupancy of these receptors by
thyroid hormone analogs correlates well with the strength
of their thyromimetic activities (6). The nuclear location
of these receptors is also consistent with the general hypothesis that many actions of thyroid hormones are mediated
by effects on the transcription of specific genes.

Although the major hormone secreted by the thyroid
gland is thyroxine (T_4), which can bind to the nuclear
receptor, triiodothyronine (T_3) occupies most of the
available sites (7). Much of the T_3 is generated by intracellular conversion of T_4 to T_3. It is not entirely
clear how T_3 reaches its receptors. In intact cells,
binding to nuclear receptors occurs at 20° or 37° but
not at $0^\circ C$, while the hormone readily binds to solubilized receptors at $0^\circ C$ (8). This implies that some transport system is required in vivo. Recent evidence suggests
that there is a 55K molecular weight plasma membrane protein involved in transport of T_3 into cells (9).

The intranuclear receptors remain associated with chromatin whether or not they are bound to the hormone. These
receptors can be extracted from chromatin by salt or other
procedures (5,8) and, once solubilized, bind to purified
DNA (10). We have been unable to demonstrate specific binding of the receptor to the cloned rat growth hormone (rGH)
gene, which is transcriptionally regulated by thyroid hormone in intact cells. However, it is possible that nuclear
proteins are also required for accurate binding of receptors
to chromatin. We have found that solubilized receptors also
bind to histones (11). When nuclei are digested with DNAse
or micrococcal nuclease, the majority of the receptors sediment in a non-nucleosomal 6.5S particle that contains some
DNA (12). This calls into question the physiologic importance of histones in chromatin localization of the receptors.

Although the data suggest strongly that the intranuclear T_3 receptor mediates most thyroid hormone responses, other receptors have been postulated (13,14). In no case has binding to these receptors been rigorously correlated with the biological actions of the hormone, as has been done for the nuclear thyroid receptors. However, there are rapid effects of thyroid hormones that appear not to involve changes in gene transcription and possibly are mediated by extranuclear receptors.

Recently, we (15) and Pascual et al. (16) have photo-affinity-labelled the nuclear thyroid receptor. This is a single polypeptide chain of approximately 47K daltons. Minor species of greater and lesser molecular weight have also been found (16).

Thyroid hormone receptors may preferentially accumulate in transcriptionally active chromatin (17-19). We have recently found that, when permissive cells are infected with the DNA tumor virus SV40, thyroid receptors preferentially associate with the episomal viral chromatin, which is transcriptionally active (20). There is no known effect of thyroid hormone on SV40 expression or replication. Furthermore, when part of the viral genome is replaced by a thyroid-responsive gene, that for human GH, there is no additional preferential association of receptor binding to viral chromatin. This is consistent with the idea that the receptor's association with active chromatin is not restricted to genes regulated by thyroid hormone.

The receptor content of cells is dynamic, and these changes may or may not coincide with changes in hormone responsiveness. In cultured rat pituitary cells, T_3 induces a decrease in the number of its own receptors, shifting the receptor occupancy curve to a form that better describes the biological response (21). More recently, we have found that, under conditions in which T_3 reduces its receptor concentration by about 50%, there is a greater decrease (up to 90%) in the capability of the hormone to induce GH precursor mRNA (22). Similar results have not been obtained in the intact rat (23). Also, in contrast, incubation of cultured pituitary cells with sodium butyrate induces an 85% diminution in the number of thyroid hormone receptors without a comparable decrease in the responsiveness of the cells to the hormone (24). This suggests that a subpopulation of the total receptors is actually involved in the response to thyroid hormone. Whether different classes of thyroid hormone receptors are determined solely by subcellular localization, by association with other macromolecules, or by covalent modification and proteolysis of the receptor itself remains unknown.

III. GLUCOCORTICOID HORMONE RECEPTORS

   Receptors for glucocorticoid hormones have been studied
in a number of laboratories (for review, see 25). In the
absence of hormones, these proteins are found in the cytosol
of fractionated cells and in cell-free conditions bind weakly
to DNA and chromatin. The hormone apparently enters the cell
by passive diffusion and forms a receptor-glucocorticoid complex that ultimately binds to the nuclear chromatin. After
the hormone binds to the receptor, the complex undergoes a
temperature- and salt-dependent change, which has been
called "activation" or "transformation," and which appears
necessary for conversion of the complex to the nuclear-bind-
ing form. Although the mechanism of the activation is not
known, prominent theories include receptor dephosphorylation
(26), disaggregation (27) and dissociation from RNA (28).
The activated receptor binds to DNA, and recent studies from
several laboratories have indicated regions of DNA located
immediately 5' to glucocorticoid-regulated genes that specifically bind hormone-receptor complex (29-31). In the case
of the mouse mammary tumor virus (MMTV) (32,33) and human
metallothionein (34) genes, these receptor-binding sequences
are the same as those required for hormone regulation in
intact cells.
   We (35) and others (36) have purified the glucocorticoid receptor to over 50% homogeneity. It has also been
studied following photoaffinity or affinity labelling (37,
38) and is a single polypeptide chain of about 97K daltons.
The steroid-binding domain appears to be on the amino-ter-
minal portion of the molecule, and the DNA-binding domain in
the middle of the molecule; another domain, critical for the
receptor's function, appears to be on the carboxy-terminal
portion. The purified receptor retains its DNA-binding
properties (29-31), and the receptor we (35) and Grandics et
al. (39) have purified retains its ability to be activated.
Our preliminary results using purified receptor suggest that
its activation does not involve removal of RNA or a disaggregation of receptors.

IV. REGULATION OF GROWTH HORMONE GENE EXPRESSION
IN CULTURED PITUITARY CELLS
BY THYROID AND GLUCOCORTICOID HORMONES

   Cultured pituitary cells of the GC, GH_1 and GH_3 sub-
lines have been useful for examining the actions of thyroid

and glucocorticoid hormones (40,41). In these cells, rGH mRNA levels are increased by both classes of hormones, and there appear to be interactions between them. Glucocorticoids, when given alone, have only a modest effect on rGH mRNA or synthesis, whereas thyroid hormone alone induces a 10- to 20-fold response (42). However, in the presence of thyroid hormone, glucocorticoids increase GH mRNA 2- to 5-fold.

The actions of T_3 and at least some of those of glucocorticoids are due to stimulation of initiation of transcription, as determined by measuring levels of precursor mRNA by hybridization to intron-specific probes or by the "polymerase run-off" assay (42). The T_3 effect on transcription rates can be observed even when protein synthesis is blocked with cycloheximide (42), suggesting that the influence is a direct one not requiring the synthesis of mediating proteins. In the presence of T_3, the effects of dexamethasone on mRNA levels exceed the increases in transcription, suggesting that at least part of the control is exerted at a post-transcriptional site, possibly on mRNA stabilization.

The synergism of the two hormones is more complex, probably involving relatively stable permissive effects. When cultured pituitary cells are incubated with dexamethasone in the absence of T_3, little or no effect on rGH synthesis is seen after 48 hr (43). If the steroid is removed at that time and replaced by T_3 for 2 days, there is a greater induction of rGH synthesis than without preincubation with dexamethasone (44). Conversely, when cells have been grown in T_3-containing medium, dexamethasone increases GH precursor mRNA at 4 to 6 hr (45). In contrast, when T_3 and dexamethasone are added to cells at the same time, there is no further increase in precursor mRNA at 4 to 6 hr than when T_3 alone is added. These data imply that T_3 and glucocorticoids each produce stable, time-dependent alterations in pituitary cells which influence the actions of the other hormone.

V. REGULATION OF TRANSFERRED GENES BY GLUCOCORTICOID AND THYROID HORMONES

Enormous advances in the understanding of glucocorticoid hormone action have been made possible by the recent development of techniques to transfer cloned genes into cells in which they are not normally expressed. By co-transferring the gene of interest with a selectable gene or covalently linking putative regulatory elements of a hormone-responsive

gene to the coding portion of a selectable gene, stable cell
lines can be derived which are useful for the study of the
minimal structural elements in DNA necessary for response
to hormones. Thus, the mRNA levels of MMTV (46), $\alpha-_{2u}-$
globulin (47), hGH (48), rGH (49), and metallothionein (50)
are all increased by glucocorticoids after transfer into
heterologous cells. This shows that the information necessary for steroid responsiveness is contained within the
cloned DNA. Furthermore, the 5'-flanking DNA of some of
these genes has been linked to genes not naturally responsive to glucocorticoids and then assayed after gene transfer
(32,33,48). These hybrids retain their regulation by glucocorticoids, implying that the site of steroid action resides
at least in part on the immediate 5'-flanking sequences. To
date, there have been no published reports of thyroid hormone regulation of transferred genes.

We have studied the expression of the hGH and and rGH
genes after transfer to several different lines of tissue
culture cells. When rGH is co-transferred with the herpes
simplex virus thymidine kinase (HSV-TK) gene into mouse
fibroblasts deficient in TK (L TK⁻ cells) and then placed
under selective pressure for expression of the TK gene, the
mouse cells also take up and integrate the rat gene into
their genome. We have been unable to detect much of the
normal 1-kb rGH mRNA in these cells, but instead find a
shorter (about 0.8 kb) transcript predominantly. Single-
stranded nuclease protection experiments indicate that the
mRNA either starts within the second intervening sequence
or has an aberrant splice acceptor site there. Dexamethasone increases the rGH gene transcript levels in these cells
3- to 5-fold without grossly altering the size of the transcript. We have been unable to demonstrate an effect on
transcription using the polymerase run-off method. This is
consistent with the idea that the steroid is acting post-
transcriptionally, possibly on mRNA stabilization.

Human GH gene expression is regulated by glucocorticoids
after transfer to mouse L TK⁻ cells (48). Furthermore,
the transferred HSV-TK gene becomes steroid-regulated when
its promoter has been replaced by the hGH gene promoter (48).
We find no regulation of the hGH gene transferred into Rat
II cells (another fibroblast line) under conditions in which
dexamethasone regulates other transferred genes (vide infra),
even though an mRNA of appropriate size is made. While the
reasons for these differences are not known, they clearly
indicate that gene-specific cellular elements, in addition
to glucocorticoid receptors, are required for regulation by

the glucocorticoid. This is supported by our recent observation that the hGH gene is regulated by both T_3 and glucocorticoids after transfer to cultured rat pituitary tumor cells. In this experiment, mRNA was measured several days after transfer of the gene, a time when the recipient cells transiently express the foreign gene. Under these conditions, the transferred gene is not integrated into the host genome. This indicates that the sites for T_3 as well as dexamethasone control reside on the cloned gene.

Metallothionein is a protein that binds heavy metals and protects cells from their toxicity. It is virtually ubiquitous in nature (51-53), and its expression in cultured cells is increased by heavy metal ions or glucocorticoids (54). In both cases, control is at the level of transcription (55). When the human metallothionein$_{IIA}$ gene (hMT$_{IIA}$) was transferred to Rat II cells, its mRNA levels were regulated by Cd^{++} as well as dexamethasone (34). In addition, three types of hybrid constructions were transferred into Rat II cells:

1. the 5'-flanking DNA of HSV-TK was replaced with that of the hMT$_{IIA}$ gene;
2. a "hybrid promoter" was constructed with elements of the hMT$_{IIA}$ gene fused to the 3'-portion of the HSV-TK gene structure beginning just upstream from the TATA box;
3. the hMT$_{IIA}$ gene 5'-flanking DNA was placed about 600 bp "upstream" of the HSV-TK gene promoter region.

In all cases, TK gene expression was regulated by glucocorticoids. In the case of the first construction, pulse-label experiments indicated that control is mediated through increases in transcription. Furthermore, in transferrants from the third construction, glucocorticoids regulate transcripts arising at the TK gene as well as the hMT$_{IIA}$ gene promoter. These data indicate that: (i) a site of glucocorticoid action is on the 5'-flanking DNA of the hMT$_{IIA}$ gene; (ii) this regulatory segment can confer steroid responsiveness on a promoter not normally regulated by glucocorticoids; and (iii) the site of glucocorticoid action is separable from the promoter and initiation site. Similar conclusions have been drawn from recent work on the regulation of the MMTV gene (56,57).

VI. SUMMARY

This report summarizes a number of our findings concerning glucocorticoid and thyroid hormone action. For both
classes of hormone, the receptors are single polypeptide
chains of 47K daltons (thyroid hormone) and 97K daltons
(glucocorticoids). They can be photoaffinity-labelled and
purified substantially. Both are DNA binding proteins and
act on a portion of hGH contained in the cloned gene.

In rat pituitary cells, both T_3 and dexamethasone
stimulate transcription of the GH gene, although the latter
may also act post-transcriptionally. Also, the two hormones
act synergistically in a time-dependent manner. At least
some of these complex relationships are preserved for the
hGH gene transferred into rat pituitary cells.

Gene transfer experiments have yielded information not
only about the structural features of a glucocorticoid-
responsive gene but also about the mechanism of hormone
action. For the few genes studied, a region that confers
steroid control of RNA transcription resides on the portion
of DNA immediately upstream from the structural gene. This
is the same general area as the promoter, but gene transfer
of chimeric genes has clearly demonstrated the hormone regulatory and promoter functions to be physically separate.
Furthermore, the glucocorticoid-responsive element (57) can
act over a distance to influence expression of genes not
normally regulated by glucocorticoids. Such a mechanism is
similar to so-called "enhancers" recently described in viral
genomes (58,59). These are elements that seem to induce
some change in chromatin structure, allowing increased transcription of neighboring genes. Enhancers are characterized
by action that is independent of orientation and effective
over relatively large distances. Viral enhancers are
generally not known to be regulated, but the regulatory region flanking the MMTV gene might be an exception. Thus,
the general model that emerges for glucocorticoid regulation
of transcription is that of a hormone-responsive enhancer
element. Whether this represents the only means for glucocorticoid control of gene expression remains unclear,
although there are data suggesting an additional post-transcriptional locus for hormone action.

REFERENCES

1. Baxter, J.D., and Rousseau, G.G. (1979) in "Glucocorticoid hormone action" (Baxter, J.D., and Rousseau, G.G., eds.), p. 1. Springer-Verlag, Heidelberg.
2. Eberhardt, N.L., Apriletti, J.W., and Baxter, J.D. (1980) in "The Biochemical Actions of Hormones" (Litwack, G., ed.), p. 311, Academic Press, New York.
3. Baxter, J.D., and Tyrrell, J.B. (1981) in "Endocrinology and Metabolism" (Felig, P., Baxter, J.D., Broadus, A.E., and Frohman, L.A., eds.), p. 385, McGraw-Hill, New York.
4. Oppenheimer, J.H., and Samuels, H.H., eds. (1983) "The Molecular Basis of Thyroid Hormone Action" Academic Press, New York.
5. Surks, M.I., Koerner, D., Dillman, W.H., and Oppenheimer, J.H. (1973) J. Biol. Chem. 248, 7066.
6. Koerner, D., Schwartz, H.L., Surks, M.I., Oppenheimer, J.H., and Jorgensen, E.C. (1975) J. Biol. Chem. 250, 6417.
7. Surks, M.I., and Oppenheimer, J.H. (1977) J. Clin. Invest. 60, 555.
8. Samuels, H.H., Tsai, J.S., Casanova, J., and Stanley, F. (1974) J. Clin. Invest. 54, 853.
9. Horiuchi, R., Johnson, M.L., Willingham, M.C., Pastan, I., and Cheng, S.-Y. (1982) Proc. Natl. Acad. Sci. U.S.A. 79, 5527.
10. MacLeod, K.M., and Baxter, J.D. (1976) J. Biol. Chem. 251, 7380.
11. Apriletti, J.W., David-Inouye, Y., Baxter, J.D., and Eberhardt, N.L. (1983) in "The Molecular Basis of Thyroid Hormone Action" (Oppenheimer, J.H., and Samuels, H.H., eds.), p. 67, Academic Press, New York.
12. Perlman, A.J., Stanley, F., and Samuels, H.H. (1982) J. Biol. Chem. 257, 930.
13. Pliam, N.B., and Goldfine, I.D. (1977) Biochem. Biophys. Res. Commun. 79, 166.
14. Sterling, K., and Milch, P.O. (1975) Proc. Natl. Acad. Sci. U.S.A. 72, 3225.
15. David-Inouye, Y., Somack, R., Nordeen, S.K., Apriletti, J.W., Baxter, J.D., and Eberhardt, N.L. (1982) Endocrinology 111, 1758.
16. Pascual, A., Casanova, J., and Samuels, H.H. (1982) J. Biol. Chem. 257, 9640.
17. Samuels, H.H., Stanley, F., and Shapiro, L.E. (1977) J. Biol. Chem. 252, 6052.

18. Charles, M.A., Ryffel, G.N., Obinata, J., McCarthy, B.J., and Baxter, J.D. (1975) Proc. Natl. Acad. Sci. U.S.A. 72, 1787.
19. Levy, B., and Baxter, J.D. (1976) Biochem. Biophys. Res. Commun. 68, 1045.
20. Savouret, J.-F., Eberhardt, N.L., Cathala, G., and Baxter, J.D. (submitted for publication).
21. Samuels, H.H., Stanley, F., and Shapiro, L.E. (1976) Proc. Natl. Acad. Sci. U.S.A. 73, 3877.
22. Lan, N.C. (unpublished observations).
23. Spindler, B.J., MacLeod, K.M., Ring, J., and Baxter, J.D. (1976) J. Biol. Chem. 250, 4113.
24. Eberhardt, N.L., Malich, N., Baxter, J.D., Nordeen, S.K., and Johnson, L.K. (submitted for publication).
25. Baxter, J.D., and MacLeod, K.M. (1980) in "Duncan's Diseases of Metabolism" (Bondy, P.K., and Rosenberg, L.E., eds.), p. 140, W.B. Saunders, Philadelphia.
26. Leach, K.L., Dahmer, M.K., Hammond, N.D., Sando, J.J., and Pratt, W.B. (1979) J. Biol. Chem. 254, 11884.
27. Higgins, S.J., Rousseau, G.G., Baxter, J.D., and Tomkins, G.M., (1973) J. Biol. Chem. 248, 5866.
28. Chong, M.T., and Lippman, M.E. (1982) J. Biol. Chem. 257, 2996.
29. Payvar, F., Wrange, O., Carlstedt-Duke, J., Okret, S., Gustafsson, J.-A., and Yamamoto, K.R. (1981) Proc. Natl. Acad. Sci. U.S.A. 78, 6628.
30. Govindan, M.U., Spiess, E., and Majors, J. (1982) Proc. Natl. Acad. Sci. U.S.A. 79, 5157.
31. Pfahl, M. (1982) Cell 31, 475.
32. Huang, A.L., Ostrowsky, M.C., Berard, D., and Hager, G.L. (1981) Cell 27, 245.
33. Lee, F., Mulligan, R., Berg, P., and Ringold, G. (1981) Nature 294, 228.
34. Karin, M., Cathala, G., Holtgreve, H., Slater, E., and Baxter, J.D. (submitted for publication).
35. Wong, J.R., Weisz, A., Lan, N.C., and Santi, D.V. (submitted for publication).
36. Wrango, O., Carlstedt-Duke, J., and Gustafsson, J.-A. (1979) J. Biol. Chem. 254, 9284.
37. Nordeen, S.K., Lan, N.C., Showers, M.O., and Baxter, J.D. (1981) J. Biol. Chem. 256, 10503.
38. Simons, S.S. Jr., and Thompson, E.B. (1981) Proc. Natl. Acad. Sci. U.S.A. 78, 3541.
39. Grandics, P., Miller, A., Schmidt, T.J., Mittman, D., and Litwack, G. (1983) Proceedings of the 65th Annual Meeting of The Endocrine Society, San Antonio, Texas, June 5-7, 1983, Abstr. No. 590.

40. Tashjian, A.H. Jr., Bancroft, F.C., and Levine, L. (1970) J. Cell Biol. 47, 61.
41. Martial, J.A., Baxter, J.D., Goodman, H.M., and Seeburg, P.H. (1977) Proc. Natl. Acad. Sci. U.S.A. 74, 1816.
42. Spindler, S.R., Mellon, S.H., and Baxter, J.D. (1982) J. Biol. Chem. 257, 11627.
43. Wegnez, M., Schachter, B.S., Baxter, J.D., and Martial, J.A. (1982) DNA 1, 145.
44. Ivarie, R.D. (personal communication).
45. Lan, N.Y.C., Gardner, D.G., Nguyen, T., Baxter, J.D., and Cathala, G. (submitted for publication).
46. Hynes, N.E., Kennedy, N., Rahmsdorf, U., and Groner, B. (1981) Proc. Natl. Acad. Sci. U.S.A. 78, 2038.
47. Kurtz, D.J. (1981) Nature 291, 629.
48. Robins, D.M., Paek, I., Seeburg, P.H., and Axel, R. (1982) Cell 29, 623.
49. Doehmer, J., Barinaga, M., Vale, W., Rosenfeld, M.G., Verma, I.M., and Evans, R.M. (1982) Proc. Natl. Acad. Sci. U.S.A. 79, 2268.
50. Mayo, K.E., Warren, R., and Palmiter, R.D. (1982) Cell 29, 29.
51. Kagi, J.H.R., and Vallee, B.L. (1961) J. Biol. Chem. 236, 2435.
52. Failla, M.L., Benedict, D.C., and Weinberg, E.D. (1976) J. Gen. Microbiol. 94, 23.
53. Rudd, C.J., and Herschman, H.R. (1979) Toxicol. Appl. Pharmacol. 47, 273.
54. Karin, M., and Herschman, H.R. (1980) J. Cell Physiol. 103, 36.
55. Hager, L.J., and Palmiter, R.D. (1981) Nature 291, 340.
56. Hynes, N., Ooyen, A.J.J. van, Kennedy, N., Herrlich, P., Ponta, H., and Groner, B. (1983) Proc. Natl. Acad. Sci. U.S.A. 80, 3637.
57. Chandler, V.L., Maler, B.A., and Yamamoto, K.R. (1983) Cell 33, 489.
58. Moreau, P., Heu, R., Wasylyk, B., Everett, R., Garib, M.P., and Chambon, P. (1981) Nucl. Acids Res. 9, 6047.
59. Banerji, J., Rusconi, S., and Schaffner, W. (1981) Cell 27, 299.

GLUCOCORTICOID REGULATION OF MOUSE MAMMARY TUMOR VIRUS GENE EXPRESSION

Gordon Ringold[1], Alger Chapman, Maureen Costello, Deborah Dobson, Carol Hall[2], J. Russell Grove, Frank Lee[2] and James Vannice

Department of Pharmacology
Stanford University
Stanford, California

I. INTRODUCTION

Glucocorticoids, as well as other classes of steroid hormones, appear to function via the "two-step" model originally proposed by Jensen and his colleagues (1). It is generally accepted that steroids interact with a soluble receptor protein inducing a structural alteration that increases the receptor's affinity for DNA or chromatin. This so-called "activated" form of the steroid-receptor complex accumulates within the nucleus of the cell leading to increased (and perhaps in some cases, decreased) transcription of specific genes. In this view, the primary role of the steroid is to act as an allosteric effector that unmasks a DNA-binding site on the receptor protein. The detailed molecular mechanisms by which the steroid-receptor complex stimulates transcription of specific genes are poorly understood.

We have previously documented the utility of glucocorticoid inducible mouse mammary tumor virus (MMTV) as a model system to study the mechanisms of steroid hormone action (2, 3). In this report we briefly summarize some of these studies and present a detailed account of the use of MMTV in furthering our understanding of the mechanisms by which glucocorticoids regulate gene expression.

---

[1]Supported by NIH Grant GM 25821 and a Basil O'Connor Grant from the March of Dimes.
[2]DNAX Research Institute, Palo Alto, CA.

II. MOUSE MAMMARY TUMOR VIRUS

As is true of all retroviruses, MMTV is an enveloped virus containing a single-stranded RNA genome (4). During infection of a cell, MMTV binds to a surface receptor, becomes internalized and the nucleoprotein core becomes "activated." Within the cytoplasm of the infected cell, a linear double-stranded DNA copy of the viral RNA is synthesized by the viral reverse transcriptase (5-9). Later, MMTV DNA becomes covalently linked to the host DNA where it resides as a stable Mendelian locus in the progeny of the infected cell. Once the DNA is integrated in the host cell's genome (in this state the DNA is refered to as a provirus) it is controlled in large part by the normal cellular machinery. Several species of RNA, including genomic-sized RNA for encapsidation into progeny virus and smaller RNAs for use as messenger RNAs are synthesized by cellular RNA polymerase II (10-12). As has been alluded to earlier, and is the major focus of our work, it is the production of these RNAs that is under glucocorticoid control. The viral life cycle is completed by assembling the appropriate RNAs into a virion precursor which buds from the cell membrane, thereby releasing an intact virus particle.

The synthesis of retroviral DNA by reverse transcription is a fascinating and remarkably complex process (13, 14). An important feature of such DNAs is that they are longer than the parental RNA; this extra length arises by duplication of sequences present at the extreme 5' and 3' ends of the viral RNA. These duplications exist at the ends of the linear viral DNA and are thus commonly refered to as the long terminal repeats or LTR's (14). In the case of MMTV DNA, the LTR's are approximately 1350 base-pairs (b.p.) in length, 130 of these arising from the 3' end (15-17). The structures of MMTV RNA and DNA are depicted in Fig. 1. For the purposes of this discussion, it is only of primary importance to note that the beginning (5') end of the viral RNA resides within the left-hand LTR; indeed, as will be discussed later, the promoter and the glucocorticoid regulatory region of the viral genome reside within the LTR.

Glucocorticoid Induction of MMTV

We have previously documented that induction of MMTV RNA is a primary response to the glucocorticoid-receptor complex (2, 3). The evidence supporting this statement includes: 1) induction of viral RNA does not require protein synthesis; 2) the effect of the hormone is to increase the rate of synthesis of RNA within 5-15 minutes; 3) induction requires functional glucocorticoid receptors. Based on these findings, it seems likely that the glucocorticoid-

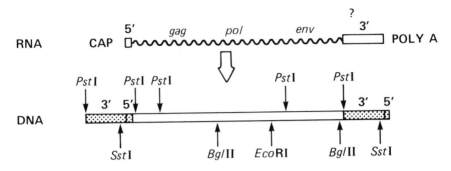

FIGURE 1. The structure of the DNA and RNA forms of the
MMTV genome. The RNA is approximately 9000 bases in length and
encodes the genes for coat proteins or group-specific antigens (gag),
envelope glycoproteins (env), reverse transcriptase (pol), and a
postulated, but as yet identified, gene product (?). The linear form
of MMTV DNA is the direct product of reverse transcription. At
each end is a long terminal repeat (LTR) consisting of sequences
derived from both the 5' and 3' ends of viral RNA; these are shown
as the boxes denoted 3' (~1200 base pairs)/5' (~130 base pairs). The
PstI fragment (stippled) containing the left-hand LTR plus 135 base
pairs coding for RNA beyond the 5' boxed region, was used in
construction of the recombinant plasmids as shown in Fig. 3.

receptor complex itself, interacting with viral DNA (and perhaps
other chromosomal proteins), is sufficient to stimulate transcription
at the MMTV promoter.

III. GENETIC APPROACH TO GLUCOCORTICOID ACTION

The ability to select mutants in a complex biochemical pathway
is often useful in delineating the components involved in a given
reaction.

The approach we have used to select glucocorticoid unresponsive cells is depicted in Figure 2. In brief, since the major MMTV
glycoprotein (gp52) is expressed on the surface of infected HTC
cells in a glucocorticoid-dependent manner (6), it seemed likely that
we could separate induced from uninduced cells in a fluorescence-
activated cell sorter (FACS). For these studies we chose two clones
of MMTV-infected HTC cells, M1-19, which contains approximately
10 proviruses and J2-17, which contains a single provirus. Our
expectations were that if we could select cells in the FACS that no
longer induce gp52, these two cell lines would give rise to hormone
unresponsive variants of different types. Since M1-19 contains

multiple copies of the provirus, inactivation of gp52 induction would have to be a consequence of a lesion that affects these genes coordinately (e.g., a receptor defect). In contrast, J2-17 has a single provirus and thus a mutation in the viral DNA itself could lead to reduced production of gp52.

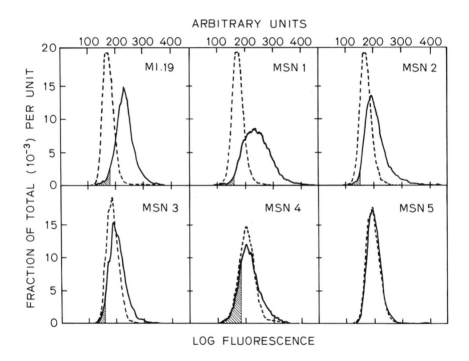

FIGURE 2: Selection of glucocorticoid unresponsive M1-19 cells. Cells were stained as described (18) and passed through a FACS. That portion of the population (+DEX) displaying the lowest fluorescence was collected under sterile conditions; this represented approximately 1-4% of the population or 5000-30,000 cells. The sorted population (MSN1) was propagated in the absence of dexamethasone for two weeks to accumulate sufficient numbers of cells for another sorting cycle. This procedure was repeated until we obtained a population (MSN5) which failed to induce gp52. The hatched area represents the population collected from the induced cells at each sort. The analyses indicate the fluorescence intensity distributions of cells grown in the presence (———) or absence (- - -) of dexamethasone.

A selection of unresponsive cells derived from M1-19 is shown in Figure 2. Cells were induced for 48 hours in dexamethasone (10^{-6} M), stained with rabbit antibody against gp52, followed by fluorescein-conjugated goat anti-rabbit IgG, and analyzed in the FACS. Those cells displaying the lowest fluorescence in the presence of hormone (typically 1-3% of the cells) were collected under sterile conditions and grown for 2-3 weeks in the absence of hormone prior to another sorting cycle. This process was repeated until no detectable induction of gp52 could be observed in the FACS. After five rounds of enrichment in the FACS such a population, designated MSN5, was obtained; MSN6 was produced as a subpopulation sorted from MSN5 (18). These populations were then cloned either in soft agar or by sorting single cells into microtiter wells.

In the case of J2-17, cells were first mutagenized with ethyl methanesulfonate to yield a population designated JZ. These cells retain hormonal responsiveness, as evidenced by their ability to induce both MMTV gp52 and the enzyme tyrosine aminotransferase in response to dexamethasone (19). A similar protocol to that for MSN was used to isolate glucocorticoid response variants of JZ cells in the FACS; in this case, three cycles of enrichment produced a population, JZN3, that displays markedly reduced levels of hormone-induced gp52 (19).

Analysis of Glucocorticoid Unresponsive Cells:
Receptor vs. Non-receptor Defects

One of the advantages to using HTC cells for our genetic studies is the availability of cellular glucocorticoid inducible genes that can be easily measured. It is, therefore, possible to approach issues related to the coordinate regulation of gene expression by glucocorticoids and to ascertain whether the defects in MSN and JZN cells are global or restricted to MMTV induction. The three cellular markers we have used are tyrosine aminotransferase (TAT), glutamine synthetase (GS), and the secreted glycoprotein known as Belt I (20).

We have used inducibility of cellular genes to analyze the defects in our variant cells in greater detail. As seen in Table IA, MSN5.3 cells (representative of all MSN cells) are incapable of inducing any glucocorticoid inducible functions, whereas the parental cells MSC-1 (a sub-fraction of the original M1-19 cells) induce all four markers. These results corroborate our previous conclusion that the unresponsiveness of MSN cells is a result of a receptor defect (18); an ancillary point of interest is that all four of the glucocorticoid inducible gene products in HTC cells thus appear to be regulated by a single receptor pathway.

Table I. Inductions of gp52, TAT, GS, and Belt I in Parental and Non-responsive Cells

		TAT fold-ind. (n)	gp52 Δ (n)	GS fold-ind. (n)	Belt I fold-ind. (n)
(A)	MSC1	4.8 (5)	105 (7)	3.1 (2)	7.9 (3)
	MSN5.3	1.0 (4)	8.8 (5)	1.0 (2)	1.3 (3)
(B)	JZ	10.6 (16)	32.7 (15)	7.0 (2)	8.7 (4)
	JZN3.7	8.3 (9)	6.4 (15)	6.4 (4)	7.6 (3)

TAT, GS, and Belt I assays and inductions were performed as described in reference 20a. MMTV gp52 was analyzed in the FACS where Δ represents the change in arbitrary logarithmic units of fluorescence (see Fig. 2) and does not reflect a fold-induction; the difference between 8.8 and 105 log fluorescence units represents at least a 20-fold change in gp52 expression. The data are presented as means, with the number of independent experiments shown in parenthesis.

(A) MSC1 is a population of cells derived from M1.19 that maintains all of its normal glucocorticoid properties.

In contrast, JZN cells, which do not induce MMTV yet contain normal levels of receptor, retain the ability to induce GS, TAT, and Belt I (Table IB). Thus, in this case, the defect appears to be specific to the MMTV genome (one is reminded that there is a single MMTV provirus in these cells). The results of these studies strongly suggest that the defect in JZN3.7 (as well as the other JZN clones) resides in the MMTV DNA itself, or possibly in a cellular factor, that is specifically required for the glucocorticoid induction of the viral genes. One method for distinguishing between these alternatives is to superinfect JZN cells with MMTV. If the defect in the unresponsive cells resides in a cellular protein that acts upon MMTV DNA (i.e. is trans acting), the newly acquired proviruses will also be unresponsive to hormone. However, if it is the original provirus that is defective (i.e. a cis acting defect), then the newly introduced viral DNA should be inducible. Such experiments clearly demonstrates that superinfected JZN3.7 cells exhibit glucocorticoid inducible gp52. Similar results have been obtained with other completely unresponsive clones such as JZN3.6 and with partially inducible clones such as JZN3.9 and JZN3.13 (20a).

IV. MAPPING A GLUCOCORTICOID REGULATORY REGION ON MMTV DNA

A. MMTV-dhfr Fusions

The results of our previous studies on integration and transcription of MMTV and our genetic studies provide strong circumstantial evidence that MMTV encodes its own glucocorticoid regulatory region. To test this directly, we have constructed hybrid genes containing the putative promoter and regulatory region from MMTV fused to the coding region of genes whose activity can be assayed conveniently and/or whose function can be selected for in vivo (21). Our initial constructions utilized a cDNA containing the coding region for mouse dihydrofolate reductase (dhfr) fused to the Pst I fragment encompassing the left-hand LTR of MMTV (see Figure 2). The plasmids we have constructed are derivatives of the SV40 eukaryotic expression vectors developed by Berg and his colleagues (22, 23). When the plasmids were introduced into dhfr⁻ CHO cells, mouse dhfr was produced under the control the MMTV promoter. Moreover, addition of glucocorticoids resulted in a 5-fold stimulation of enzyme production (21).

Similar experiments have recently been performed using an analogous plasmid (Figure 3) containing the E. coli gene encoding xanthine guanine phosphoribosyl transferase (XGPRT) (24). This plasmid designated PSVMgpt was used to transform mouse 3T6 cells using the dominant selection scheme described by Mulligan and Berg. We have quantitated the amount of XGPRT RNA and determined that the message initiates at the known start site of MMTV transcription using the procedure of Berk and Sharp (36). The hybrid band detected by autoradiography is ~ 400 b.p. in length (Figure 4) indicating that the predominant 5' end of the XGPRT RNA maps to a site within the MMTV LTR, ~ 275 bases upstream of the XGPRT insert; this corresponds to the 3'-5' border of the LTR (i.e. the start site for MMTV transcription). Moreover, the production of this RNA is increased in dexamethasone-treated cells 5-15 fold.

B. MMTV-β-galactosidase Fusions

As described in the dhfr and XGPRT experiments, expression of foreign genes encoded on plasmids has generally been studied in stable transformants arising either from direct selection for the functional gene or from co-transfection with another selectable marker (26). A general shortcoming of this approach is the length of time required to grow sufficient numbers of cells from individual clones for analysis. A very useful alternative is provided by experiments in which expression of plasmid genes is assayed within the first few days following DNA infection. These so-called "transient-expression assays" offer not only a time advantage, but since the average level of gene expression from the transfected population is measured, the considerable variability typically observed among individual clones can be avoided.

The gene we have utilized for this series of experiments is the E. coli lac Z gene, which encodes the enzyme β-galactosidase. Quantitation of the enzyme is performed by a very simple, reproducible, and extremely sensitive colorimetric assay. The plasmid we have constructed, pCH105 (27), is again a derivative of the pSMVgpt plasmid (Figure 3) in which the XGPRT gene has been replaced by the E. coli lac Z gene obtained originally as a fusion gene product (28). A similar plasmid, pCH110, containing the SV40 promoter, rather than the MMTV promoter, was also constructed (27). As shown in Table II, when these plasmids are introduced into mouse L cells using the DEAE-dextran procedure (29), the levels of β-galactosidase detected in cell extracts three days after DNA infection was approximately the same as mock infected cells. However, when dexamethasone (10^{-6} M) was added to the trans-

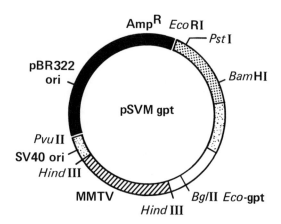

FIGURE 3. Structure of the fusion plasmid containing E. coli gpt DNA linked to the MMTV LTR. The solid black segment is a 2.3 Kb fragment of the plasmid pBR322 (from the EcoRI site to the PvuII site) containing the ampicillin-resistance gene and the origin of replication. The stippled regions are derived from SV40 virus and provide signals for processing of mRNA transcripts (22, 23, 25). The hatched region represents the MMTV LTR, derived from the Pst fragment shown in Fig. 1. The open region is the Eco gpt DNA. Transcription from the MMTV promoter is in the counterclockwise direction as is the coding region for gpt. See Refs. 21 and 24 for further description of the construction of this plasmid.

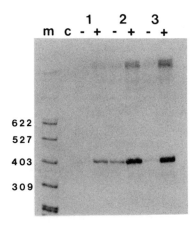

FIGURE 4. Glucocorticoid induction and mapping of gpt RNA in 3T6 cells transformed with pSVM gpt. Mouse 3T6 cells were transfected with plasmid DNA using $CaPO_4$ (35); transformants expressing gpt were selected by their ability to grow in the presence of mycophenolic acid and xanthine (25). Three such transformants were grown in the presence (48 hours) or absence of dexamethasone (10^{-6} M) and cytoplasmic RNA was isolated. Poly(A)–containing; RNA was prepared by chromatography on oligo dT–cellulose and approximately 1 μg was hybridized with a probe end labeled with [^{32}P] ATP at the BglII site within the gpt gene (see Fig. 3). Hybridization was performed at 50°C for ~16 hours in 80% formamide according to the procedure of Berk and Sharp (36). RNA-DNA hybrids were treated with S_1 nuclease and run on a 6% acrylamide gel which was autoradiographed for 4 days. Left lane: size marker of [^{32}P]pBR322 DNA digested with Hinf L. RNA from cells grown in the absence (–) or presence (+) of dexamethasone. The band migrating at a size of ~410 base pairs corresponds to a gpt RNA that is initiated at the proper MMTV promoter.

fected cells 24 hours prior to assaying the enzyme, the levels were at least 25 times above background when pCH105 was used. In contrast, β-galactosidase production from the SV40 promoter is not glucocorticoid inducible.

C. Deletion Mapping Studies of the MMTV LTR

The results of our gene fusion experiments clearly demonstrate that the MMTV LTR contains a region that confers glucocorticoid responsiveness on the expression of any linked gene. To further delineate the sequences of importance for hormonal regulation, we

TABLE II. Glucocorticoid Induction of β–galactosidase in Transient Expression Experiments

Plasmid	β–galactosidase Specific Activity		
	−DEX	+DEX	Fold Induction
mock	0.67 (4)	0.95 (4)	1.4
pCH110 (SV40- βgal)	11.8 (2)	8.6 (2)	0
pCH105 (MMTV-β gal)	0.7 (4)	18.3 (4)	26

Infections with DNA were performed by incubating mouse L Tk⁻
cells with 10-20 μg plasmid in the presence of 200 μg/ml DEAE-
dextran for 4 hours. Cells were washed and then incubated for 2
days in growth medium. Dexamethasone (10^{-6}M) was added for 1
day and cells were collected, pelleted, and resuspended in 0.25M
sucrose, 10mM Tris-HCl pH 7.4 and 10 mM EDTA. Cells were lysed
by freeze-thawing and debris was removed by a 5 minute centrifugation in a microfuge.   β-galactosidase activity is expressed as n
moles ONPG cleaved per minute per mg protein.

have constructed deletion mutants that remove portions of the LTR
in either the XGPRT plasmid (PSVMgpt) or the β–galactosidase
plasmid (pCH 105). Data from the XGPRT deletions was obtained
by RNA mapping studies in transformed 3T6 cells as described above;
from the β–gal plasmids, data was obtained using the transient
expression assay. A summary of a large set of such studies is
presented in Figure 5.

The result of these experiments allow three major conclusions
to be made. The first is that one can eliminate inducible expression
without interfering with basal promoter function; moreover, the
sequences important for regulation must reside (at least in part)
upstream of nucleotide -109, since deletion of such sequences
abolishes hormonal responsiveness. Second, the left hand (upstream)
border of the glucocorticoid regulatory region must be downstream
of nucleotide -224, since plasmids in which the entire left end of the
LTR up to -224 respond to hormone. Third, the right hand boundary
of the regulatory region must be upstream of nucleotide -141, since
plasmids in which the sequence between -109 and -141 is deleted
retain inducibility. Deletion of the nucleotides between -210 and
-109 eliminates glucocorticoid responsiveness corroborating these
points. In the aggregate, these studies strongly suggest that the
major region of the MMTV LTR responsible for glucocorticoid sensitivity resides between nucleotides -210 and -141 relative to the
start of transcription.

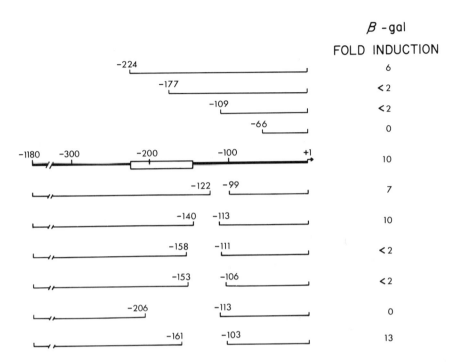

FIGURE 5. Mapping the glucocorticoid regulatory region of the MMTV LTR by deletion analysis. Construction of the indicated molecules was accomplished either by removal of specific restriction endonuclease fragments or by digestion with Bal 31 exonuclease. In some cases the deletions were reconstructed so as to replace sequences between -110 and +1 as shown in the diagram. Analysis of β-galactosidase activity was as described in Table II. The end points of the deletions were determined by direct sequencing analysis of the DNA.

A further, and perhaps subtle, point that can be made from analysis of some of the internal deletions is that the absolute spacing between the promoter and regulatory region need not be constant. In fact, we have also found that insertion of 4 nucleotides at position -109 does not interfere with induction by dexamethasone. Since this is a minor alteration, we are currently determining the maximum distance by which the promoter and regulatory region can be separated by inserting larger fragment at position -109.

A point must be made of the anomalous behavior of a deletion mutant in which the sequence between -103 and -161 have been removed. Although we currently have no explanation for the ability of this mutant to respond normally to hormone, we hypothesize that a fortuitous regulatory region may have been reconstructed in this molecule.

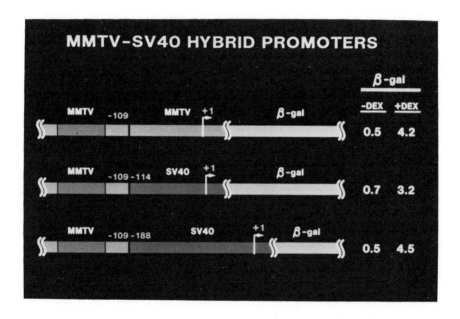

FIGURE 6.   Glucocorticoid induction from SV40 promoters fused to the hormone regulatory region.   The sequences in the MMTV LTR upstream of residue -109 were fused to portions of the SV40 early promoter provided by M. Fromm and P. Berg (37).   These molecules were then inserted into a plasmid of the type described in Fig. 4; in this case, as in Table II and Fig. 6, the gene assayed was E. coli β-galactosidase as described (27).

D. The Hormone Regulatory Region Confers Glucocorticoid Responsiveness on a Heterologous Promoter

Analysis of a deletion mutant that removes all but 66 nucleotides upstream of the start of MMTV transcription revealed that such a mutant contains the DNA required for appropriate basal level of expression (30). We have recently asked whether these so-called promoter sequences can be replaced with similar regions from a non-glucocorticoid regulated promoter. The constructions entailed fusing a portion of the MMTV LTR containing the regulatory region to a series of fragments containing all or part of the SV40 early promoter region. Results of two such constructions are depicted in Figure 6 and document that the glucocorticoid regulatory region will indeed confer hormonal responsiveness on a heterologous promoter. Moreover, as indicated above, the absolute spacing between the regulatory region and the start of transcription does not need to be constant.

V. SUMMARY

We have analyzed the glucocorticoid responsive transcription of MMTV DNA using genetic and molecular techniques. The major conclusions we can draw are: 1) induction is at the transcription level and is dependent on functional glucocorticoid receptors; 2) sequences within MMTV DNA are required for hormone responsiveness; 3) at least one glucocorticoid regulatory domain resides within a 50-60 nucleotide region of the MMTV LTR. It is noteworthy that this region has been shown by other groups to contain a high affinity binding site for the glucocorticoid-receptor complex (31-35); speculations on the function of receptor binding to the regulatory region must take into account the facts that the position of these sequences need not be fixed with respect to the start of transcription and that heterologous promoters are suitable substrates for activation of transcription by this regulatory machinery.

REFERENCES

1. Jensen, E.V., Suzuki, T., Kawashima, T., Strumpf, W.E., Jungblut, P.W., and DeSombre, E.R. Proc. Natl. Acad. Sci. 59: 632 (1968).
2. Ringold, G., Yamamoto, K., Tomkins, G., Bishop, J.M., and Varmus, H. Cell 6: 299(1975).
3. Ringold, G., Yamamoto, K., Bishop, J.M., and Varmus, H. Proc. Natl. Acad. Sci. 74: 2879 (1977).
4. Cardiff, R. and Duesberg, P. Virology 36: 696 (1968).

5. Vaidya, A. Lasfargues, E., Henkel, G., Lasfargues, J., and Moore, D. J. Virol. 18: 911 (1976).
6. Ringold, G., Cardiff, R., Varmus, H., and Yamamoto, K. Cell 10: 11 (1977).
7. Ringold, G., Yamamoto, K., Shank, P., and Varmus, H. Cell 10: 19 (1977).
8. Ringold, G., Shank, P., and Yamamoto, K. J. Virol. 26: 93 (1978).
9. Bishop, J.M. Ann. Rev. Biochem. 47: 35 (1978).
10. Stallcup, M., Ring, J., and Yamamoto, K. Biochemistry 17: 1515 (1978).
11. Robertson, D. and Varmus, H. J. Virol. 30: 576 (1979).
12. Groner, B., Hynes, N., and Diggelman, H. J. Virol. 30: 417 (1979).
13. Temin, H. Cell 27: 1 (1981).
14. Varmus, H. Science 216: 812 (1982).
15. Ringold, G., Shank, P., Varmus, H., Ring, J., and Yamamoto, K. Proc. Natl. Acad. Sci. 76: 665 (1979).
16. Majors, J. and Varmus, H. Nature 289: 253 (1981).
17. Donehower, L., Huang, A., and Hager, G. J. Virol. 37: 226 (1981).
18. Grove, J.R., Dieckmann, B., Schroer, T., and Ringold, G.M. Cell 21: 47 (1980).
19. Grove, J.R. and Ringold, G.M. Proc. Natl. Acad. Sci. 78: 4349 (1981).
20. Ivarie, R. and O'Farrell, P. Cell 13: 41 (1978).
20a. Vannice, J.L., Grove, J.R., and Ringold, G.M. Mol. Pharmacol. 23:779 (1983).
21. Lee, F., Mulligan, R., Berg, P., and Ringold, G. Nature 294: 228 (1981).
22. Mulligan, R. and Berg, P. Science 209: 1423 (1980).
23. Subramani, S., Mulligan, R., and Berg, P. Molec. Cell. Biol. 1: 854 (1981).
24. Chapman, A.B., Costello, M.A., Lee, F., and Ringold, G.M. Mol. Cell Biol., in press.
25. Mulligan, R. and Berg, P. Proc. Natl. Acad. Sci. 78: 2072 (1981).
26. Perucho, M., Hanahan, D., Wigler, M. Cell 22: 309 (1980).
27. Hall, C.V., Jacob, P.E., Ringold, G.M., and Lee, F. J. Mol. Appl. Genet. 2:101 (1982).
28. Casadaban, M. and Cohen, S. J. Mol. Biol. 138: 179 (1980).
29. Sompayrac, L. and Danna, K. Proc. Natl. Acad. Sci. 78: 7575 (1981).
30. Dobson, D. E., Lee, F., and Ringold, G.M. In Gene Expression, UCLA-CETUS Symposium (Homer, D., ed.), in press.
31. Payvar, F., Firestone, G.L., Ress, S.R., Chandler, V.C., Wrange, O., Carlstedt-Duke, J., Gustafson, J.-A., and Yamamoto, K.R. J. Cell. Biochem. 19:241 (1982).

32. Govindan, M.V., Spiess, E., and Majors, Proc. Natl. Acad. Sci. 79: 5757 (1982).
33. Geisse, S., Scheiderist, C., Westphal, H.M., Hynes, N.E., Groner, B., and Beato, M. EMBO J. 1:1613 (1982).
34. Pfahl, M. Cell 31:475 (1982).
35. Graham, F. and van der Eb, A. Virology 52: 456 (1973).
36. Berk, A. and Sharp, P. Cell 12: 721 (1977).
37. Fromm, M. and Berg, P. J. Mol. Appl. Genet. 1:457 (1982).

DRUG RESISTANCE AND GENE AMPLIFICATION IN EUKARYOTIC CELLS[1]

Robert T. Schimke, Stephen Beverley, Peter Brown, Richard Cassin, Nancy Federspiel, Charles Gasser, Anna Hill, Randal Johnston, Brian Mariani, Elise Mosse, Heidi Rath, David Smouse, and Thea Tlsty

The Department of Biological Sciences
Stanford University
Stanford, CA 94305

INTRODUCTION

The finding that a specific gene can increase in copy number when cells in culture are placed under selective conditions (1) has considerably extended our understanding of the process of gene amplification. The frequency at which gene amplification occurs can be much greater than standard mutation frequencies, suggesting that this is a likely strategy of cells for the overproduction of specific proteins necessary to their survival. This paper will review the current status of gene amplification, in particular in cultured eukaryotic cells, and will focus on recent attempts in the author's laboratory to manipulate frequencies of gene amplification in an effort to better understand the mechanisms by which amplification may occur.

[1]Supported by grants from the National Institute of General Medical Sciences (GM 14931), the National Cancer Institute (CA 16318), and the American Cancer Society (NP 148).

RESULTS

Properties of Gene Amplification in Methotrexate-resistant Cultured Cells.

Resistance to methotrexate (MTX), a 4-amino analog of folic acid, in cultured animal cells results from three mechanisms which are not mutually exclusive: altered transport of MTX (2); reduced affinity for MTX by dihydrofolate reductase(DHFR), the target enzyme of MTX inhibition (3); and overproduction of DHFR (4). In every case where it has been investigated, the overproduction of DHFR enzyme has been achieved by virtue of amplification of the gene for DHFR. Indeed, there is a close correspondence between the degree of overproduction of DHFR and the gene copy number, i.e., a gene dosage effect.

The general properties of MTX resistance due to DHFR gene amplification include the following points. (a) Resistance is most often obtained by step-wise, incremental increases of MTX in the medium. Recent studies in our laboratory indicate that a selection protocol employing multiple small increments in MTX concentration yields highly resistant cells much more rapidly than do single-step selections at the same final concentration of MTX (Rath et al, manuscript in preparation). We have interpreted this phenomenon to indicate that amplifications occur in small increments; that is, step-wise selection permits the progressive selection of cells with gradually increasing numbers of DHFR genes. (b) Resistance is associated with overproduction of a normal protein (although, see Haber et al, (3), the result of which is the overcoming of selection pressure. Thus, at any intracellular MTX level, the elevated levels of DHFR allow for sufficient free enzyme to carry out the conversion of dihydrofolate to tetrahydrofolate. (c) The resistant phenotype and genotype can be either stable or unstable. Typically cells that are newly resistant to MTX have unstably amplified genes (5,6). For example, such cells may lose 50% of their amplified genes in approximately 20 cell doublings (7,8) when removed from MTX selection. However, when cells are grown in MTX for long time periods the emerging variants will often have stably amplified genes and, even when grown in the absence of MTX, will retain amplified genes for as long as two years.

The stability of amplified DHFR genes is related to their localization (9). When the genes are stable, the DHFR genes reside on one or more chromosomes (6,10-13). Thus, a frequent consequence of stable gene amplification is the presence of an expanded chromosome, generally involving only one of the two homologous chromosomes. Even so, extensive chromosomal amplification of genes need not result in a visible karyological abnormality (14, and Fougere-Deschatrette et al, manuscript to be published). The presumed reason for this is that the unit length of amplified DNA may vary; the length of an expanded region of a chromosome is then a function of the length of the amplified sequence times the number of amplified sequences. In at least three cases of stable amplifications, i.e., DHFR (10), CAD (15), and HPRT (16), the amplified genes reside in a single chromosome in the vicinity of the non-amplified gene. Our current hypothesis is that initial chromosomal amplifications occur at the site of the resident gene. Nevertheless, amplified DHFR genes are sometimes found on a number of different chromosomes; we consider these to be most likely a result of secondary translocations-rearrangements occurring during multiple step selections (Fougere-Deschatrette et al, manuscript to be published).

In cell lines with unstably amplified genes, metaphase chromosome spreads generally contain double minute chromosomes (DMs) in a number proportional to the degree of DHFR gene amplification (8,17). Double minute chromosomes are self-replicating (18,19), and do not contain centromeres (20). Thus DMs can redistribute unequally into daughter cells at mitosis. When cells are grown in the absence of MTX, those cells with progressively fewer DMs grow more rapidly and, hence, become dominant in the cell population (9).

How Widespread is Gene Amplification?

When first documented in 1978 (7) gene amplification in somatic cells was considered to be an unusual phenomenon. In subsequent years an increasing number of examples of amplification have been reported, including the CAD gene (15), the metallothionine gene (21), the HPRT gene (22), thymidylate synthetase (23,24), hydroxymethylglutaryl-CoA reductase (25,26), adenosine deaminase(27), ribonucleotide reductase (28), asparagine synthetase (29), glutamine synthetase, (30), and ornithine decarboxylase (P. Caffino, personal communication). In all such cases, a specific enzyme inhibitor was employed to obtain resistant cell variants. Of considerable interest are a number of cell variants selected for resistance to vinca alkaloids that also show cross resistance to multiple drugs, including actinomycin D, puromycin, and cycloheximide, (31–33). These cells have karyotypes suggestive of gene amplification, i.e., expanded chromosomes or DMs. Resistance results from an inhibition of drug transport, and may be associated with an increased concentration of a particular cell surface protein. In our laboratory we have obtained a number of methotrexate resistant cell variants which do not have amplified DHFR genes. However, they grow poorly, are unstably resistant, and are killed by folate antimetabolites that enter cells by circumventing normal MTX uptake mechanisms. Such cell lines have chromosomal aberrations consistent with gene amplification, and we believe that many of the MTX transport variants may also be the result of amplification of presently unidentified genes, the consequence of which is a reduced intracellular concentration of MTX (R. Cassin, to be published).

Dihydrofolate reductase gene amplification is not limited to cultured mammalian cells. Gene amplification and MTX resistance have been documented in two instances where MTX resistance has been found in tumor cells following the clonogenic assay procedure (34,35), as well as in the entire tumor cell population of a patient treated with MTX for chronic myeloid leukemia (36). The human blood parasite, Leishmania, also develops resistance to MTX as a result of gene amplification (37). Thus gene amplification may well underlie many types of resistance phenomena observed clinically.

How Frequent is Gene Amplification?

In order to study the mechanism of gene amplification (see Schimke et al, (9), for a review of alternate mechanisms for amplification), it is first necessary to determine the frequency at which this process occurs. As a first approximation we determined the frequency with which resistant colonies emerge following a single step of MTX selection. Brown et al, (38) have estimated that approximately 5×10^{-5} mouse 3T6 cells become resistant when selected at 120 nM MTX (approximately 6 times normal half-killing), and that 1/3 to 1/2 of the colonies that arise have amplified DHFR genes; presumably the remainder are transport or enzyme variants. This frequency is a minimal estimate of the frequency of DHFR gene amplification since for a single cell to generate a visible colony requires some 2–3 weeks of growth, during which time a number of initially unstably amplified cells may lose genes and hence not survive as colonies under prolonged MTX selection. In addition, substantial amplification (5-10 fold) of DHFR is necessary for growth of colonies at this concentration of MTX. Thus, weakly amplified cells, which are likely to be more frequent, are not readily detected in this assay. These experiments, however, do not allow us to distinguish whether the observed amplification events arise as a consequence of MTX mutagenesis, or may occur independently of drug exposure.

In an effort to resolve these issues, we have used the Fluorescence Activated Cell Sorter (FACS) in conjunction with a fluorescein conjugate of MTX (39), to determine the frequency of spontaneous DHFR gene amplification under conditions that do not involve perturbation with MTX (40). By repeatedly sorting and growing (in the absence of MTX) those cells within the population that spontaneously display high DHFR enzyme content (i.e., high fluorescence), we obtained successive cell populations with gradually increasing DHFR enzyme levels and DHFR gene copy numbers. After 10 such sorting cycles, the cells are highly fluorescent, and contain on an average 50 copies of the DHFR gene. We calculate that the frequency of gene amplification in such cell populations is approximately 1×10^{-3} cells per cell generation. This number is far greater than the 5×10^{-5} obtained by clonal analysis of MTX-resistant cells, and likely reflects both the instability of such amplified genes in most of the newly amplified cells, and also the ability of the FACS to detect small variations in the degree of amplification. In addition, we conclude from this study that DHFR gene amplification can occur spontaneously, that is, even in the absence of overt drug mutagenesis and cytotoxicity.

Can we Vary the Frequency of Gene Amplification?

Although we estimate that the spontaneous rate of gene amplification in the CHO cells is 1×10^{-3} per cell generation, this frequency remains too low to study the initial events of gene amplification at a biochemical level. We have therefore sought ways of treating cells that increase the frequency of gene amplification and MTX resistance. We have employed two general means for enhancing such amplification events: (a) The use of a number of treatments of cells that result in partial and/or transient inhibition of DNA replication. Among the agents employed are hydroxyurea, an inhibitor of ribonucleotide reductase (38), methotrexate (Beverley and Johnston, to be published), and aphidicolin, an inhibitor of DNA polymerase alpha (Brown, to be published). (b) The use of agents that introduce DNA damage, including ultraviolet light (Tlsty and Schimke, to be published) and N-acetoxy acetoaminofluorene (41). Our results are encouraging: in randomly growing 3T6 and CHO cells, transient inhibition of DNA synthesis and introduction of DNA damage (approximately a 20-30% killing dose) result in a 10-100 fold increase in the number of cells subsequently determined to be resistant to MTX by single step clonal analysis.

Our most recent studies on the mechanism of gene amplification have involved the use of CHO cells synchronized in the cell cycle. Mariani et al, (42), showed that the expression of the DHFR gene is regulated during the cell cycle; the rate of DHFR synthesis declines during G1 and then increases markedly in the 2nd hour of S-phase. More recently Mariani and Schimke (to be published) have shown that the DHFR gene is both replicated and transcribed during the first 1-2 hours in S-phase. When synchronized cells are treated during G1 with hydroxyurea (at a concentration sufficient to reduce thymidine incorporation by 95% in S-phase control cells), the subsequent frequency of DHFR gene amplification is not altered. In contrast, when the hydroxyurea is added for a period of 6 hours beginning 2 hours after the initiation of S phase, following which the cells are allowed to recover and resume DNA replication, we observe that:

1.   The subsequent frequency of resistance to high levels of MTX increases as much as 1000 fold, compared to cells not subjected to the S-phase block.

2.   Extensive over-replication of DNA occurs as monitored by incorporation of bromodeoxyuridine. Indeed, it appears that essentially all of the DNA replicated prior to the hydroxyurea block is rereplicated. Thus, the rereplication of DNA involves not only the DHFR gene, but also all of the DNA that is normally replicated in the first two hours of S-phase.

3.   Finally, a large fraction of the cell population (variable from experiment to experiment, 10 to 40%) displays a 3-5 fold increase in DHFR enzyme content as monitored in the FACS by staining with fluoresceinated MTX, compared to cells normally progressing through a cell cycle. When the cells with high DHFR enzyme content are sorted and plated in concentrations of MTX 100 times normal half-killing concentrations, essentially all of the viable cells display a resistant phenotype.

We conclude that inhibiting DNA replication in mid S-phase followed by relief of inhibition can result in over replication of a portion of the genome. Such "extra" DNA is highly unstable, and most is rapidly lost from the cell. Nevertheless, some rearrangements and/or recombination events may occur such that some of the additional DNA is retained in the genome. Under appropriate selection conditions, those cells retaining the additional (i.e., amplified) DNA corresponding to a necessary gene product will survive.

We believe that the same general process underlies amplifications induced by DNA damaging agents. For instance, we find that the timing of the introduction of DNA damage by ultraviolet light is critical in enhancing MTX resistance. Thus, it is only during the 3-6th hour of the S phase in CHO cells that ultraviolet light enhances MTX resistance (Tlsty, to be published). This suggests that only in cells undergoing active DNA synthesis will DNA damaging agents promote gene amplification.

Consistent with these proposals, we have recently found a variety of chromosomal aberrations in metaphase spreads of cells, fixed while progressing through the first mitosis following treatment with hydroxyurea or UV light (as above). These include (Hill, to be published): (a) metaphase cells that have essentially undergone endoreduplication, i.e., have gone from 2N to 4N in which the chromosomes appear normal; (b) metaphase cells with a normal 2N chromosome complement but in which there is a large amount of small sized, but clearly visible extrachromosomal DNA, and (c) metaphase cells with varying degrees of fragmented chromosomes.

DISCUSSION

It is clear that gene amplification can occur with a very high frequency in cultured cells of many types. Even cells lines that do not readily amplify are able to do so when appropriately selected with MTX in a slow stepwise fashion (Fougerre-Deschatrette, to be published).

Since malignant cells appear to use gene amplification as a common strategy for survival during selection by chemo-therapeutic drugs, then conditions of chemotherapy that might minimize gene amplification are of special interest. Our studies in cultured cells would suggest that DNA damaging treatments, i.e., radiation and alkylating agents, may be hazardous when applied to cells actively synthesizing DNA, as it is in this situation that introduction of DNA damage enhances gene amplification. Our studies would also suggest that antimetabolite drugs will be relatively ineffective in selectively killing tumor cells (when used alone) since it is extremely difficult to completely inhibit DNA replication in all tumor cells. Indeed, it is in the instances of partial transient inhibition of DNA replication that we observe the greatest enhancement of gene amplification. Our studies instead support the use of an alternate protocol of drug therapy in which cells are first prevented from entering S-phase, then treated with radiomimetic agents, and subsequently released from the cell cycle block. This experimental protocol is based on an attempt to kill cells with minimal risk of the emergence of drug resistance as a result of gene amplification. In addition, different sets of drugs with different potential resistance mechanisms should be alternated, thereby, hopefully, preventing the emergence of stable resistances. Clearly the clinical setting differs from that of cultured cells, making it difficult to translate protocols from the laboratory directly to the clinic.

The DNA damaging agents we have employed which enhance the frequency of MTX resistance, i.e., ultraviolet light and N-acetoxy-acetoaminofluorene are themselves carcinogenic. This suggests that gene amplification may actually play a role in the genesis and/or progression of tumors. In the past several years, an increasing number of reports have, in fact, indicated the presence of different "oncogenes" in high gene copy number in various cell lines derived from tumors (43-45). It is tempting to speculate that carcinogens that damage DNA may facilitate the amplification of genes, whose products when present in increased amounts overcome normal growth constraints on cells, i.e., cancer. Our observations of cell populations, heterogeneous with respect to DHFR gene copy number and DNA content, are consistent with the heterogeneity and instability of cellular phenotypes within tumors. Further study of mechanisms of gene amplification should continue to contribute to our understanding of the generation and progression of tumors, and the drug resistance properties they display.

REFERENCES

1. Schimke, R.T., Kaufman, R.J., Alt, F.W., and Kellems, R.F. Science 202:1051 (1978).
2. Sirotnak, F.M., Moccio, D.M., Kelleher, L.E., and Goutas, L.J. Cancer Research 41:4447 (1981).
3. Haber, D.A., Beverley, S.M., Kiely, M.L., and Schimke, R.T. J. Biol. Chem. 256:9501 (1981).
4. Alt, F.W., Kellems, R.E., and Schimke, R.T. J. Biol. Chem. 251:3063 (1976).
5. Kaufman, R.J., and Schimke, R.T. Mol. Cell. Biol. 1:1069 (1981).
6. Kaufman, R.J., Brown, P.C., and Schimke, R.T. Mol. Cell. Biol. 1:1084 (1981).
7. Alt, F.W., Kellems, R.E., Bertino, J.R., and Schimke, R.T. J. Biol. Chem. 253:1357 (1978).
8. Brown, P.C., Beverley, S.M., and Schimke, R.T. Mol. Cell. Biol. 1:1077 (1981).
9. Schimke, R.T., Brown, P.C., Kaufman, R.J., McGrogan, M., and Slate, D.L. Cold Spring Harbor Symp. on Quant. Biol. Vol. XLV, pp. 785 (1981).
10. Nunberg, J.N., Kaufman, R.J., Schimke, R.T., Urlaub, G., and Chasin, L.A. Proc. Natl. Acad. Sci. 75:5553 (1978).
11. Biedler, J.L., and Spengler, B.A. J. Natl. Cancer Inst. 57:683 (1976).
12. Milbrandt, J.D., Heintz, N.H., White, W.C., Rothman, S.M., and Hamlin, J.L. Proc. Natl. Acad. Sci. 78:6043 (1981).
13. Dolnick, B.J., Berenson, R.J., Bertino, J.R., Kaufman, R.J., Nunberg, J.H., and Schimke, R.T. J. Cell. Biol. 83:394 (1979).
14. Fougere-Deschatrette, C., Schimke, R.T., Weil, D., and Weiss, M.C. in Gene Amplification, edited by R.T. Schimke. Cold Spring Harbor Laboratory, New York. pp. 29-31 (1982).
15. Wahl, G.M., Padgett, R.A., Stark, G.R. J. Bio. Chem. 254:8679 (1979).
16. Melton, D.W., Brennand, J., Ledbetter, D.H., Konecki, D.S., Chinault, A.C., and Caskey, C.T. in Gene Amplification, edited by R.T. Schimke. Cold Spring Harbor Laboratory, New York. pp. 59-65 (1982).
17. Kaufman, R.J., Brown, P.C., and Schimke, R.T. Proc. Natl. Acad. Sci. 76:5669 (1979).
18. Barker, P.E., Drwinga, H.L., Hittelman, W.N., and Maddox, A.M. Exp. Cell Res. 130:353 (1980).
19. Haber, D.A., and Schimke, R.T. Cell 26:355 (1981).
20. Levan, A., and Levan, G. Hereditas 88:81 (1978).

21. Beach, L.R., and Palmiter, R.D. Proc. Natl. Acad. Sci. 78:2110 (1981).
22. Brennard, J., Chinault, A.C., Konecki, D.S., Melton, D.W., and Caskey, C.T. Proc. Natl. Acad. Sci. 79:1950 (1982).
23. Baskin, F., Carlin, S.C., Kraus, P., Friedkin, M., and Rosenberg, R.N. Molecular Pharmacology 11:105 (1975).
24. Rossana, C., Rao, L.G., and Johnson, L.F. Mol. Cell. Biol. 2:1118 (1982).
25. Chin, D.J., Luskey, K.L., Anderson, R.G.W., Faust, J.R., Goldstein, J.L., and Brown, M.S. Proc. Natl. Acad. Sci. 79:1185 (1982).
26. Ryan, J., Hardeman, E.C., Endo, A., and Simoni, R.D. J. Biol. Chem. 256:6762 (1981).
27. Yeung, C-Y., Ingolia, D.E., Bobonis, C., Dunbar, B.S., Riser, M.E., Siciliano, M.J., and Kellems, R.E. J. Biol. Chem. (in press)
28. Lewis, W.H., and Srinivasan, P.R. Mol. Cell. Biol. 3:1053 (1983).
29. Andrulis, I.L., and Siminovitch, L. in Gene Amplification, edited by R.T. Schimke. Cold Spring Harbor Laboratory, New York. pp. 75-80 (1982).
30. Young, A.P., and Ringold, G.M. J. Biol. Chem. (in press).
31. Baskin, F., Rosenberg, R.N., and Dev, V. Proc. Natl. Acad. Sci. 78:3654 (1981).
32. Biedler, J.L. in Gene Amplification, edited by R.T. Schimke. Cold Spring Harbor Laboratory, New York. pp.39-45 (1982).
33. Kuo, T., Pathak, S., Ramagli, L., Rodriguez, L., and Hsu, T.C. in Gene Amplification, edited by R.T. Schimke Cold Spring Harbor Laboratory, New York. pp. 53-57. (1982).
34. Curt, G.A., Carney, D.N., Cowan, K.H., Jolivet, J., Bailey, B.D., Drake, J.C., Kao-Shan, C.S., Minna, J.D., and Chabner, B.A. N. Engl. J. Med. 308:199 (1983).
35. Trent, J.M., Buick, R.N., Olson, S., Horns, R.C., Jr., and Schimke, R.T. J. Clinical Oncology (in press).
36. Horns, R.C., Jr., Dower, W.J., and Schimke, R.T. J. Clinical Oncology (in press).
37. Coderre, J.A., Beverley, S.M., Schimke, R.T., and Santi, D.V. Proc. Natl. Acad. Sci. 80:2132 (1983).
38. Brown, P.C., Tlsty, T.D., and Schimke, R.T. Mol. Cell. Biol. 3:1097 (1983).
39. Kaufman, R.J., Bertino, J.R., and Schimke, R.T. J. Biol. Chem. 253:5852 (1978).

40. Johnston, R.N., Beverley, S.M., and Schimke, R.T. Proc. Natl. Acad. Sci. 80:3711 (1983).
41. Tlsty, T., Brown, P.C., Johnston, R., and Schimke, R.T. in Gene Amplification, edited by R.T. Schimke. Cold Spring Harbor Laboratory, New York. pp. 231–238 (1982).
42. Mariani, B.D., Slate, D.L., and Schimke, R.T. Proc. Natl. Acad. Sci. 78:4985 (1981).
43. Chattopadhyay, S.K., Chang, E.H., Lander, M.R., Ellis, R.W., Scolnick, E.M., and Lowy, D.R. Nature 296:361 (1982).
44. Collins, S., and Groudine, M. Nature 298:679 (1982).
45. Schwab, M., Alitalo, K., Varmus, H.E., Bishop, J.M., and George, D. Nature 303:497 (1983).

III ANTIPARASITIC AGENTS

GLYCOLYSIS AS TARGET FOR THE DEVELOPMENT OF NEW TRYPANOCIDAL DRUGS[1]

Fred R. Opperdoes

Research Unit for Tropical Diseases
International Institute of Cellular and Molecular Pathology
Brussels, Belgium

I. INTRODUCTION

Trypanosomatids are protozoan hemoflagellates responsible for a number of serious diseases of man and his domestic animals. Human trypanosomiases, sleeping sickness caused by Trypanosoma rhodesiense and T. gambiense in tropical Africa and Chagas' disease caused by T. cruzi in South America, affect many millions of people. Trypanosomiasis of livestock (nagana) is caused by T. brucei, T. congolense and T. vivax in tropical Africa and is responsible for the death of 3 million heads of cattle each year.

Kala azar, oriental sore and visceral and (muco)cutaneous leishmaniasis are all caused by other Trypanosomatids belonging to the species Leishmania. It is estimated that in total a hundred million people suffer from these different forms of one disease.

In general, if untreated, most of the diseases caused by Trypanosomatids run a fatal course. Drugs when available are not very effective. They are too toxic or their use is restricted because of the spreading occurrence of resistance of the parasite to them. Trypanosomiases are clearly a class of diseases where better and new drugs are needed; however, in

---

[1] This investigation received financial support from the UNDP/World Bank/WHO Special Programme for Research and Training in Tropical Diseases.

the last three decades no new drugs have been developed for the treatment of African trypanosomiasis whereas for Chagas' disease, there exists no reliable treatment at all.

II. GLYCOLYSIS

In the bloodstream form of the best studied African trypanosome, Trypanosoma brucei, the single mitochondrion has been reduced to a peripheral canal containing no cytochromes and no functional Krebs'cycle thus resembling the promitochondria of anaerobically grown yeast (1). The bloodstream form therefore is entirely dependent on glycolysis for its production of energy and glucose is the preferred energy source. The trypanosome relies entirely on an exogenous source of carbohydrate. Fructose, mannose and glycerol can replace glucose in that they all support motility and respiration. Removal of exogenous substrate results in a rapid loss of respiratory activity and motility and the cells disintegrate (2) due to the absence of significant polysaccharide reserves or "high energy phosphate" stores like creatine phosphate, or polyphosphates (3).

Glucose metabolism in Trypanosoma brucei bloodstream forms differs from glycolysis in other eukaryotes in a number of respects (Fig. 1): i) lactate dehydrogenase is absent and, therefore, the reducing equivalents generated in glycolysis are indirectly reoxidized by molecular oxygen via a dihydroxy-acetone phosphate : glycerol-3-phosphate shuttle plus a cyanide-insensitive mitochondrial terminal oxidase : glycerol-3-phosphate-oxidase (4); ii) under aerobiosis pyruvate is the sole end-product of glycolysis and is excreted into the hosts bloodstream; iii) under anaerobic conditions glucose is quantitatively converted into equimolar amounts of pyruvate and glycerol which are excreted (2). This glucose dismutation proceeds with net ATP synthesis (4), an observation which could not readily be explained until recently (see below).

Glycolysis in T. brucei proceeds at an extremely high rate: 85 nmol glucose/min/mg protein. The rate of glycolysis is directly coupled to the rate of ATP production (5) and calculations indicate that such a high rate of glycolysis is required to enable the trypanosome to divide every 7 h (6). Therefore, even an incomplete inhibition of glycolysis will lead to an increase in division time of the trypanosome and would help the host to overcome the infection by its natural defence systems.

Another advantage of using the only energy-generating pathway of the bloodstream trypanosome as target for the development of new drugs would be the following : a drug that

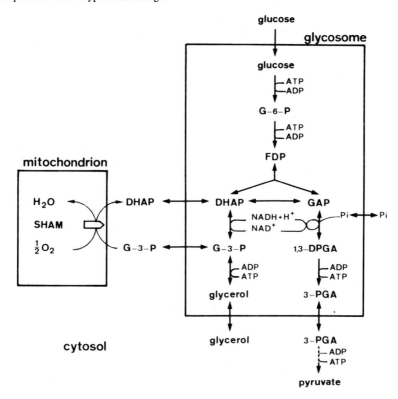

FIGURE 1. Compartmentation of glycolysis in T. brucei bloodstream forms.

interferes directly with the energy production of the organism would rapidly kill it . This would drastically shorten the duration of treatment and thus the chance that the organism will develop resistance.

How vulnerable a trypanosome is to inhibition of its glycolytic pathway is demonstrated by the fact that 2 drugs (suramin and melarsen oxide), currently used in the treatment of sleeping sickness, inhibit glycolysis and energy production in T. brucei. Although the trivalent organic arsenical, melarsen oxide, inhibits several enzymes of carbohydrate metabolism it has been shown that in intact cells only the enzyme pyruvate kinase is selectively inhibited as phosphoenol pyruvate accumulates within cells treated with concentrations of the drug that have negligible effects on rate of respiration or glucose consumption (1).

Suramin interferes with the reoxidation of glycolytically produced NADH by inhibition in vitro of the glycerol-3-phosphate dehydrogenase and glycerol-3-phosphate oxidase, two enzymes of the dihydroxyacetone phosphate : glycerol-3-phosphate shuttle. It has recently been shown that in intact cells respiration is inhibited after exposure of the cells to the drug for several hours and that consequently there is a shift from an aerobic to an anaerobic type of glycolysis leading to the formation of glycerol in addition to pyruvate and a reduction in the rate of ATP synthesis (5).

Finally a single administration of the experimental drug combination salicylhydroxamic acid (SHAM) and glycerol, inhibitors of the aerobic and anaerobic glycolytic pathways, respectively, blocks glycolysis completely in vitro (7) and in vivo eliminates the trypanosomes from the bloodstream of an infected host within minutes (8).

III : THE GLYCOSOME

Some six years ago we discovered that in the bloodstream form of T. brucei a number of glycolytic enzymes (i.e. hexokinase, phosphoglucose isomerase, phosphofructokinase, aldolase,

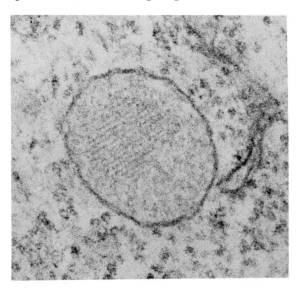

FIGURE 2. Glycosome in situ displaying a dense core with a lamellar structure.

triosephosphate isomerase, glycerol kinase, glycerol-3-phosphate dehydrogenase, glyceraldehyde-phosphate dehydrogenase and phosphoglycerate kinase) all involved in the conversion of glucose and glycerol to 3-phosphoglycerate are localized in special membrane-bounded microbody-like organelles with a diameter of 0.3 μm, which contain sometimes a crystalloid core. We have called these organelles "glycosomes" (Fig.2) (9). The glycosomes of T. brucei have a density of 1.087 g/cm$_3$ in isotonic sucrose (10) and equilibrate at 1.23 g/cm^3 in sucrose gradients (Fig. 3). They can be isolated almost pure by sequential Percoll - and sucrose-gradient centrifugation.

The presence of glycosomes is not a special form of adaptation of T. brucei to its stay in the glucose-rich bloodstream of its host, since evidence for their presence has now also been found in insect stages of T. brucei (11) and in all major representatives of the other Trypanosomatids like Crithidia spp (12,13), T. cruzi (12,14) and Leishmania mexicana (15). This renders the presence of glycosomes a general property of all Trypanosomatids. Therefore, any drug that will be developed as a specific inhibitor of glycolysis in T. brucei bloodstream forms might also be effective against the causative agents of Leishmaniasis or Chagas'disease, alone or in combination with other drugs.

In general glycosomes do not contain hydrogen peroxide-producing oxidases, nor catalase like the microbodies of other eukaryotic cells, although some catalase was found in the microbodies of Crithidia spp (16) as well as peroxidase in those of T. cruzi (17). In addition to the early enzymes of the glycolytic sequence the last two enzymes of the pyrimidine biosynthetic pathway : orotate phosphoribosyl transferase and orotidine carboxylase (18) and the enzymes adenylate kinase, malate dehydrogenase (11) and phosphoenolpyruvate carboxykinase (19) have been demonstrated in glycosomes.

The presence of a number of glycolytic enzymes inside an organelle, is a property unique to Trypanosomatids. In any other organism studied so far, prokaryote or eukaryote, the glycolytic reactions proceed in the soluble portion of the cell. This, for Trypanosomatids unique property, suggested to us that the glycolytic enzymes, present inside the glycosome, might exhibit physical and chemical characteristics which are different from their soluble counterparts present in the host cells, rendering them excellent targets for future chemotherapy. Apart from the fact that in trypanosomes the glycolytic enzymes are located in a glycosome recently evidence has been obtained that even inside the glycosome a number of the enzymes are associated with each other. In contrast to the interactions between glycolytic enzymes that have been described for the enzymes of bacteria (20) and higher eukaryotes

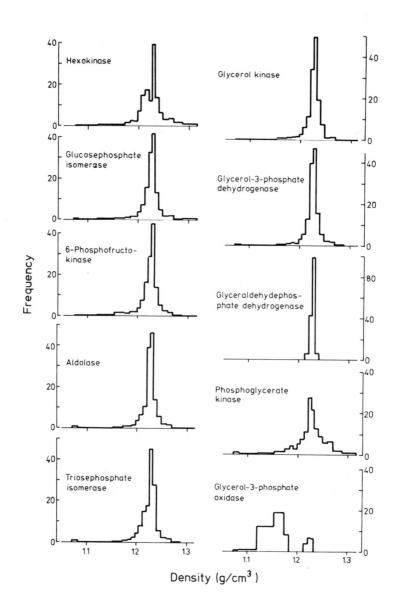

FIGURE 3. Distribution of 9 enzymes involved in glycolysis and the mitochondrial marker glycerol-3-phosphate oxidase from a T. brucei large-granule fraction after isopycnic centrifugation in a linear sucrose gradient. From ref. 9.

(21), which are weak interactions, the interactions between the trypanosoma enzymes seem to be much stronger. Irrespective of the homogenization procedure or of the detergent used, the majority of the enzymes behave as members of a big multi-enzyme complex (22,23).

In T. brucei and other Trypanosomatids a number of enzymes of glycolysis and some enzymes related to this pathway have already been purified and partially characterized and clear differences between the trypanosoma enzymes and their mammalian counterparts have been found (unpublished results).

IV. COMPARTMENTATION OF GLYCOLYSIS

In freshly isolated T. brucei glycosomes, the glycolytic enzymes exhibit latency (as high as 95 %), which can be abolished in part by freezing and thawing, sonication, osmotic shock or by treatment with phospholipase or detergent. This indicates that the membrane has a limited permeability to the phosphorylated intermediates of glycolysis and that the glycosome probably constitutes a separate pool of glycolytic intermediates within the cell. This was confirmed by pulse-labeling experiments with [14C] glucose on intact T. brucei cells clearly showing the existence of two separate compartments for glycolytic intermediates (24). One which is rapidly labeled and most likely represents the glycosomal compartment, and another compartment where label slowly appears, which represents the rest of the cell. It has been speculated that the glycosomal membrane acts as a permeability barrier preventing dilution of glycolytic intermediates into the cytosol and so enabling T. brucei to maintain an extremely high glycolytic flux. Opperdoes and Borst (9) have proposed a model (Fig. 1) for the glycolytic reactions occurring in the glycosome. This organelle catalyzes the following net reactions:

$$Glucose + [2] Pi + [2] DHAP \rightarrow [2] 3PGA + [2] G3P$$
$$Glycerol + \quad Pi + [2] DHAP \rightarrow \quad 3PGA + [2] G3P$$

It is interesting to note that in this model the production and consumption of ATP and NAD are balanced and that, therefore, the glycosome itself is not involved in net ATP synthesis. This occurs in the cytosol when phosphoglyceric acid is converted to pyruvate.

V. ANAEROBIC GLYCOLYSIS

Under anaerobic conditions, when the glycerol-3-phosphate oxidase is inhibited by SHAM, glucose is metabolized at the same rate as under aerobic conditions, forming equimolar amounts of pyruvate and glycerol. If glycerol production would be the result of the action of a phosphatase on glycerol-3-phosphate anaerobic glycolysis could not lead to a net synthesis of ATP and consequently the trypanosome would not survive anaerobiosis. A thermodynamic calculation shows that the free energy change of the overall dismutation of glucose into pyruvate and glycerol is negative enough to allow for the synthesis of 1 mole of ATP.

$$\text{Glucose} \rightarrow \text{pyruvate} + \text{glycerol} - 77 \text{ KJ/mole}$$
$$\text{ADP} + \text{Pi} \rightarrow \text{ATP} + H_2O \qquad\qquad + 31 \text{ KJ/mole}$$

$$\text{glucose} + \text{ADP} + \text{Pi} \rightarrow \text{pyruvate} + \text{glycerol} + \text{ATP} + H_2O$$
$$- 46 \text{ KJ/mole}$$

Assuming that net ATP synthesis occurs in the cytosol when 3-phosphoglyceric acid is converted to pyruvate glycosomal ATP consumption and production should again be balanced. Several hypothetical schemes have been proposed to account for the fact that trypanosomes are capable of synthesis of ATP in the absence of oxygen. Additional glycolytic enzymes were proposed (8, 25) but none of these were found. With their discovery of the glycosome Opperdoes and Borst (9) hypothesized that the production of glycerol with concomitant ATP synthesis had to be the result of special conditions existing under anaerobiosis inside the glycosome . Fig. 1 shows how this occurs. For each mole of triosephosphate converted to pyruvate one mole of NAD^+ is reduced to NADH which in its turn is reoxidized by DHAP to glycerol-3-phosphate. It has been shown that in the presence of SHAM the concentration of glycerol-3-phosphate is drastically increased (26). If due to the glycosomal permeability barrier all the glycerol-3-phosphate would be restricted to the glycosomal matrix, this would lead to a high intraglycosomal concentration of glycerol-3-phosphate and thus to a reversal of the glycerol kinase reaction and the formation of ATP and glycerol from ADP and glycerol-3-phosphate (24)

$$\text{G-3-P} + \text{ADP} \rightarrow \text{glycerol} + \text{ATP} + 20.4 \text{ KJ/mole.}$$

Recently evidence was obtained that such conditions exist inside the glycosome and that glycerol-3-phosphate is indeed the direct precursor of glycerol (24). Hammond and Bowman (27) described a glycerol-3-phosphate : ADP transphosphorylase activity which could be attributed to glycerol kinase and they measured in pulse-labeling experiments with [^{14}C] glycerol (28) that under anaerobiosis glycerol is incorporated into glycerol-3-phosphate at a much higher rate than the net production of glycerol (Fig.4). Since this would imply a rate of ATP break-down largely exceeding that of ATP synthesis by the pyruvate kinase reaction and since net consumption of glycerol does not occur in the absence of oxygen this means that the glycerol kinase reaction is at equilibrium. When now under such conditions glycerol is added, the reversed glycerol kinase reaction is blocked due to mass action leading to a complete inhibition of anaerobic glycolysis and the subsequent death of the trypanosome (7, 8), by which the mode of action of the SHAM-glycerol combination is explained. This pathway is unique to the bloodstream African trypanosomes and not found in other Trypanosomatids.

The latter example shows how insight in trypanosome metabolism can lead to the development of combinations of drugs which would not have been detected in a conventional screen for trypanocidal drugs, because neither of the drugs alone has measurable trypanocidal activity.

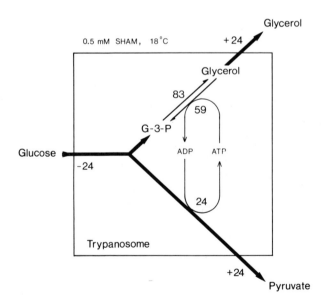

FIGURE 4. The involvement of glycerol kinase in anaerobic glycolysis of T. brucei. Figures indicate the rate of metabolite fluxes in nmol/min/mg protein at 18°C. Drawn from data by Hammond and Bowman (28).

VI. CONCLUSION

Glycolysis in Trypanosomatids has unique properties resulting from the presence of glycosomes. The differences that exist between parasite and host should be exploited for the development of new trypanocidal drugs. Features that lend themselves well for further study are : 1) the mechanism of glucose transport into the trypanosome; 2) the properties of the individual glycolytic enzymes and the development of specific inhibitors of these; 3) the development of an inhibitor of glycerol kinase in combination with an inhibitor of respiration; 4) the properties of the glycosomal membrane and the development of compounds that might interfere with its integrity and 5) the interference with possible carriers of glycolytic intermediates in the glycosomal membrane.

ACKNOWLEDGMENT

I thank miss Isabelle Coppens for preparing Fig. 2.

REFERENCES

1. Bowman, I.B.R., and Flynn, I.W. (1976). In "Biology of the Kinetoplastida (W.H.R. Lumsden & D.A. Evans, eds), vol. I, p 435-476. Academic Press, New York.
2. Ryley, J.F. (1956), Biochem. J. 62:215.
3. Visser, N. Ph.D. Thesis, University of Amsterdam (1981).
4. Grant, P.T., and Sargent, J.R. (1960). Biochem. J. 76:229
5. Fairlamb, A.H., and Bowman, I.B.R. (1980). Molec. Biochem. Parasitol. 1:315.
6. Brohn, F.H., and Clarkson, A.B. (1980). Molec. Biochem. Parasitol. 1:291.
7. Fairlamb, A.H., Opperdoes, F.R., and Borst, P. (1977). Nature 256:270.
8. Clarkson, A.B., and Brohn, F.H.(1976). Science 194:204.
9. Opperdoes, F.R., and Borst, P. (1977). FEBS Lett. 80:360.
10. Opperdoes, F.R. (1981). Molec. Biochem. Parasitol. 3:181.
11. Opperdoes, F.R., Markos, A. and Steiger, R.F. (1981). Mol. Biochem. Parasitol. 4:291.
12. Taylor, M.B., Berghausen, P., Heyworth, P., and Gutteridge, W. (1980). Int. J.Biochem. 11:117.
13. Opperdoes, F.R. (1981). In: Klein, R.A. and Miller, P.G.E. Parasitol. 82:1

14. Cannata, J.J.B., Valle, E., Docampo, R. and Cazzulo, J.J. (1982). Mol. Biochem. Parasitol. 6:151.
15. Hart, D.T., and Coombs, G.H. (1980). Abstr.16, Proc. 3rd Europ. Multicolloquium Parasitol., Cambridge.
16. Opperdoes, F.R., Borst, P., Bakker, S., and Leene, W. (1977). Eur. J. Biochem. 76:29.
17. Docampo,R., Deboiso, J.F., Boveris, A., and Stoppani, A.O.M. (1976). Experientia 32:972.
18. Hammond, D.J., Guttcridge, W.E., and Opperdoes, F.R. (1981). FEBS Letters 128:27.
19. Opperdoes, F.R. and Cottem, D. (1982). FEBS Letters 143:60.
20. Mowbray, J.,and Moses, V. (1976). Eur. J. Biochem. 66:25.
21. Ottaway, J.H., and Mowbray, J. (1977). In "Current Topics in Cellular Regulation," 12:107.
22. Opperdoes, F.R., and Nwagwu, M. (1980). In "The Host-Invader Interplay" (Van den Bossche, H., ed.) p. 683, Elsevier/North Holland Biochemical Press, Amsterdam.
23. Oduro, K.K., Bowman, I.B.R., and Flynn, I.W. (1980). Exp. Parasitol. 50:240.
24. Visser, N., Opperdoes, F.R., and Borst, P. (1981). Eur. J. Biochem. 118:521.
25. Opperdoes, F.R., Borst, P., and Fonck, K. (1976). FEBS Letters 62:169.
26. Visser, N., and Opperdoes, F.R. (1980). Eur. J. Biochem. 103:623.
27. Hammond, D.J., and Bowman, I.B.R. (1980). Mol. Biochem. Parasitol. 2:77.
28. Hammond, D.J., and Bowman, I.B.R. (1980). Mol. Biochem. Parasitol. 2:63.

PURINE AND PYRIMIDINE METABOLISM IN TRICHOMONADIDAE AND GIARDIA: POTENTIAL TARGETS FOR CHEMOTHERAPY[1]

Ching Chung Wang

Department of Pharmaceutical Chemistry
University of California, School of Pharmacy
San Francisco, California

I. INTRODUCTION

Hexamitidae and Trichomonadidae are two families of anaerobic protozoan flagellates responsible for a number of diseases among humans and animals. The former is commonly represented by Giardia lamblia, a universal inhabitant of human intestine transmitted mainly by ingestion of the cysts in contaminated food or water. The infection causes diarrhea, abdominal pain, weight loss and retarded growth in children. There are no good methods for diagnosis of giardiasis or effective chemoprophylactic drugs for prevention. The two drugs for treating the infection, metronidazole (Flagyl) and atabrine, are known to have many undesirable side effects (1). Trichomonas vaginalis, a member of the Trichomonadidae family, is also world-wide in distribution, and the incidence of trichomonal vaginitis affects 20 to 40% of the female population (2). Its recommended treatment is by using metronidazole; yet recent emergence of drug-resistant strains of T. vaginalis (3) cast doubt on its future effectiveness. There is thus a genuine need for new, safer but effective agents for controlling giardiasis and trichomoniasis.

Recent biochemical studies of various protozoan parasites have revealed that all of them thus far investigated are incapable of de novo synthesis of purine nucleotides (4),

[1]This investigation received financial support from the National Institute of Health grant AI-19391.

although the ability of de novo synthesis of pyrimidines
appears to be intact. This metabolic deficiency has been
successfully exploited for opportunities of antiparasitic
chemotherapy, and is best examplified by the activities of
pyrazolopyrimidines on the hemoflagellates discussed by J. J.
Marr in another chapter of this book.

Similar studies have been directed recently toward Giardia
and Trichomonas (5). Because of the relative ease in cultiva-
ting G. lamblia (6) and T. vaginalis (7) in vitro in axenic
media and the well controlled harvest of large numbers of log-
phase cells for further studies, rapid progress has been made
in recent time. Trichomonas foetus, a cattle parasite
closely related to T. vaginalis, has been also added to the
list for investigation because it has been the one species
studied in greatest biochemical details (8) among the
anaerobic flagellates. It can be cultivated in vitro axeni-
cally (7), and grown at a fast rate to high cell densities to
allow extensive investigations with minimal technical diffi-
culties.

II. THE ABSENCE OF DE NOVO SYNTHESIS OF BOTH PURINE AND
PYRIMIDINE NUCLEOTIDES

Heyworth et al. (9) first observed in T. vaginalis the
total lack of incorporation of radiolabeled purine ring precursors glycine, bicarbonate, formate and serine, into the
nucleic acid fraction. Similar studies in our laboratory on
radioactive precursor incorporation into nucleotide pool of
log-phase G. lamblia trophozoites (10), T. vaginalis
(unpublished) and T. foetus (11) in buffered saline over one
to two hours also indicated no detectable incorporation of any
of the precursors into the purine nucleotides analyzed in high
pressure liquid chromatography (HPLC). It is apparent that
all the three species of anaerobic flagellates are incapable
of de novo synthesis of purine nucleotides.

Five of the six enzymic activities of pyrimidine biosynthesis have been measured in T. vaginalis by Hill et al. (12);
they found only the carbamoylphosphate synthetase activity.
Lindmark and Jarroll (13) examined carbamoylphosphate synthetase, aspartate transcarbamylase, dihydroorotase and dihydro-
orotate dehydrogenase activities in G. lamblia trophozoite
homogenates, and could not detect any of them. We have investigated the possible incorporation of radiolabeled aspartate
and orotate into the nucleotide pool as well as the nucleic
acids in the three parasites at their log-phase, and could not
detect any incorporation of these pyrimidine precursors
(5,15). Assays for orotate phosphoribosyl transferase

activity in the crude extracts of the three parasites also
turned out negatively (5,15). Apparently, the parasites are
lacking the capability of de novo synthesis of pyrimidines and
pyrimidine nucleotides.
    These double deficiencies in de novo synthesis of both
purines and pyrimidines in G. lamblia, T. vaginalis and T.
foetus distinguish them from the rest of the protozoan parasites. These anaerobic protozoa are clearly representing a
group of living organisms with the most deficient nucleic acid
metabolism known to date. They must be dependent exclusively
on the salvage of purines, pyrimidines or their nucleosides
from the living environment for survival and growth. These
salvaging activities are thus of great interest for further
investigation in view of possible rational approach to antiparasitic chemotherapy.

III. MORE DEFICIENCY IN PYRIMIDINE NUCLEOTIDE METABOLISM

    Our further studies demonstrated that radiolabeled uracil
and uridine were incorporated into the RNA fraction of T.
vaginalis (15) and T. foetus (5) to very high levels. But the
labels were never transferred into the DNA fraction despite of
prolonged incubation. On the other hand, labeled thymidine
was found readily incorporated into the DNA fraction. There
was thus the likelihood that UMP was not converted to TMP in
the parasites. This probability was supported by our further
discoveries that [1] in the crude extracts of G. lamblia , T.
vaginalis and T. foetus, no dihydrofolate reductase or thymidylate synthetase activity could be detected (5,15); [2] all
three parasites grew normally in the in vitro axenic cultures
in the presence of millimolar concentrations of potent anti-
folates or thymidylate synthetase inhibitors such as methotrexate, pyrimethamine, trimethoprim and 6-azauridine (5,15); [3]
T. foetus could be cultured in a semi-defined medium (14) in
which folic acid and p-aminobenzoic acid have been omitted.
These findings further pointed out the uniqueness of the three
parasites in which the ubiquitous enzymes dihydrofolate reductase and thymidylate synthetase, commonly found in all the
wild-type living organisms, are missing. This additional
deficiency discovered in the pyrimidine nucleotide metabolism
may suggest another point of vulnerability among the three
parasites. But, ironically, it also renders the organisms
resistance toward methotrexate, one of the most potent antifo-
lates toxic to all known living cells.
    T. foetus contained high ribonucleotide reductase activity
(15 nmoles/hr/mg protein). This high activity apparently
enabled T. foetus to grow in the medium (14) where deoxyribose

was absent. The enzyme recognized CDP as substrate, did not act on ribonucleoside triphosphates and showed no dependence on coenzyme B_{12}. On the other hand, however, the enzyme activity was totally resistant to hydroxyurea up to 0.1 M concentration (Figure 1). T. foetus grew well in the presence of similarly high concentrations of hydroxyurea (Figure 1).

This property of the enzyme distinguishes itself from the mammalian ribonucleotide reductase (16) but bears resemblance to that of Epstein-Barr viral ribonucleotide reductase (17). It could be a potential target for selective chemotherapeutic attack.

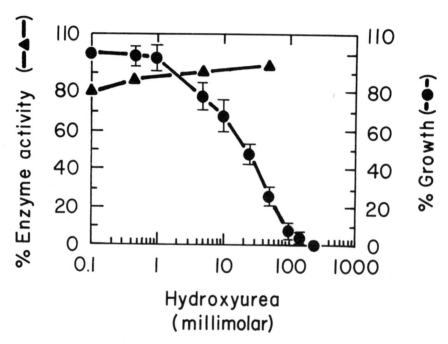

FIGURE 1. Effects of hydroxyurea on the growth and ribonucleotide reductase activity of T. foetus (strain KV_1). The culturing medium was as described previously (7). Incubation was at 37°C for 24 hr, and the cell density was estimated in a ZF Coulter counter. Ribonucleotide reductase activity was assayed according to the procedure by Steeper and Steuart (18).

IV. PATHWAYS OF PYRIMIDINE SALVAGE

The detailed pyrimidine salvage pathways in T. vaginalis

(15) and T. foetus (5) have been thoroughly analyzed. Data in
Figures 2 and 3 indicate that only uracil, uridine, cytidine
and thymidine can be incorporated into the nucleotide pools of
the two parasites. Preference for the four substrates
differs, however, between the two species; while uracil is
most actively incorporated into T. foetus (Fig. 2), cytidine
is preferentially incorporated into T. vaginalis (Fig. 3).

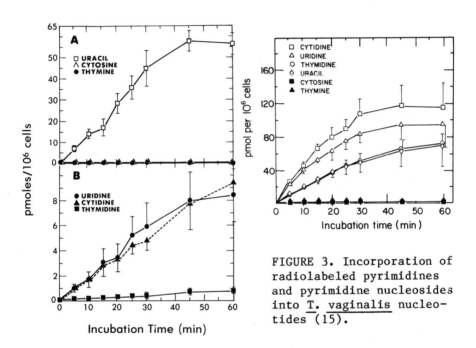

FIGURE 3. Incorporation of
radiolabeled pyrimidines
and pyrimidine nucleosides
into T. vaginalis nucleo-
tides (15).

FIGURE 2. Incorporation of
radiolabeled pyrimidines
and pyrimidine nucleosides
into T. foetus nucleo-
tides (5).

The profile of enzyme activities in crude extracts of the
two parasites indicates that T. foetus has very high uracil
phosphoribosyl transferase activity in its cytoplasm, whereas
T. vaginalis (strain ATCC 30001) has very little such activity
(Table I). There is no detectable pyrimidine nucleoside
kinase, but plenty of uridine, cytidine and thymidine phospho-
transferases are found in both species. These enzymes
transfer phosphate group from artificial phosphate donors such
as p-nitrophenylphosphate or purine and pyrimidine nucleotides
to the 5'-position of pyrimidine nucleoside. They constitute

essentially the only means of providing T. vaginalis with
pyrimidine nucleotides. Thymidine phosphotransferase is the
only enzyme found supplying both Trichomonas spp. with TMP;
HPLC analysis of the nucleotide pool pulse-labeled by radioactive thymidine and chased by unlabeled thymidine suggested
that thymidine is first converted to TMP, then to TDP, TTP and
finally incorporated into DNA. There is no label from thymidine transferred into other nucleotides, nor is there any
label from other nucleotides transferred into TMP, TDP or
TTP. The thymidine phosphotransferase pathway is thus isolated from the other salvage activities, and it may be essential for DNA synthesis in T. vaginalis and T. foetus. This
enzyme is associated with the 10^5xg pellet fraction of the
cells (see Table I), and has a high substrate specificity with
an estimated K_m value of 10 mM for thymidine. Among the
compounds tested, guanosine and 5-fluorodeoxyuridine are found
inhibitory to the enzyme as well as to the in vitro growth of
T. vaginalis and T. foetus.

Table I. Pyrimidine Salvage Enzymes in T. vaginalis and T.
          foetus

| Enzymes | Specific Activities (nmoles/min/mg protein) | | | |
| | T. vaginalis | | T. foetus | |
	Supernatant	Pellet	Supernatant	Pellet
Uracil phosphori- bosyl transferase	ND	ND	0.516	ND
Uridine phospho- transferase	1.63	0.13	ND	0.254
Cytidine phosphotrans- ferase	0.99	0.29	ND	0.039
Thymidine phospho- transferase	ND	0.99	ND	0.144
Cytidine deaminase	156	ND	1.84	ND
Uridine phosphorylase	477	45	1.64	ND

ND, not detectable. The supernatant and pellet fractions
of crude extracts were separated by 10^5xg centrifugation
for one hour (5,15).

The enzyme profile in Table I also indicate that cytidine
deaminase and uridine phosphorylase are extraordinarily high
in T. vaginalis and very substantial in T. foetus. These
enzymes catalyze the conversions of cytidine → uridine ↔

uracil. Our HPLC data indicated that cytidine was incorporated into both cytosine and uracil nucleotides whereas uracil
and uridine were predominantly converted to uracil nucleotides
in two parasites. Prolonged chase of incorporated radiolabels
showed a limited conversion of UTP to CTP in T. foetus but
none in T. vaginalis. This information enables construction
of pyrimidine salvage networks in T. vaginalis and T. foetus
as following;

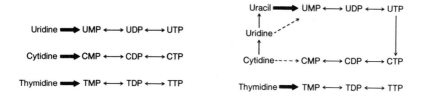

FIGURE 4. Pyrimidine Salvage   FIGURE 5. Pyrimidine Salvage
Pathways in T. vaginalis   Pathways in T. foetus

Detailed knowledge on pyrimidine salvage in G. lamblia has
not yet been available. Our preliminary findings, however,
suggest a very similar network in G. lamblia as in T. vaginalis.

V. PATHWAYS OF PURINE SALVAGE

Heyworth et al. (9) investigated incorporation of preformed
purines into the cold trichloroacetic acid-insoluble fraction
of T. vaginalis, analyzed hydrolysates of the fraction in
thin-layer chromatography and examined the potential purine
salvage enzymes in high-speed supernatants of T. vaginalis.
They concluded that hypoxanthine did not become incorporated
into nucleic acid of T. vaginalis and that there were no
detectable purine phosphoribosyl transferase in T. vaginalis. There were, however, high levels of purine nucleoside
phosphorylases and kinases which apparently provided the
purine salvage for T. vaginalis. Miller and Linstead (19)
indicated the absence of inosine kinase and purine nucleoside
phosphotransferase in T. vaginalis extracts. We have demonstrated (unpublished observation) the total lack of incorporation of hypoxanthine, xanthine and inosine into the nucleotide
pool of T. vaginalis. We also found that adenosine and
adenine were only incorporated into adenine nucleotides,
whereas guanosine and guanine were converted only to guanine

nucleotides. There was no detectable interconversion between adenine and guanine nucleotides in T. vaginalis. Its scheme of purine salvage thus can be simply summarized as follows:

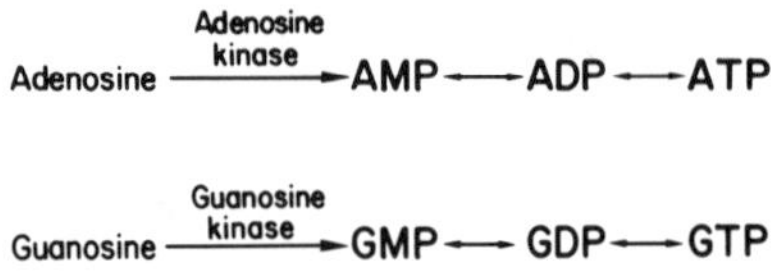

$$\text{Adenosine} \xrightarrow[\text{kinase}]{\text{Adenosine}} \text{AMP} \longleftarrow \text{ADP} \longleftarrow \text{ATP}$$

$$\text{Guanosine} \xrightarrow[\text{kinase}]{\text{Guanosine}} \text{GMP} \longleftarrow \text{GDP} \longleftarrow \text{GTP}$$

FIGURE 6. Purine Salvage Pathways in T. vaginalis

The purine salvage activities in T. foetus (11) and G. lamblia (10) have been thoroughly examined in our laboratories. Data in Figure 7 indicate that essentially all the naturally occurring purines and purine nucleosides can be incorporated into the nucleotides of T. foetus at varying rates. Adenine, hypoxanthine and inosine are among the most actively incorporated substrates; HPLC profiles indicate that they are incorporated about equally into adenine and guanine nucleotides. G. lamblia salvages purines like T. vaginalis; no hypoxanthine, xanthine or inosine can be incorporated into its nucleotide pool (Figure 8). HPLC studies indicate exclusive incorporation of adenosine and adenine into adenine nucleotides and guanosine and guanine into guanine nucleotides. There is no interconversion between the two kinds of purine nucleotides in G. lamblia. However, purine salvage in G. lamblia is different from that in T. vaginalis, in which radioactivity from [5'-^{3}H]guanosine is not appreciably incorporated into G. lamblia guanine nucleotides (10), suggesting that guanosine has to be converted to guanine before being incorporated into GMP.

This finding has been confirmed by studies of purine salvage enzyme profile in G. lamblia (see Table II). Among all the enzyme activities, only four enzymic activities have been identified in the crude extract; adenosine and guanosine hydrolases and adenine and guanine phosphoribosyl transferases. Apparently, G. lamblia converts the nucleosides to purine bases by its overwhelming hydrolase activities and then incorporates purine bases through the actions of its phosphoribosyl transferases (see Figure 9).

The enzyme profile in T. foetus is much more complicated. There are high levels of hypoxanthine and guanine phosphoribosyl transferases, but no adenine phosphoribosyl transferase. Adenosine kinase and guanosine phosphotransferase are found in T. foetus which suggest the possibility of direct incorporation of the two nucleosides. However, the overwhel-

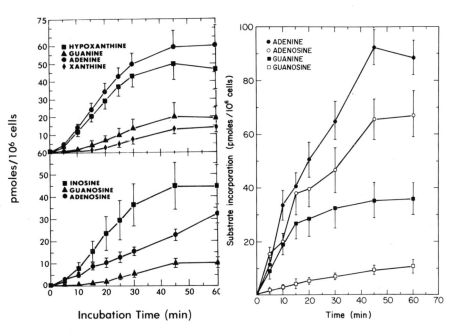

FIGURE 7. Incorporation of radiolabeled purines and purine nucleosides into the nucleotide pool of T. foetus (11).

FIGURE 8. Incorporation of radiolabeled purines and purine nucleosides into the nucleotide pool of G. lamblia (10).

mingly high activities of adenosine phosphorylase, guanosine phosphorylase, inosine phosphorylase, adenine deaminase and adenosine deaminase suggest that most of the purine nucleosides and purine bases are first converted to hypoxanthine before incorporation into nucleotides. This is best illustrated by the facts that adenine is among the most actively incorporated substrates (Figure 7) but there is no adenine phosphoribosyl transferase activity found in T. foetus (Table II). HPLC analysis of T. foetus nucleotide pool indicated identical profiles of radioactivities between hypoxanthine- and adenine-pulse-labeled samples. Apparently, adenine must be converted to hypoxanthine by the adenine deaminase in T. foetus before its incorporation into nucleotide pool. The direct salvage of hypoxanthine thus could be the major route of purine salvage in T. foetus (Figure 10).

The summaries presented in Figures 6, 9 and 10 thus give us a most interesting comparison among the three parasites. Each parasite has a totally unique and simple network for

purine salvage. The formation of IMP as the precursor of AMP
and GMP, observed among all the known prokaryotes and eukaryotes, is only found in T. foetus . T. vaginalis and G.
lamblia have no such common presursor of purine nucleotides,
and, consequently, represent the ultimate simplicity of purine
metabolism among all the living organisms.

From the point of interest on potential chemotherapeutic
control of the three parasites, it appears that an effective
inhibition of hypoxanthine phosphoribosyl transferase in T.
foetus, of adenosine or guanosine kinase in T. vaginalis and
of adenine or guanine phosphoribosyl transferase in G. lamblia

Table II. Purine Salvage Enzymes in G. lamblia and T.
           foetus

| Enzymes | Specific Activities (nmoles/min/mg protein) | |
	G. lamblia	T. foetus
Hypoxanthine phosphoribosyl transferase	ND	$0.92 \pm 0.01^*$
Guanine phosphoribosyl trans-ferase	$5.40 \pm 1.61^*$	$1.14 \pm 0.05^*$
Adenine phosphoribosyl trans-ferase	$3.16 \pm 0.52^*$	ND
Adenosine kinase	ND	$0.92 \pm 0.10^*$
Guanosine phosphotransferase	ND	$0.57 \pm 0.03^{\ddagger}$
Inosine phosphorylase	ND	$44.0 \pm 5.0^*$
Adenosine phosphorylase	ND	$16.0 \pm 1.5^*$
Guanosine phosphorylase	ND	$21.8 \pm 2.0^*$
Adenosine hydrolase	$967.7 \pm 32.4^*$	ND
Guanosine hydrolase	$970.6 \pm 23.5^*$	ND
Adenosine deaminase	–	$29.0 \pm 2.0^*$
Adenine deaminase	–	$0.66 \pm 0.07^*$

ND, not detectable. *, supernatant; ‡, pellet fraction of
the crude extract separated by 10^5xg centrifugation for one
hour (10,11).

would achieve the purpose. Although none of these enzymes has
yet been purified or chracterized, the G. lamblia guanine
phosphoribosyl transferase seems to be a particularly interesting enzyme because it does not recognize either hypoxanthine

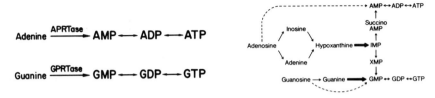

FIGURE 9. Purine Salvage
Pathways in G. lamblia

FIGURE 10. Purine Salvage
Pathways in T. foetus.

or xanthine as substrate. Since the human host enzyme takes
both hypoxanthine and guanine as substrates (20), a difference
in substrate specificity may exist between the parasite and
host enzymes which may allow specific inhibitor design for the
former.

On the other hand, the plainly presented purine salvage
pathways may suggest some known enzyme inhibitors as possible
controlling agents of growth of the parasites. For instance,
the inhibitor of hypoxanthine-guanine phosphoribosyl transferase 8-azaguanine (21), the inhibitor of IMP dehydrogenase
mycophenolic acid (22) and the inhibitor of succino-AMP synthetase formycin B (23) should block the purine salvage in T.
foetus without affecting those in T. vaginalis and G.
lamblia. Our results from in vitro cultures indicated that
these three compounds were indeed inhibitors of T. foetus
growth in vitro with IC_{50} values ranging from 10^{-5} to 10^{-4}M
(24). They had, however, absolutely no effect on the growth
of T. vaginalis or G. lamblia up to 10^{-3}M in the culturing
media (24). Conversely, adenosine analogs such as tubercidin,
sangivamycin, toyocamycin and adenine arabinoside, known to be
phosphorylated by adenosine kinase (25), were found inhibitory
to T. vaginalis in vitro growth ($IC_{50} \sim 1-5 \times 10^{-5}$M) without
appreciable effect on T. foetus (24). Thus the different
purine salvage pathways make selective killings of the three
parasites possible.

CONCLUSION

The studies on purine and pyrimidine metabolism in G.
lamblia, T. vaginalis and T. foetus have yet to be completed
in the near future. But, from what has been learned already,
this investigation may be developed into an ideal model for
rational approach to antiparasitic chemotherapy. By classical
comparative biochemical approaches, we were able to demon-

strate, first, the metabolic deficiencies in the parasites which are expected because of their parasitic nature. We then identified the crucial pathways for salvaging pyrimidines and purines whose functions are likely to be essential for the survival of the parasites. Some known inhibitors of these pathways were then tested to see if they indeed inhibit the parasite growth. Once this correlation is verified, the future will depend on isolation, purification and characterization of some of the pivotal enzymes for possible specific inhibitor design.

REFERENCES

1. Smith, J. W., and Wolfe, M. S. (1980). Ann. Rev. Med. 35:373.
2. Gardner, H. L. (1962). Obstet. Gynecol. 1:279.
3. Meingassner, J. G., and Thurner, J. (1979). Antimicrobial Agents Chemother. 15:254.
4. Wang, C. C. and Simashkevich, P. M. (1981). Proc. Natl. Acad. Sci. USA 78:6618.
5. Wang, C. C., Verham, R., Tzeng, S., Aldritt, S., and Cheng, H-W. (1983). Proc. Natl. Acad. Sci. USA 80:2564.
6. Diamond, L. S., Harlow, D. R., and Cunnick, C. C. (1978). Trans. Roy. Soc. Trop. Med. Hyg. 72:431.
7. Diamond, L. S. (1957). J. Parasitol. 43:488.
8. Müller, M. (1980). Symp. Soc. Gen. Microbiol. 30:127.
9. Heyworth, P. G., Gutteridge, W. E., and Ginger, C. D. (1982). FEBS Letters 141:106.
10. Wang, C. C., and Aldritt, S. (1983). J. Exp. Med. (in press).
11. Wang, C. C., Verham, R., Rice, A., and Tzeng, S. (1983). Mol. Biochem. Parasitol. (in press).
12. Hill, B., Kilsby, J., Rogerson, G. W., McIntosh, R. T., and Ginger, C. D. (1981). Mol. Biochem. Parasitol. 2:123.
13. Lindmark, D. G., and Jarroll, E. L. (1982). Mol. Biochem. Parasitol. 5:291.
14. Wang, C. C., Wang, A. L., and Rice, A. (1984). Exp. Parasitol. (in press).
15. Wang, C. C., and Cheng, H-W. (1983). Mol. Biochem. Parasitol. (in press).
16. Frenkel, E. P., and Arthur, C. (1967). Cancer Res, 27:1016.
17. Henry, B. E., Glaser, R., Hewetson, J., and O'Callaghan, D. J. (1978). Virology 89:262.
18. Steeper, J. R., and Steuart, C. D. (1970). Anal. Biochem. 34:123.
19. Miller, R. and Linstead, D. (1983). Mol. Biochem. Para-

sitol. 7:41.
20. Murray, A. W., Elliot, D. C., and Atkinson, M. R. (1970) Prog. Nucleic Acid Res. Mol. Biol. 10:87.
21. Elion, G. (1969). Cancer Res. 29:2448.
22. Snyder, F. F., Henderson, J. F., and Cook, D. Z. (1972). Biochem. Pharmacol. 21:2351.
23. Carson, D. A., and Chang, K-P. (1980). Biochem. Biophys. Res. Comm. 100:1377.
24. Wang, C. C., Verham, R., Cheng, H-W., Rice, A., and Wang, A. L. (1984). Biochem. Pharmacol. (in press).
25. Bloch, A., Leonard, R. J., and Nichol, C. A. (1967). Biochim. Biophys. Acta 138:10.

PYRAZOLOPYRIMIDINE METABOLISM
IN THE PATHOGENIC HEMOFLAGELLATES

J. Joseph Marr[1,2]

Division of Infectious Diseases
Departments of Medicine and Microbiology
University of Colorado Health Sciences Center
Denver, Colorado

I. INTRODUCTION

The hemoflagellates that infect man have proven recalci-
trant to effective chemotherapy since the specificity found in
agents used in the treatment of bacterial diseases is lacking
in these protozoan diseases. A high therapeutic index for a
given antimicrobial usually requires a specific, although not
necessarily major, difference in the metabolism between the
host and the parasite. Leishmania and trypanosomes metabolize
the pyrazolopyrimidine nucleus as a purine base, whereas mammalian cells cannot. Mammalian cells synthesize purines de
novo and have the capacity to salvage purine bases and nucleosides for nucleic acid and coenzyme synthesis. Leishmania
spp. and Trypanosoma spp. cannot synthesize purines de novo
and use salvage mechanisms for purine incorporation (1-5).
These differences and those in the specificities of enzymes in
the purine salvage pathways, with respect to pyrazolopyrimidines, have led to a more comprehensive understanding of the

---

[1]Present address: Div. of Infectious Diseases B-168, Univ. of
Colorado Health Sci. Ctr., 4200 E. 9th Ave., Denver, CO 80262

[2]This investigation received financial support from UNDP/World
Bank/WHO Special Program for Research and Training in Tropi-
cal Diseases (T16/181/T8/30), the National Institutes of
Health (AI1566309), and the Burroughs Wellcome Co.

147

biochemistry of these organisms and raised some exciting questions of basic biochemistry and chemotherapy.

II. CHEMISTRY

Pyrazolopyrimidines are structural analogues of purines in
which there is an inversion of the nitrogen from the seven
position of the purine ring to what would correspond to position eight. This makes the compound a pyrazolo (3,4-d) pyrimidine and substantially alters its metabolic fate (Fig. 1).
Allopurinol (4-hydroxypyrazolo(3, 4-d)pyrimidine; HPP) is a
structural analogue of hypoxanthine. It is a substrate for
and an inhibitor of xanthine oxidase.

The metabolism of HPP in man differs from that in the
hemoflagellates (Fig. 2). About 60% is rapidly converted to
oxipurinol. Thirty percent, in the steady state, will be excreted in the urine as allopurinol and the remaining 10% as
allopurinol-1-ribonucleoside (HPPR)(6). Besides HPPR, two
other ribonucleosides are formed as minor metabolic products
(7,8). The ribonucleotides formed from these are potential
inhibitors of orotidylate decarboxylase (9) but there is
little or no effect on pyrimidine metabolism in man or animals
(10). The possible effects of allopurinol on purine metabolism has been subject to considerable investigation but none
have been noted (11-13) nor is there evidence for incorporation of any allopurinol derivative into nucleic acid (14).

III. METABOLISM OF PYRAZOLOPYRIMIDINES
IN LEISHMANIA

Allopurinol inhibition of the growth of leishmania was
first demonstrated in L. braziliensis (15), and subsequently
in L. donovani and L. mexicana (16). The investigation
developed from an observation by Frank et al. (17) that allopurinol could inhibit the growth of Crithidia fasciculata.

Subsequent investigations documented the metabolic conversions of allopurinol in these organisms (Fig. 2). The
promastigotes concentrate HPP from the medium and form allopurinol ribonucleoside-5'-monophosphate (HPPR-MP)(18). The
intracellular concentration of HPPR-MP is 2-3 mM, approximately the same as ATP, indicating that the purine economy of the
cell has been altered greatly. HPPR-MP is aminated to 4-
aminopyrazolopyrimidine-5'-monophosphate (APPR-MP), converted
to the di- and triphosphates, APPR-DP and APPR-TP, respectively, and the latter is incorporated into the cellular RNA (18)

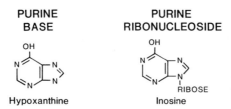

PURINE BASE

Hypoxanthine

PURINE RIBONUCLEOSIDE

Inosine

PYRAZOLOPYRIMIDINE ANALOGUE

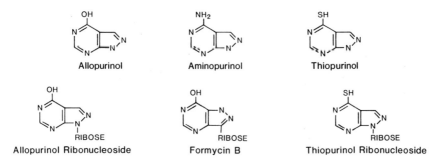

Allopurinol

Aminopurinol

Thiopurinol

Allopurinol Ribonucleoside

Formycin B

Thiopurinol Ribonucleoside

Figure 1. Structures of certain purines and pyrazolopyrimidines. (Reproduced with permission from Marr, J.J., Berens, R.L. (1983). Mol. Biochem. Parasitol. 7: 339-357.

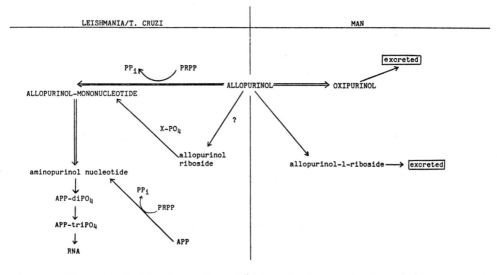

Figure 2. Metabolic transformations of allopurinol and its ribonucleoside in pathogenic hemoflagellates and man.

(Fig. 2). This incorporation of APPR-TP into RNA of the parasite is unique.

The important feature which distinguishes the metabolism of pyrazolopyrimidines in these parasitic protozoans from that in man is the accumulation of large quantities of HPRR-MP. This accumulation is due to the substrate specificities of the PRTases in these organisms. The pyrazolopyrimidines, HPP and 4-thiopyrazolopyrimidine (TPP) are less efficient substrates than normal purines, but are more efficient substrates for the HGPRTase from this organism than for the enzyme from human erythrocytes by a factor of ten. This is consistent with the observations that promastigotes accumulate large quantities of HPPR-MP and human cells do not (19).

Approximately 10% of HPPR-MP is converted to APPR-MP via the succino-AMP synthetase (EC 6.3.4.4) and the succino-AMP lyase (EC 4.3.2.2)(20). This compound is not a substrate of succino-AMP synthetase from a mammalian source (21). The protozoan enzymes may be unique in their abilities to accept HPPR-MP as an alternate substrate for IMP. There is no evidence for this transformation in mammalian tissues (8,22). The amination of HPPR-MP, despite the unfavorable kinetic constants, is due to the high concentration of this compound within the cell, about 100-fold higher than that of IMP. A similar situation exists in T. cruzi.

The GMP reductase (EC 1.6.6.8) is inhibited by both HPPR-MP and TPPR-MP (23). This is a major difference between the GMP reductase of the parasite and that derived from a human source (24). That from human erythrocytes is unresponsive to pyrazolopyrimidines.

IV.   ALLOPURINOL RIBONUCLEOSIDE

In man, about 10% of HPP is converted to allopurinol ribonucleoside (22). HPPR is not oxidized by xanthine oxidase but only by aldehyde oxidase, which is present in low levels in humans (25,26). It is approximately 10-fold more active against L. braziliensis and 300-fold more active against L. donovani than the parent compound (27). HPPR-MP is formed in large amounts from HPPR and the aminopyrazolopyrimidine ribonucleotides are made and incorporated into RNA. The direct phosphorylation of HPPR is due to a nucleoside phosphotransferase, rather than a nucleoside kinase, and the product was a 5'-ribonucleotide (Fig. 2).

V. OTHER PURINE ANALOGUES

These results prompted an investigation of other pyrazolopyrimidines and related compounds. Of these, only thiopurinol
and its ribonucleoside showed promise (28). TPP and HPP are
of approximately equivalent antileishmanial activities. The
ribonucleosides are also of essentially equal activities and
are more active than the bases, except in L. mexicana where
HPP and HPPR are of equal potency (27). The organisms did not
metabolize TPP beyond the 5'-monophosphate stage (TPPR-MP).
The thiol group was stable for the duration of the experiment
(24 hours) and no radiolabeled sulfate was found. The ribose
remained with the pyrazolopyrimidine.

TPP was a substrate for the HGPRTase of L. donovani (19)
but studies with the succino-AMP synthetase showed that the
possible product, succino-APPR-MP, was not formed (28). The
inability of TPPR-MP to serve as a substrate corroborated the
studies in vivo which did not detect the formation of APPR-MP.
Although TPPR-MP was unable to substitute for IMP in the reaction, it did inhibit the conversion of IMP. TPPR was phosphorylated by a nucleoside phosphotransferase and the kinetic
data were similar to those found previously for HPPR (27,28).

The related inosine analogue, formycin B (7-hydroxy-3-β-
D-ribofuranosylpyrazolo[4,3-d]pyrimidine; FORB), also has
antileishmanial activity (Fig. 1). This C-nucleoside analogue
of inosine is neither phosphorylated nor cleaved in mammalian
cells (29,30). A study of the effects of FORB on leishmania
was published by Carson and Chang (31). They showed that FORB
inhibited the growth of L. donovani and L. mexicana promastigotes. The promastigotes produced formycin B monophosphate
(FORB-MP). A subsequent study (32) confirmed that FORB was an
effective antileishmanial agent but also demonstrated that
these organisms converted FORB to the ribonucleotides of FORA,
the AMP analogue, indicating that the metabolic pathway is
exactly the same as that for HPPR. The conversion of FORB to
FORA ribonucleotides was confirmed by Rainey and Santi (33).

VI. EFFECT OF PYRAZOLOPYRIMIDINES
ON AMASTIGOTES OF L. DONOVANI

Since the intracellular parasite, or amastigote, is the
pathogenic form in man, it is imperative to demonstrate that
HPP and HPPR have similar effects on it. Experiments to compare HPP metabolism included: exposure of free amastigotes,
and minced, infected, hamster spleen preparations, infected

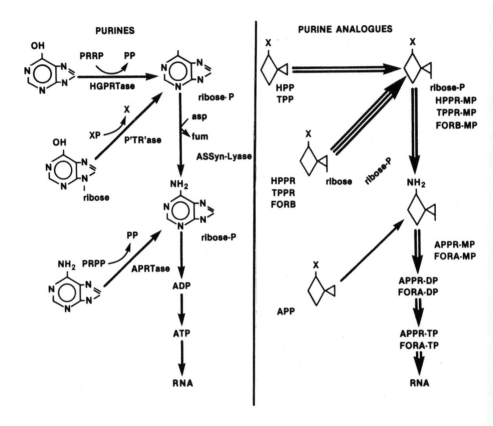

Figure 3. Comparison of purine and pyrazolopyrimidine meta-
           bolism in hemoflagellates. The major salvage
           pathways for purines are depicted on the left and
           the corresponding transformations of the pyra-
           zolopyrimidine analogues on the right. The abbre-
           viations are as follows: HGPRTase - hypoxanthine-
           guanine-phosphoribosyltransferase; P'T'ase-nucleo-
           side phosphotransferase; ASSYN/lyase - succinyl-
           AMP synthetase/lyase. Abbreviations for the
           pyrazolopyrimidine analogues are given in the text.
           All of the analogues are metabolized to the corres-
           ponding aminopyrazolopyrimidine triphosphate except
           for TPP and TPPR which are halted at the thiopyra-
           zolopyrimidine ribonucleotide. (Reproduced with
           permission from Marr, J.J., Berens, R.L. (1983).
           Mol. Biochem. Parasitol. 7:339-357.

388D, macrophage cultures with radiolabeled HPP. All produced
HPPR-MP as well as the three ribonucleotides of APP. Under
identical conditions uninfected spleen and macrophages yielded
only radiolabeled HPPR-MP; no APP ribonucleotides were formed.
When HPP, TPP, HPPR or TPPR were added to infected P388D$_1$ cultures, all compounds eliminated the intracellular parasites
(34,28). None of these agents inhibited the growth of uninfected macrophages. FORB at a concentration of 1 μM inhibited
the growth of amastigotes of L. mexicana in J774G8 macrophages
by approximately 50%. When the concentration was increased to
10 μM the macrophages were inhibited by approximately 30%.
FORB markedly decreased the number of amastigotes in the
livers of hamsters infected with L. donovani when the drug was
given for five days (31).

VII.   THE METABOLISM OF PYRAZOLOPYRIMIDINES
       IN TRYPANOSOMA CRUZI

A. Similarities to Leishmania

The growth of the culture (epimastigote) form of Trypanosoma cruzi is inhibited by HPP (35). Subsequent studies
showed that epimastigotes of the Costa Rica, CL, Peru and Y
strains (35) (Berens and Marr, unpublished results), as well
as the Ma and F$_1$ (36) strains of T. cruzi, converted HPP to
APP ribonucleotides and incorporated the latter into RNA.
After incubation with HPP, the intracellular concentrations
of HPPR-MP were similar to those found with leishmania.
    The enzymes responsible for these conversions have not
been studied in as much detail as have those of L. donovani.
Gutteridge et al. (37) reported that T. cruzi contains the
same PRTases that were described for L. donovani. Presumably
the HGPRTase is responsible for the conversion of HPP to HPPR-
MP while the APRTase converts APP to APPR-MP. Spector et al.
(38) described the kinetic properties of succino-AMP synthetase and lyase from T. cruzi. The substrate specificity and
the K$'_m$ of succino-AMP synthetase were essentially identical to
those of L. donovani (20).

B. Differences from Leishmania

While the effects and metabolism of HPP in T. cruzi are
similar to those found for leishmania, there are some differences with respect to other pyrazolopyrimidines. HPPR has
little effect on the growth of the Costa Rica (CR) and the CL
strains of T. cruzi and only small amounts of the compound are

converted to HPPR-MP and APP ribonucleotides (35, and Berens, Marr, Nelson, LaFon, unpublished results). There are strain differences, however, since the Peru and Y strains of T. cruzi are sensitive to HPPR. The biochemical data suggest that this is related to the relative inabilities of some strains to metabolize the ribonucleoside. In general, T. cruzi shows the same response to FORB as it does to HPPR. Those strains which are sensitive to the latter also respond to the former; those resistant to one are resistant to both. As was found for L. donovani, sensitive strains of T. cruzi convert FORB to FORB-MP. This is followed by amination to FORA-MP and the di- and triphosphates (39-41).

C. Comparison of epimastigotes, trypomastigotes and amastigotes

Bloodstream trypomastigotes (Peru strain), isolated from infected chinchillas, amastigote-infected spleen cells from infected chinchillas, and transformed human diploid lung cells (VA-13) infected with T. cruzi produce significant amounts of HPPR-MP, APPR-MP, APPR-DP and APPR-TP. Thus, both the amastigotes and trypomastigotes possess the same metabolic sequence described for epimastigotes. Treatment of infected VA-13 cultures with HPP (25 μg/ml) eradicated the infection (42). This agrees with the findings of Avila and Avila that T. cruzi infected mice treated with allopurinol showed a very significant increase in survival time compared to infected controls (43,44).

VIII. CHEMOTHERAPEUTIC POTENTIAL

Metabolism of pyrazolopyrimidines by enzymes of the purine salvage pathways is a characteristic common to all of the hemoflagellates studied thus far. This metabolic peculiarity may offer opportunities for chemotherapy of diseases caused by some of them. Although the biochemistry of purine and pyrazolopyrimidine metabolism is relatively well understood, the potential chemotherapeutic benefits remain to be demonstrated. To date, there have been relatively few studies in animals. A study in mice using L. major and L. mexicana amazonensis demonstrated that allopurinol was an effective agent in this model (45). A study in the Aotus monkey demonstrated that allopurinol, given orally, was an effective agent against L. braziliensis panamensis (46). A small clinical study documented some efficacy of allopurinol in humans with antimony-resistant, visceral leishmaniasis (47). However, these patients have not had prolonged follow-up and more time must pass before this study can be evaluated critically. One animal study by Avila and Avila (44) demonstrated that allopurinol was effective in treating acute Chagas' disease in mice. All of these studies were done with allopurinol and initiated before it was recognized that allopurinol riboside was much more active in vitro. At this writing a clinical trial of the ribonucleoside is being organized which will clarify the role that it may have in the management of leishmaniasis.

REFERENCES

1. Marr, J.J., Berens, R.L., Nelson, D.J. (1978). Biochem. Biophys. Acta. 44:360.
2. Trager, W. (1974). In Ciba Symposium 20, pp. 225-245.
3. Gutteridge, W.E., Gaborek, N. (1979). Int. J. Biochem. 10:415.
4. Ceron, C.R., Caldas, R.A., Feliz, C.F., Mundim, M.H., Roitman, I. (1979). J. Protozool. 26:479-483.
5. Berens, R.L., Marr, J.J., LaFon, S.W., Nelson, D.J. (1981). Mol. Biochem. Parasitol. 3:187-196.
6. Elion, G.B., Kovensky, A., Hitchings, G.H. (1966). Biochem. Pharmacol. 15:863.
7. Krenitsky, T.A., Strelitz, R.A., Hitchings, G.H. (1967). J. Biol. Chem. 242:2675-2682.
8. Nelson, D.J., Bugge, C.J.L., Krasny, H.C., Elion, G.B. (1973). Biochem. Pharmacol. 22:2003-2022.
9. Beadmore, T.D., Kelley, W.N. (1971). J. Lab. Clin. Med. 78:696-704.
10. Fyfe, J.A., Nelson, D.J., Hitchings, G.H. (1974). In Sperling, O., Devries, A., Wyngaarden, J.B. pp. 621-628. Plenum, New York.
11. Fox, I.H., Wyngaarden, J.B., Kelley, W.N. (1970). N. Engl. J. Med. 283:1177-1182.
12. Krenitsky, T.A., Papaioannou, R., Elion, G.B. (1969). J. Biol. Chem. 244:1263-1270.
13. Elion, G.B., Nelson, D.J. (1974). "Ribonucleotides of allopurinol and oxypurinol in rat tissues and their significance in purine metabolism." In Sperling, O., DeVries, A., Wyngaarden, J.B. pp. 639-652. Plenum, New York.
14. Hitchings, E.H. (1975). Arthritis and Rheumatism 18: 863-870.
15. Pfaller, M.A., Marr, J.J. (1974). Antimicrob. Agents Chemother. 5:469-472.

16. Marr, J.J., Berens, R.L. (1977). J. Infect. Dis. 136:
    724-732.
17. Frank, O., Baker, H., Hutner, S.H. (1970). J. Protozool.
    17:153-158.
18. Nelson, D.J., Bugge, C.J.L., Elion, G.B., Berens, R.L.,
    Marr, J.J. (1979). J. Biol. Chem. 254:3954-3959.
19. Tuttle, J.V., Krenitsky, T.A. (1980). J. Biol. Chem. 255:
    909-916.
20. Spector, T., Jones, T.E., Elion, G.B. (1979). J. Biol.
    Chem. 254:8422-8426.
21. Spector, T., Miller, R.L. (1976). Biochem. Biophys. Acta
    455:509-517.
22. Elion, G.B. (1978). In "Handbook of Experimental Pharma-
    cology." (Kelley, W.N., Weiner, I.M., eds.), pp. 485-514.
    Springer-Verlag, New York.
23. Spector, T., Jones, T.E., Miller, R.L. (1980). J. Biol.
    Chem. 54:2308-2315.
24. **Spector, T., Jones, T.E., Miller, R.L. (1982). J. Biol.
    Chem. 54:2308-2315.**
25. Krenitsky, T.A., Neil, S.M., Elion, G.B., Hitchings, G.H.
    (1972). Arch. Biochem. Biophys. 150:585-599.
26. Krenitsky, T.A., Tuttle, J.V., Cattau, E.L., Wang, P.
    (1974). Comp. Biochem. Physiol. 49B:687-703.
27. Nelson, D.J., LaFon, S.W., Tuttle, J.V., Miller, W.H.,
    Miller, R.L., Krenitsky, T.A., Elion, G.B., Berens, R.L.,
    Marr, J.J. (1979). J. Biol. Chem. 254:11544-11549.
28. Marr, J.J., Berens, R.L., Nelson, D.J., Krenitsky, T.A.,
    Spector, T., LaFon, S.W., Elion, G.B. (1982). Biochem.
    Pharmacol. 31:143-148.
29. Umezawa, H., Sawa, T. Fukagawa, Y., Homma, I., Ishizuka,
    M., Takeuchi, T. (1967). J. Antibiotics (Tokyo) 20:308-
    316.
30. Sheen, M.R., Kim, B.K., Parks, R.E. (1968). Mol. Pharma-
    col. 4:293-299.
31. Carson, B.A., Change, K-P. (1981). Biochem. Biophys. Res.
    Commun. 100:1377-1383.
32. Nelson, D.J., LaFon, S.W., Jones, T.E., Spector, T.,
    Berens, R.L., Marr, J.J. (1982). Biochem. Biophys. Res.
    Commun. 108(1):349-354.
33. Rainey, P., Santi, D.V. (1983). Proc. Natl. Acad. Sci.
    80:288-292.
34. Berens, R.L., Marr, J.J., Nelson, D.J., LaFon, S.W.
    (1980). Biochem. Pharmacol. 29:2397-2398.
35. Marr, J.J., Berens, R.L., Nelson, D.J. (1978). Science
    201:1018-1020.
36. Avila, J.L., Avila, A., Casanova, M.A. (1981). Biochem.
    Parasitol. 4:265-272.

37. Gutteridge, W.E., Davies, M.J. (1982). FEMS Microbiol. Let. 13:207-212.
38. Spector, T., Berens, R.L., Marr, J.J. (1982). Biochem. Pharmacol. 31:225-229.
39. Marr, J.J. (1983). Cell Biochem. Supplement 7A, 4.
40. Berens, R.L., Marr, J.J., Nelson, D.J. (1983). J. Cell Biochem. Supplement 7A, 28.
41. Rainey, P., Garrett, C.E., Santi, D.V. (1983). Biochem. Pharmacol. 32:749-753.
42. Berens, R.L., Marr, J.J., Cruz, F.S., Nelson, D.J. (1982). Antimicrob. Agents Chemother. 22:657-661.
43. Avila, J.L., Avila, A., Minoz, E. (1981). Am. J. Trop. Med. Hyg. 30:744-769.
44. Avila, J.L., Avila, A. (1980). Exp. Parasitol. 51:204-208.
45. Peters, W., Trotter, E.R., Robinson, B.L. (1980). Ann. Trop. Med. Parasitol. 74:321-355.
46. Walton, B.C., Harper, J., Neal, R.A. (1983). Am. J. Trop. Med. Hyg. 32:46-50.
47. Kager, P.A., Rees, P.H., Wellde, B.T., Hockemeyer, W.T., Lyerly, W.H. (1981). Trans. Roy. Soc. Trop. Med. Hyg. 75:556-559.

DIFLUOROMETHYLORNITHINE AND THE RATIONAL DEVELOPMENT OF POLYAMINE ANTAGONISTS FOR THE CURE OF PROTOZOAN INFECTION

Peter P. McCann, Cyrus J. Bacchi*, Henry C. Nathan*
and Albert Sjoerdsma

Merrell Dow Research Center
Cincinnati, Ohio

and

*Haskins Laboratories and
Department of Biology, Pace University
New York, New York

I. INTRODUCTION

The definitive and somewhat ambitious title of this paper when taken in a historical and chronological aspect is, in fact, quite accurate. Whether or not all the results described herewith were done in the exact sequence given is not particularly relevant. The fact remains that antagonism of polyamine metabolism was specifically investigated as a means of restricting cell proliferation, and the ultimate use of such inhibitors as a means of curing protozoan infections did follow a rational sequence of events.

All cells from unicellular organisms to highly differentiated mammalian tissues contain significant amounts of the di- and polyamines, putrescine (1,4-diaminobutane) and spermidine, and, in most higher eukaryotes, spermine (1). All of the physiological functions of these amines are not

Supported by N.I.H. grant AI17340 and a grant from the UNDP/World Bank, WHO Special Programme for Research and Training in Tropical Diseases. (C.J.B.)

well understood at the molecular level but recent studies have
shown that their cellular levels are highly regulated and that
normal cellular proliferation and differentiation require
polyamines (2). Asking what is "the physiological role of
polyamines" is almost the same as asking what is the specific
cellular role of cations such as calcium or magnesium. As is
the case with the above two cations, the polyamines have many
roles and only in certain experimental circumstances is a
particular requirement for a parameter under investigation
made apparent. (For reviews see: 1-7).

II. MAMMALIAN CELL ORNITHINE DECARBOXYLASE AND POLYAMINES

A. Polyamines and Cell Growth

Ornithine decarboxylase (ODC) the enzyme that controls the
formation of putrescine in mammalian cells is a pyridoxal
phosphate-dependent enzyme and is present at very low levels
in quiescent cells. It is a unique mammalian enzyme because
of several unusual properties, including its striking
inducibility and very short half-life (8). Many different
stimuli have been shown to cause early and large increases of
ODC in numerous eukaryotic cells, often concurrently with the
onset of cell proliferation (8). Factors which influence ODC
activity in different cell types include RNA synthesis (8,9),
induction of a regulatory protein or antizyme (10), changes in
enzyme turnover (8), and transition between an active and less
active form (11). The existence of such a number of complex
ODC regulatory mechanisms is certainly related to the ubiquity
of the polyamines themselves.

De novo synthesis of polyamines has been associated for
some time with the induction of cell proliferation and the
traverse of the cell cycle, even apart from the phenomena of
induction of ODC during cell proliferation (2). Correlative
studies, however, could never answer the question of the true
relationship between the availability of polyamines and the
cell growth and division processes. The discovery and
synthesis of inhibitors of the biosynthetic pathways allowed
much more conclusive experiments to be done.

B. MGBG and α-Methylornithine

Several groups, particularly Morris and his colleagues,
utilized methylglyoxal bis(guanylhydrazone) or MGBG, a somewhat non-specific and cytotoxic inhibitor of S-adenosyl-

methionine decarboxylase, to block the synthesis of spermidine
from putrescine in activated lymphocytes. They postulated
that increased levels of spermidine and spermine generally
seen in rapidly proliferating eukaryotic systems are necessary
for enhanced rates of DNA synthesis (12). Subsequently,
definitive experiments were done by Mamont et al. (13) with
α-methylornithine, a specific competitive inhibitor of
ornithine decarboxylase. These clearly demonstrated that
in situ inhibition of ODC in rat hepatoma cells induced to
proliferate causes a rapid fall in the levels of putrescine,
which is followed by a striking decrease of spermidine. DNA
synthesis and cell proliferation were inhibited precisely in
parallel with the depletion of spermidine. Addition of
exogenous polyamines back to the cells resulted in an
immediate resumption of cell proliferation. Furthermore, no
deleterious effects resulted from use of the inhibitor and
consequent depletion of polyamines.

C. α-Difluoromethylornithine (DFMO)

The results with MGBG and α-methylornithine indicated that
there was indeed a strong link between cell proliferation and
polyamine biosynthesis, and consequently new emphasis was
placed on the discovery or, more precisely, the synthesis of
specific irreversible inhibitors of the polyamine biosynthetic
enzymes. Several have been characterized which are analogues
of both the substrate and product of ornithine decarboxylase.
These were effective against a broad spectrum of ODC's from
a number of mammalian and bacterial enzymes (see 14-16).
These compounds were synthesized by a team of chemists at
the Centre de Recherche Merrell International in Strasbourg,
France led by B.W. Metcalf and P. Bey (14). DL-α-difluoro-
methylornithine (DFMO) has been the most widely used. DFMO,
as an analogue of ornithine, has very high specific affinity
for mammalian ODC and significantly reduces putrescine
synthesis in vivo. DFMO binds so specifically that labeled
DFMO can be used to titrate the number of active ornithine
decarboxylase molecules, to localize the enzyme in the cell,
and to label it both in vitro and in vivo since it forms a
stable covalent bond with ornithine decarboxylase and no other
protein (17,18).
Biological experiments with DFMO confirmed earlier studies
with α-methylornithine and showed that exposure to the inhibitor restricted growth in HTC cells, L1210 mouse leukemia
cells, and MA 160 human prostate adenoma cells with the
effects again completely reversible by the addition of exogenous polyamines (19). A subsequent finding was the striking

effect of DFMO on the survival of human small-cell lung carci-
nomas in culture (20,21). After the onset of decreased proliferation caused by polyamine depletion, there was a pro-
nounced cell loss directly related to viability. These data
and subsequent in vivo studies with these tumor cells in nude
mice (22) suggest that such cells are among the most sensitive
to the effects of polyamine depletion, a fact which may prove
useful in the therapy of the human tumor (2,23).

Other in vivo studies have been done with DFMO in various
animal tumor cell models and even preliminary human clinical
trials. While it is somewhat early to say, it would seem that
the use of DFMO as a biological modulating agent increasing
the clinical effectiveness of known cytotoxic drugs will, in
all likelihood, become a widely used chemotherapeutic regimen
(23,24). Studies too numerous to detail here have already
shown enormously enhanced efficacy of a combination of DFMO
with, e.g., MGBG (25), 1,3-bis(2-chloroethyl)-1-nitrosourea
(BCNU) (26), vindesine or Adriamycin (27) and interferon (28).

III. POLYAMINES AND PROTOZOA

A. Polyamines in Trypanosomes

As extensive studies were succeeding in linking the
biosynthesis of polyamines and mammalian cell proliferation,
another aspect of polyamine function was being investigated in
the parasitic hemoflagellate protozoan, Trypanosoma brucei
brucei. This organism, a veterinary parasite, and the closely
related human parasites T. b. gambiense and T. b. rhodesiense
are important medical and economic problems in Africa.
Studies on pathogenic bloodstream forms of T. b. brucei had
demonstrated that an α-glycerophosphate shuttle system was
responsible for reoxidation of NADH in glycolysis (review:
29). The shuttle is composed of a mitochondrial α-glycero-
phosphate oxidase and an extra-mitochondrial NAD-linked
α-glycerophosphate dehydrogenase (αGPDH: EC 1.1.1.8). Studies
on purified trypanosomatid αGPDH's revealed that Mg^{++} was
required for activation and that spermidine or spermine, but
not diamines could replace Mg^{++} (30). Initial analysis of
insect, reptilian and mammalian trypanosomatids for polyamines
determined that putrescine and spermidine formed the major
pool of polyamines and, analogous to mammalian cells, their
levels fluctuated during growth (31). In later studies using
more sensitive HPLC techniques, spermine was detected in low
levels in pathogenic bloodstream and culture forms of T. b.
brucei (32). Synthesis of putrescine and spermidine occurred

rapidly in bloodstream T. b. brucei from ^{3}H-ornithine and methionine, although uptake of extracellular polyamines took place more slowly than in mammalian cell lines (33).

B. Polyamines as Drug Targets

As it became clear that polyamines played an important role in the cellular metabolism of the parasitic trypanosomatids, the cationic nature of most trypanocides, due to the predominance of amine groups in these molecules, suggested investigation for evidence of interaction with polyamines. Indeed, evidence of interactions was found in early studies in which: a) cationic trypanocides displaced polyamines from trypanosomatid ribosomal preparations; b) ethidium and Antrycide, as well as other trypanocides replaced polyamines in activation of trypanosomatid GPDH (reviewed in 6); c) ethidium displaced polyamines bound to purified E. coli tRNA (34). Stronger evidence for the "antipolyamine" nature of cationic trypanocides was the blockade by spermidine or spermine of curative doses of pentamidine, Berenil, Antrycide (quinapyrimine) and prothidium (35). An intracellular mode of action, such as drug displacement of bound polyamines, as opposed to a simple competition for drug uptake was indicated since uptake of ^{3}H-pentamidine in vitro by bloodstream trypomastigotes of T. b. brucei was not affected by coincubation with 1000-fold higher levels of putrescine, spermidine, or spermine (35).

C. DFMO: In Vivo Activity Against African Trypanosomes

The development of the specific ODC inhibitor DFMO (14) and demonstration of its antiproliferative properties (19) prompted trials in T. b. brucei (36). In these initial studies, an acute model infection was used (EATRO 110 isolate) in which mice died 4-6 days after infection.

DFMO was highly effective in this model; animals receiving the drug as a 1% or 2% solution in the drinking water for 3 days, 24 h. post-infection remained aparasitic more than 30 days after controls died. The blood of these animals was also non-infective to naive animals (36). Proof of its antagonism of polyamine biosynthesis was demonstrated by coadministration of diamines or polyamines with curative doses of DFMO. Animals receiving putrescine, spermidine or spermine with 1% or 2% DFMO retained the infection and eventually died, while those receiving the non-physiological diamines, cadaverine

TABLE 1. **Effects of** α**-DFMO and Polyamines on T. b. brucei**
infections in mice[a]

Polyamines	mg/kg	Average survival in days[b]
		2% α-DFMO
None		>30.0 (15)
Spermine 4 HCl	50[c]	7.0 (6)
Spermidine 3 HCl	100	14.1 (6)
Putrescine 2 HCl	500	13.4 (6)
Cadaverine 2 HCl	500	>30.0 (3)
1,3-Diaminopropane 2 HCl	500	>30.0 (3)

[a] Groups of 5 mice were infected with 2 X 10^5 trypanosomes.
Treatment was begun 24 h after infection. DFMO was
administered as a 2% solution in the drinking water for
3 days. Polyamines were administered concurrently as
separate i.p. injections.
[b] Average survival in days beyond control deaths. Cures
are indicated by >30. Parentheses indicate number of
experiments.
[c] Polyamines or diamines, given alone to infected animals,
had no effect on the course of infection.

(1,5-diaminopentane) or 1,3-diaminopropane recovered (Table 1;
see Ref. 37). The amines alone had no effect on the course of
infection.

DFMO (2%) was also curative for an acute strain of the
human parasite T. b. rhodesiense. In trials against a chronic
T. b. rhodesiense isolate, 2% DFMO administered for 8 days
initially cleared the blood of parasites but reoccurrence of
infection occurred in at least half of the infected animals
(38).

DFMO was curative in an acute mouse model of another
veterinary parasite T. congolense. The minimal curative dose
in this case was 2% for 5 days. Lower doses or shorter dose
schedules resulted in aparasitemic periods but eventual
resurgence of the infection in most animals (39). DFMO was
also active in the chronic rodent Microtus montanus model of
the human parasite T. b. gambiense. A 70% survival rate (at
40 days) was obtained if treatment was begun during the early
stage of infection (2% DFMO for 21 days beginning 7 days post-
infection), however only 37% survived if initiation of treatment was delayed until day 21 (40). These studies clearly
demonstrated that polyamine metabolism was critical for the

parasites, and indicated that while DFMO alone could cure
acute infections of these trypanosomes it could suppress, but
not eliminate, chronic infections.

It appears that an antibody response to the surface
antigen of trypanosomes is necessary for the elimination, i.e.
cure, of parasites after DFMO treatment (41). The effects of
DFMO were greatly reduced in immunosuppressed mice infected
with T. b. rhodesiense (EATRO 1886), a clone which produces
chronic relapsing parasitemias. Furthermore, only DFMO-
treated immunocompetent mice were completely cured of the
infection, again suggesting that the overall effect of DFMO
is cytostatic rather than cytolytic. These experiments also
indicated that DFMO may prevent the normally numerous
antigenic variants in the infected host from replicating and
therefore may provide the host with sufficient time to mount
effective immunity to the restricted number of variants (41).

D. DFMO: Effects on Parasite Metabolism

With the development of significant in vivo evidence for
susceptibility of trypanosomes to polyamine inhibition, there
was a need to examine the metabolic consequences of DFMO
treatment in the parasite. Large quantities of drug-treated
bloodstream trypomastigotes for in vitro studies were obtained
using an acute T. b. brucei model in rats (32); purified
preparations of drug-treated parasites exposed to DFMO for 12
or 36 h were then examined for effects of polyamine depletion
(summarized in Table 2; see Ref. 32). Parasites were rapidly
depleted of polyamines, i.e. putrescine was depleted by more
than 90% within 12 h., while spermidine levels declined
approximately 70% by 36 h. ODC activity was completely absent
after 12 h. of treatment (32).

The rapidity with which ODC inactivation and polyamine
depletion took place can be explained by a major difference
between mammalian cells and trypanosomes in terms of their
susceptibility to DFMO. The parasites actively transport DFMO
(32), while mammalian cells take up DFMO by a passive
diffusion mechanism which is not affected by either polyamines
or basic amino acids (42).

Polyamine uptake by intact, treated parasites also
increases 2- to 4-fold after 12 h. of treatment. Increased
polyamine transport has also been found in DFMO-treated
mammalian tumor cell lines (43), and has formed the rationale
for a novel combination chemotherapy of human leukemia. After
DFMO treatment an increased uptake of the spermine-like analog
MGBG by polyamine-depleted leukemic cells results in their
rapid, selective destruction (25).

TABLE 2.   Effects of DFMO on the Metabolism and Morphology of T.b. brucei EATRO 110*

Morphological Changes	Production of multiple nuclei and kineto-plasts, enlarged organisms (up to 40 μ long)
ODC Activity	> 90% inhibition of ODC activity in cells treated for 12 h
Polyamine Levels	Putrescine was > 90% depleted within 12 h post-treatment. Spermidine levels decreased ~60% at 12 h and 70% after 36 h
Polyamine Uptake	Putrescine, spermidine and spermine increased 2- to 4-fold in 12 h treated cells
Polyamine Synthesis by Intact Treated Cells	Putrescine synthesis from [^{3}H]ornithine decreased > 95% in 12 h treated cells. Spermi-dine synthesis from [^{3}H]putrescine + methio-nine increased 3- to 4-fold in treated cells
dSAM Levels	Increased >1000-fold in 12 h treated trypanosomes
Synthesis of Macromolecules	100% inhibition of DNA synthesis and 50-80% inhibition of RNA synthesis resulted after 36 h. Protein synthesis increased up to 4-fold in 36 h treated cells.

*Trypanosomes were harvested from 200g rats treated with 4% DFMO in the drinking water at 60 h post-infection. DFMO was given for 12 or 36 h; treatment resulted in average serum DFMO levels of 45 μM. Data from treated trypanosomes were compared to control, untreated trypanosomes obtained from concurrently infected rats with a 72 h infection.

DFMO also rapidly affects synthesis of macromolecules in T. b. brucei: DNA synthesis ceased in 36 h. treated cells, while RNA synthesis decreased more than 50%. Incorporation of ^{3}H-leucine into protein, however, increased 2- to 4-fold in these same cells.

A major finding of this study was that decarboxylated S-adenosylmethionine (dSAM) increased more than 1000-fold in 12 h. treated cells. dSAM, the product of S-adenosylmethio-nine decarboxylase, which controls the formation of spermidine from putrescine, is believed to be metabolically inert unless used for aminopropyl group transfer in spermidine and/or

spermine production (44). Accumulation of dSAM, and the
resultant sequestering of adenine in an unrecoverable form, as
in the case of mammalian cell lines (45), may account in part
for the rapid effect of DFMO therapy on DNA synthesis,
especially as trypanosomes cannot synthesize adenine de novo
(46). Mammalian cells convert methylthioadenosine (MTA),
the product of n-aminopropyl group transfer from dSAM, to
methylthioribose-1-PO_4 and adenine via a MTA-phosphorylase
(44). Significant MTA phosphorylase activity is present in
T. b. brucei bloodstream forms [specific activity 25-50
nmoles/mg protein/h. (C.J. Bacchi, unpub.)], increasing the
likelihood that the enzyme is involved in adenine salvage.

In addition to these biochemical effects, DFMO induces
morphological changes and aberrations in T. b. brucei: within
12 h. after exposure trypanosomes cease to divide and, after
36 h. exposure, they become elongated with multiple nuclei
and kinetoplasts. Similar effects on cytokinesis were
observed in Chinese Hamster Ovary cells depleted of polyamines
by α-methylornithine (47) or by starvation of polyamine auxo-
trophs (48). The blockade of cytokinesis observed in both
studies was attributed to interference with microfilament
organization and disappearance of actin filaments.
Trypanosomes are endowed with a subpellicular longitudinal
layer of microtubules which serve as means of support (49)
and these structures may be similarly affected by polyamine
depletion.

E. DFMO and Other Parasitic Protozoa

DFMO has also been investigated for activity against a
number of other parasitic protozoa. Striking effects were
noted in vivo against Eimeria tenella in chickens. Eimeria
spp. cause coccidiosis in a number of vertebrates with the
disease being a particular economic problem for poultry.
Concentrations as low as 0.0625% DFMO in drinking water
completely suppressed E. tenella infective lesions and allowed
development of an acquired immunity to reinfection. Negation
of the anticoccidal activity of DFMO was seen with co-administration of putrescine (38,50).

DFMO also blocked in vitro schizogony (replication) in
Plasmodium falciparum, a major cause of human malaria. The
resultant depletion of polyamines arrests DNA synthesis in a
manner similar to effects in mammalian cells. Low concentrations of polyamines again completely blocked the effects
of DFMO (38). Subsequent in vivo studies with P. berghei, a
rodent malarial parasite, showed that DFMO inhibited the

initial infective cycle (exoerythrocytic schizogony) of the
parasite in mice but had little or no action on the succeeding
erythrocytic infection (51).

Another parasite, <u>Giardia</u> <u>lamblia</u>, the cause of human
intestinal giardiasis, is effectively inhibited by DFMO in
culture. The antiproliferative effect is again reversed by
addition of polyamines to the medium. DFMO appeared
essentially cytostatic as irreversible growth inhibition was
observed only after prolonged incubation (52).

F. Combination Chemotherapy: Bleomycin + DFMO

In 1977, Lapi and Cohen (53) reported that the cytotoxic
effects of the antitumor antibiotic bleomycin were abolished
by inclusion of polyamines in the growth medium. The
Bleomycins are a group of glycopeptide antibiotics which
differ with respect to the type of polyamine or other amine
present at the active site. These amine moieties facilitate
binding of the drug(s) to DNA (54). Commercially available
bleomycin (Blenoxane: Bristol Laboratories) was found to be
curative at 3.5-14 mg/kg for the acute <u>T. b. brucei</u> EATRO 110
isolate in mice. Moreover, spermidine or spermine, co-admin-
istered with Blenoxane, blocked cures (55). Subsequently, a
combination of DFMO and bleomycin was tried and a dramatic
synergism was found; use of the combination resulted in cures
with 1/4 and 1/12 the amount of the individual curative
dosages of DFMO and bleomycin, respectively (0.25% and 0.25
mg/kg). Moreover, co-administration of polyamines with
curative combinations negated any drug effects and resulted
in normal increases in parasite populations (56).

Recently, the efficacy of the DFMO/bleomycin combination
was extended to a long-term central nervous system (CNS)
infection (57). The TREU 667 isolate of <u>T. b. brucei</u> has been
developed as a model CNS infection by Jennings and coworkers
(58,59). In this model animals are refractory to drugs such
as Berenil at 21 days post-inoculation, but remain sensitive
to Melarsoprol, an effective but toxic agent used for CNS
trypanosomiasis chemotherapy. Dramatically, combinations of
bleomycin at 3.5 or 7 mg/kg and DFMO (1% or 2%) administered
concurrently in 8 different regimens for 7 to 14 days cured
all mice of the infection. No reoccurrence of parasitemia in
blood was found in animals observed for more than 200 days,
and inoculation of brain homogenates of "cured" animals into
lethally irradiated mice did not result in subinfections (57).

Although the basis for this synergism is not clear, it is
evident from earlier studies on acute and chronic infections,
as well as the more recent studies with the CNS model (57)

TABLE 3. Combination Chemotherapy of an Acute, T.b. brucei Laboratory Infection (EATRO 110) Using DFMO and Standard Trypanocides*

Drug Treatment		No. Cured/Total Treated
DFMO	0.5%	0/5
	2.0%	5/5
Suramin	5.0 mg/kg	5/5
	0.5 mg/kg	0/5
DFMO	0.5%	
+ Suramin	0.5 mg/kg	5/5
Pentamidine	2.0 mg/kg	5/5
	0.1 mg/kg	0/5
DFMO	0.5%	
+ Pentamidine	0.1 mg/kg	4/10
Melarsoprol	5.0 mg/kg	5/5
	0.1 mg/kg	0/5
DFMO	0.5%	
+ Melarsoprol	0.1 mg/kg	3/5
Berenil	1.0 mg/kg	5/5
	0.1 mg/kg	0/5
DFMO	0.5%	
+ Berenil	0.1 mg/kg	4/5

*
Studies were conducted as in Table 1. Trypanocides were administered concurrently with DFMO as single daily i.p. injections.

that DFMO is not cytotoxic and that it often does act synergistically with cytotoxic agents. Furthermore, as mentioned above, the immunocompetence of the host is ultimately responsible for clearing the blood of parasites during DFMO-treatment (41). This presents another argument for the potential utility of combination chemotherapy since chronic trypanosome infections often compromise the host immune system (60). The optimal use of DFMO in combination with other agents must also reflect the timing of the DFMO dose with respect to the cytotoxic agent. For example, treatment of acutely infected animals with low doses of DFMO prior to and concurrent with administration of bleomycin doubled longevity over animals in which the dosage sequence had been reversed, again indicating that polyamine depletion plays an important role in enhancing the effect of bleomycin (40).

It may well be feasible to use DFMO to augment treatment with standard trypanocides as such combinations may permit enhanced CNS activity of those trypanocides now effective only

in early stages of the disease. Several trypanocides have
been tested in combination with DFMO at subcurative doses and
evidence of synergism has been found (Table 3). As noted
earlier, curative doses of both pentamidine and Berenil are
blocked by polyamines, and there is now evidence that
spermidine interferes with suramin in curing acute infections
of <u>T. b. brucei</u> (H.C. Nathan and C.J. Bacchi, unpub.).

IV. CONCLUSION

The general development of a rational approach to chemotherapy of parasitic diseases has been urged for some time
(61,62). The success of DFMO, alone and in combination with
other drugs, represents the culmination of a rational, progressive approach to treatment of trypanosomiasis. Furthermore, because of the potency of the DFMO bleomycin combination
against both the acute and chronic or CNS infections of <u>T. b.
brucei</u>, and since so many standard trypanocides are enhanced
by the use of DFMO, polyamine metabolism clearly represents a
unique and feasible target for treatment of African
trypanosomiasis and most likely a number of other protozoan
diseases.

REFERENCES

1. Tabor, C.W., and Tabor, H. (1976). Annu. Rev. Biochem.
   45, 285.
2. Pegg, A.E., and McCann, P.P. (1982). Am. J. Physiol. 243,
   C212.
3. Janne, J., Poso, H., and Raina, A. (1978). Biochim.
   Biophys. Acta 473, 241.
4. Heby, O. (1981). Differentiation 14, 1.
5. Bitonti, A.J., Kallio, A., McCann, P.P., and Sjoerdsma, A.
   (1983). Adv. Polyamine Res. 4, 495.
6. Bacchi, C.J. (1981). J. Protozool. 28, 20.
7. Pegg, A.E., and Williams-Ashman, H.G. (1981). In
   "Polyamines in Biology and Medicine" (D.R. Morris and
   L.J. Marton, eds.), p. 3, Marcel Dekker, New York.
8. McCann, P.P. (1980). In "Polyamines in Biomedical
   Research" (J.M. Gaugas, ed.), p. 109, John Wiley, New
   York.
9. McCann, P.P., Tardif, C., Duchesne, M.C., and Mamont, P.S.
   (1977). Biochem. Biophys. Res. Commun. 76, 893.
10. Heller, J.S., Fong, W.F., and Canellakis, E.S. (1976).
    Proc. Natl. Acad. Sci. USA 73, 1858.

11. Mitchell, J.L.A. (1981). Adv. Polyamine Res. 3,15.
12. Fillingame, R.H., Jorstad, C.M., and Morris, D.R. (1975). Proc. Natl. Acad. Sci. USA 72, 4042.
13. Mamont, P.S., Bohlen, P., McCann, P.P., Bey, P., Schuber, F., and Tardif, C. (1976). Proc. Natl. Acad. Sci. USA 73, 1626.
14. Metcalf, B.W., Bey, P., Danzin, C., Jung, M.J., Casara, P., and Vevert, J.P. (1978). J. Am. Chem. Soc. 100, 2551.
15. Kallio, A., and McCann, P.P. (1981). Biochem. J. 200, 69.
16. Kallio, A., McCann, P.P., and Bey, P. (1982). Biochem. J. 204, 771.
17. Pegg, A.E., Seely, J.E., and Zagon, I.S. (1982). Science 217, 68.
18. Seely, J.E., Poso, H., and Pegg, A.E. (1982). J. Biol. Chem. 257, 7549.
19. Mamont, P.S., Duchesne, M.C., Grove, J., and Bey, P. (1978). Biochem. Biophys. Res. Commun. 81, 58.
20. Luk, G.D., Goodwin, G., Marton, L.J., and Baylin, S.B. (1981). Proc. Natl. Acad. Sci. USA 78, 2355.
21. Luk, G.D., Goodwin, G., Gazdar, A.F., and Baylin, S.B. (1982). Cancer Res. 42, 3070.
22. Luk, G.D., Abeloff, M.D., Griffin, C.A., and Baylin, S.B. (1983). Proc. Am. Assoc. Cancer Res., 24, 318.
23. Sjoerdsma, A. (1981) Clin. Pharmacol. Ther. 30, 3.
24. Koch-Weser, J., Schechter, P.J., Bey, P., Danzin, C., Fozard, J.R., Jung, M.J., Mamont, P.S., Prakash, N.J., Seiler, N., and Sjoerdsma, A. (1981) In "Polyamines in Biology and Medicine" (D.R. Morris and L.J. Marton, eds.) p. 437, Marcel Dekker, New York.
25. Janne, J., Alhonen-Hongisto, L., Seppanen, P., and Siimes, M. (1981). Med. Biol. 59, 448.
26. Marton, L.J., Levin, V.A., Hervatin, S.J., Koch-Weser, J., McCann, P.P., and Sjoerdsma, A. (1981). Cancer Res. 41, 4436.
27. Bartholeyns, J., and Koch-Weser, J. (1981). Cancer Res. 41, 5158.
28. Sunkara, P.S., Prakash, N.J., Mayer, G.D., and Sjoerdsma, A. (1983). Science 219, 851.
29. Bowman, I.B.R., and Flynn, I.W. (1976). In "Biology of the Kinetoplastidae" (W.H.R. Lumsden and D.H. Evans, eds.), 1, 435, Academic Press, New York.
30. Bacchi, C.J., Hutner, S.H., Lambros, C., and Lipschik, G.Y. (1978). Adv. Polyamine Res. 2, 129.
31. Bacchi, C.J., Lipschik, G.Y., and Nathan, H.C. (1977). J. Bacteriol. 131, 657.

32. Bacchi, C.J., Garofalo, J., Mockenhaupt, D., McCann, P.P.,
    Diekema, K.A., Pegg, A.E., Nathan, H.C.,
    Mullaney, E.A., Chunosoff, L., Sjoerdsma, A., and
    Hutner, S.H. (1983). Mol. Biochem. Parasitol. 7, 209.
33. Bacchi, C.J., Vergara, C., Garofalo, J., Lipschik, G.Y.,
    and Hutner, S.H. (1979). J. Protozool. 26, 484.
34. Sakai, T.T., Torget, R.I.J., Freda, C.E., and Cohen, S.S.
    (1975). Nucl. Acids Res. 2, 1005.
35. Bacchi, C.J., McCann, P.P., Nathan, H.C., Hutner, S.H.,
    and Sjoerdsma, A. (1983). Adv. Polyamine Res. 4, 221.
36. Bacchi, C.J., Nathan, H.C., Hutner, S.H., McCann, P.P.,
    and Sjoerdsma, A. (1980). Science 210, 332.
37. Nathan, H.C., Bacchi, C.J., Hutner, S.H., Rescigno, D.,
    McCann, P.P., and Sjoerdsma, A. (1981). Biochem.
    Pharmacol. 30, 3010.
38. McCann, P.P., Bacchi, C.J., Hanson, W.L., Cain, G.D.,
    Nathan, H.C., Hutner, S.H., and Sjoerdsma, A. (1981).
    Adv. Polyamine Res. 3, 97.
39. Karbe, E., Bottger, M., McCann, P.P., Sjoerdsma, A., and
    Freitas, E.K. (1982). Tropenmed. Parasit. 33, 161.
40. McCann, P.P., Bacchi, C.J., Clarkson, A.B., Seed, J.R.,
    Nathan, H.C., Amole, B.O., Hutner, S.H., and
    Sjoerdsma, A. (1981). Med. Biol. 59, 434.
41. deGee, A.L.W., McCann, P.P., and Mansfield, J.M. (1983).
    J. Parasitol., 69, in press.
42. Erwin, B.G., and Pegg, A.E. (1982). Biochem. Pharmacol.
    31, 2820.
43. Alhonen-Hongisto, L., Seppanen, P., and Janne, J. (1980).
    Biochem. J. 192, 941.
44. Williams-Ashman, H.G., Seidenfeld, J., and Galletti, P.
    (1982). Biochem. Pharmacol. 31, 277.
45. Pegg, A.E., Poso, H., Shuttleworth, K., and Bennett, R.A.
    (1982). Biochem. J. 202, 519.
46. Fish, W.R., Marr, J.J., and Berens, R.L. (1982). Biochim.
    Biophys. Acta 714, 422.
47. Sunkara, P.S., Rao, P.N., Nishioka, K., and Brinkley, B.R.
    (1979). Exp. Cell Res. 119, 63.
48. Pohjanpelto, P., Virtanen, I., and Holtta, E. (1981).
    Nature 293, 475.
49. Vickerman, K., and Preston, T.M. (1976). In "Biology of
    the Kinetoplastidae" (W.H.R. Lumsden and D.H. Evans,
    eds.) 1, 35, Academic Press, New York.
50. Hanson, W.L., Bradford, M.M., Chapman, W.L., Waits, V.B.,
    McCann, P.P., and Sjoerdsma, A. (1982). Am. J. Vet.
    Res. 43, 1651.
51. Gillet, J.M., Bone, G., and Herman, F. (1982). Trans. R.
    Soc. Trop. Med. Hyg. 76, 776.

52. Gillin, F.D., Reiner, D.S., and McCann, P.P. (1983).,
    J. Protozool., in press.
53. Lapi, L., and Cohen, S.S. (1977). Cancer Res. 37, 1384.
54. Muller, W.E.G. (1980). In "Inhibitors of DNA and RNA
    Polymerases" (P.S. Sarin and R.C. Gallo, eds.), 207,
    Pergamon Press, New York.
55. Nathan, H.C., Bacchi, C.J., Sakai, T.T., Rescigno, D.,
    Stumpf, D., and Hutner, S.H. (1981). Trans. R. Soc.
    Trop. Med. Hyg. 75, 394.
56. Bacchi, C.J., Nathan, H.C., Hutner, S.H., McCann, P.P.,
    and Sjoerdsma, A. (1982). Biochem. Pharmacol. 31,
    2833.
57. Clarkson, A.B., Bacchi, C.J., Mellow, G.H., Nathan, H.C.,
    McCann, P.P., and Sjoerdsma, A. (1983). Proc. Natl.
    Acad. Sci. USA, in press.
58. Jennings, F.W., Whitelaw, D.D., Holmes, P.H.,
    Chizyuka, H.G.B., and Urquhart, G.M. (1979). Int. J.
    Parasitol. 9, 381.
59. Murray, P.K. and Jennings, F.W. (1983). In "Animal Models
    for Experimental Bacterial and Parasitic Infection"
    (G. Keusch and T. Wadstrom, eds.), 343, Elsevier,
    New York.
60. Mansfield, J.M. (1981). In "Parasitic Diseases",
    (J.M. Mansfield, ed.) 1, 167, Marcel Dekker, New York.
61. Cohen, S.S. (1979). Science 205, 964.
62. Wang, C.C. (1982). Trends Biochem. Sci. 82, 354.

MATERIALS WHICH PROMOTE AND INHIBIT THE BIOSYNTHESIS OF CACHECTIN, A MACROPHAGE PROTEIN WHICH INDUCES CATABOLIC STATE: A REVIEW[1]

Anthony Cerami

Laboratory of Medical Biochemistry
The Rockefeller University
New York, New York

I. INTRODUCTION

For the past several years, we have been investigating the biochemical basis for the cachectic state that is observed frequently in animals in response to various invasions, e.g., bacterial, protozoal, viral, and neoplastic. This cachectic state is characterized by loss of appetite, weight loss, a catabolic metabolism, and anemia. If not corrected, this can proceed to severe wasting, shock and eventually death of the animals (for review, see 1). In some of these situations, (for example, trypanosomiasis of cattle or endotoxin administration to mice) the response of the animal is out of proportion to the actual threat posed by the number of invading organisms or the toxicity of the material. We recently have found that immune cells, presumably macrophages, can produce a product(s) in response to various stimuli which can affect dramatically a number of anabolic activities of several cell lines in culture. Utilizing these cell culture systems, we have begun to unravel the complex communication system between the immune system and energy storage and production tissues of the body. This factor(s) presumably plays a role in mobilizing energy for the immune system to combat the invasion.

---

[1]This review discusses work that has been carried out over the past three years in collaboration with Drs. M. Kawakami, P. Pekala, N. Le Trang, S. Sassa, C. Rouzer, D. Lane, W. Vine, Y. Ikeda, and W. Angus.

A. Loss of Lipoprotein Lipase in Tissues of Rabbits
Infected with T. brucei

Our work in this area began with a study of rabbits
infected with the protozoa, Trypanosoma brucei. This work
(2) was prompted by the observation that cattle infected
with trypanosomes frequently developed a cachectic state and
died without having the swarming parasitemia that is associated with experimental infections in mice. Rabbits, like
cattle, also have less protozoa than mice and demonstrate a
cachectic response. During the course of these studies, it
was noted that the rabbits, although extremely cachectic
from loss of muscle and adipose tissue, had lipemic sera.
This was the result of the accumulation of VLDL (very light
density lipoprotein). Further analyses of this phenomenon
revealed that the production of VLDL remained normal during
the course of the infection, but that there was a severe
impairment of the removal rate. This defect was caused by
loss of the enzymatic activity, lipoprotein lipase, from
the peripheral tissues. This enzyme, with a very short
half-life, is responsible for the uptake of lipid by
adipocytes and peripheral tissue. In addition to
trypanosome-infected rabbits, we observed that a similar
defect in lipoprotein lipase activity occurred in rabbits
bearing the V2 carcinoma.

B. Endotoxin Induces Macrophages to Produce Factor
Which Inhibits Lipoprotein Lipase

In order to advance these studies with a more standard
model system, we studied (3) the effect of the administration of bacterial endotoxin in mice. It was observed that
the administration of lipopolysaccharide (LPS) to mice led
within 20 hours to a significant decrease in lipoprotein
lipase activity in the adipose tissue and a rise in serum
triglyceride concentrations (Figure 1). The degree of the
loss of enzymatic activity was related to the amount of LPS
that was administered. Besides being more uniform and standard, the endotoxin mouse model also offered the advantage
of being able to study the effect of LPS on endotoxin sensitive C3H/HeN and resistant C3H/HeJ mice (4). As with other
effects of endotoxin, the lipoprotein lipase activity of
the LPS-resistant mice was found not to be as susceptible
to LPS inhibition as it was in the sensitive mice. However,
it was possible to decrease the lipoprotein activity in the
endotoxin resistant mice by administering sera which had
been removed from sensitive mice 2 hours after LPS injec-

tion. A similar mediator activity could also be prepared
by incubating in vitro thioglycolate-induced exudate cells
from sensitive mice with LPS. Administration of conditioned media from the exudate cells to resistant animals
showed a dramatic decrease in the lipoprotein lipase
activity in the adipose tissue. Since the majority of the
adherent cells used in this preparation are macrophages
(5), we presume that the mediator is a macrophage product
which is produced in response to the addition of endotoxin.

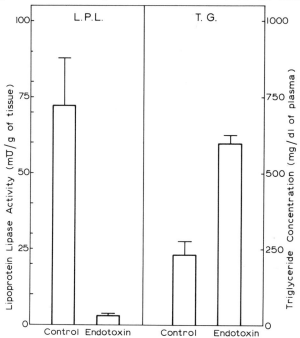

FIGURE 1. Effect of endotoxin on serum triglyceride
(TG) and adipose tissue LPL activity in endotoxin-sensitive
mice, 100 μg of endotoxin dissolved in 0.2 ml of saline was
injected into C3H/HeN mice. Serum and tissue were obtained
16 h after the injection. Plasma triglyceride and tissue
LPL were assayed. Control mice were injected with pyrogen
free saline. Data are expressed as the mean (+ SEM) of six
mice for each group. Reproduced from J. Exp. Med. 154:631, 1981.

C. Macrophage Factor Inhibits Lipoprotein Lipase
in 3T3-L1 cells

In order to study the biochemical events surrounding
the inhibition of lipoprotein lipase activity in adipocytes, we have studied the effect of the macrophage factor

on 3T3-L1 cells (6). This cell line, which is a fibroblast-
like cell line, can be induced to assume most of the properties of adipocytes (7,8,9). Following differentiation,
these cells exhibit copious amounts of three lipid biosynthetic enzymes - lipoprotein lipase, necessary for bringing
exogenous lipid into the cell, and acetyl-CoA carboxylase
and fatty acid synthetase which are essential for endogenous
fatty acid synthesis. The addition of conditioned media
from endotoxin-incubated exudate cells of sensitive mice to
induced 3T3-L1 cells led to a rapid decrease in lipoprotein
lipase activity (Figure 2). Endotoxin by itself had no
effect on these cells. For these studies, three compartments were analyzed for enzymatic activity: soluble enzyme

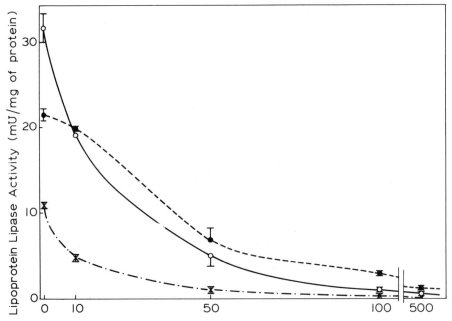

FIGURE 2. Dependence of lipoprotein lipase activity on
the concentration of lipoprotein lipase suppression mediator. Ten to 1000 µl of conditioned medium from endotoxin-
treated exudate cells was added to 3T3-L1 cell cultures in
3.5 cm dishes with 1.5 ml of DME medium. Conditioned
medium added was supplemented with fresh DME to make the
final volume of medium 2.5 ml in all dishes. The lipoprotein lipase activity in the medium (X), on the cell
surface (0), and in cell sap (●), was assessed after 20 h
incubation. The data represent mean + SEM (n = 4).
Reproduced from Proc. Natl. Acad. Sci. 79:912, 1982.

found in the media, enzyme activity released from the cell
membrane by the addition of heparin, and that found within
the cell. Enzyme activity in all compartments was
decreased. The fall in activity was rapid and occurred
within 5 hours. The loss of activity was not the result of
inactivation by the macrophage factor since incubation of
the conditioned media with lipoprotein lipase did not alter
the normal decay of enzyme activity.

D. Macrophage Factor Inhibits Biosynthesis of Fatty Acid Synthetase and Acetyl-CoA Carboxylase

These results implied that the mediator effected the
biosynthesis of lipoprotein lipase. When ^{35}S-methionine
incorporation studies were carried out with and without the
addition of the mediator, it was observed that no significant alteration in total protein synthesis occurred (10).
However, when the ^{35}S pulse-labelled soluble membrane proteins were subjected to SDS electrophoresis it was observed
that although the general protein labelling of the cells
with and without factor remained constant, there were
several bands which disappeared or appeared in the presence
of the mediator. One of the protein bands which disappeared
had a molecular weight of approximately 220,000 daltons.
Since the band undoubtedly corresponded to the enzymes -
fatty acid synthetase and acetyl-CoA carboxylase, immuno-
precipitation of these enzymes was undertaken. As can be
seen in Figure 3, the amount of immunoprecipitable radioactivity over time associated with these two enzymes is
severely decreased by the presence of the factor. From
these results, it appears that the macrophage factor has
the selective ability to turn off the synthesis of key
enzymes involved in the anabolic activity of the cell.

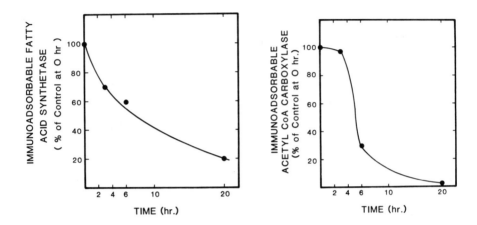

FIGURE 3. Effect of mediator that suppresses the synthesis of acetyl-CoA carboxylase and fatty acid synthetase.
At the indicated times after exposure of the 3T3-L1 cells
to the mediator (300 ml of conditioned medium), the cells
were pulse-labelled with 0.5 mCi of ^{35}S-methionine for 1 h.
Cytosolic fractions were obtained by digitonin treatment of
the monolayer. Aliquots of the cytosolic fractions (2 x
10^5 cpm for all determinations) were incubated with antibodies against fatty acid synthetase or acetyl-CoA carboxylase and the immunoprecipitable material isolated and
characterized by electrophoresis. Panel A: results of a
densitometric scan of the autoradiogram, indicating percent
of immunoadsorbable material (fatty acid synthetase)
remaining relative to control after exposure to mediator.
Panel B: same as Panel A except representing acetyl-CoA
carboxylase. Reproduced from Proc. Natl. Acad. Sci.
80:2743, 1983.

E.   Inability of Insulin to Overcome Effect
of Macrophage Factor

The mechanism for the selective inhibition of protein
synthesis is unknown. One of the possibilities that we
have examined in detail (11) is that the mediator interferes
with the action of insulin. Since the activity of all three

of these anabolic enzymes is dependent on the presence of
insulin, it seemed possible that the mediator had a direct
effect on this process. When several thousand-fold more
insulin was added to the 3T3-L1 cells in the presence of
the mediator, the insulin was unable to overcome the
depression of lipoprotein lipase activity (Table I).

TABLE I. Effect of Insulin on the Mediator Suppression
of Lipoprotein Lipase in 3T3-L1 Cells

Insulin µg	Mediator[*]	Lipoprotein lipase[+], mU/mg protein		
		In medium	Cell surface	Intracellular
0.050	+	0.3 + 0.2	1.0 + 0.2	1.3 + 0.2
	–	25.2 + 2.9	68.5 + 5.4	8.8 + 0.3
1	+	0.2 + 0.1	1.6 + 0.2	1.9 + 0.2
	–	22.0 + 2.3	54.9 + 3.6	8.2 + 0.8
50	+	0.3 + 0.2	0.9 + 0.2	0.8 + 0.1
	–	34.0 + 5.9	68.2 + 9.5	11.2 + 1.2

[*]3T3-L1 cells were incubated with 100 µl of mediator in
3.5 cm plates containing 1.5 ml of DME medium supplemented
with insulin at the indicated levels.
[+]Lipoprotein lipase activity was assessed after a 20 h
incubation. Data are expressed as mean + SEM (n = 6).
Reproduced from Proc. Natl. Acad. Sci. 79:912, 1982.

The inability of insulin to overcome the effect of the
macrophage factor may have reflected 1) a lack of insulin
receptors, 2) an uncoupling of the insulin receptor from
the glucose transport system, 3) a competition of the
macrophage factor for either glucose or insulin or 4) a
post-receptor defect. Measurement of the number of insulin
receptors on the cells with and without mediator did not
reveal any alteration (Figure 4). In addition, we observed
that insulin was able to promote a two-fold increase in a
transport of 3'-0-methyl glucose into the cells with or
without the mediator. Thus, the insulin receptor which has
a short half-life (12) continues to be synthesized in the
presence of the factor and the glucose transport unit is
still effectively coupled to the insulin receptor. The
macrophage factor also did not compete with either glucose
or insulin. This leaves the fourth possibility as a
potential explanation for the insulin resistance.

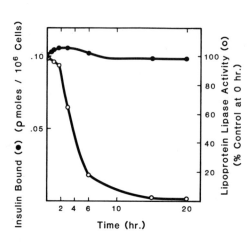

FIGURE 4. Effect of
conditioned medium from
endotoxin-treated mouse
peritoneal exudate cells
on the insulin binding
capacity and the lipo-
protein lipase activity of
3T3-L1 adipocytes. 300 µl
of conditioned medium was
added to cultures of 3T3-L1
cells (4.2 x 10^6 cells/
dish) in 6 cm dishes con-
taining 3.5 ml of DME
medium and 10% fetal calf
serum. After the indicated
periods of incubation, cell
surface insulin binding
capacity (●) and lipopro-
tein lipase activity (O)
were determined. Repro-
duced from J. Exp. Med.
157:1360, 1983.

These results suggest a possible explanation for the
hyperinsulinemia frequently observed in various invasive
states such as septicemia. Insulin, which is released from
the β-cells of the pancreas in response to hyperglycemia,
stimulates peripheral cells, such as adipocytes, to take up
glucose. Once inside the cell, however, glucose will diffuse out again if it is not utilized. As demonstrated
above, cells which normally utilize glucose for the synthesis of fat are incapable of synthesizing fatty acids in the
presence of mediator, because of the lack of appropriate
enzymatic activity. This impairment in total body glucose
disposal rate could stimulate increased insulin secretion.

F. Differentiation of Friend Erythroid Cells

As noted above, one of the hallmarks of the response of
mammals to chronic invasion is an anemic state (1). The
anemia of chronic diseases is thought to result in part
from three pathological processes: 1) an increase in blood
volume with a concomitant decrease in hematocrit; 2) a
hemolytic component which is believed to be the result of
reticulo-endothelial (RE) cell hyperplasia; and 3) a
dyserythropoiesis which is believed, in part, to be the

result of an iron blockade within the RE system. Reasoning
that the macrophage factor described above for the adipocyte
could likewise modulate the anabolic activity of the
erythroid cell, we have utilized the Friend leukemia cell
line that can be induced to differentiate into hemoglobin
containing cells by the addition of dimethylsulfoxide or
other factors (13). As can be seen in Figure 5, the addition of media of endotoxin-induced exudate cells to DMSO-
induced Friend cells brought about a significant reduction
in the number of cells produced and the percent that contained hemoglobin, compared to cells not receiving the
macrophage factor (14). Thus, the factor inhibits the DMSO-
induced cells from dividing and differentiating. Of obvious
interest is whether this mediator is the same or similar to
that involved in decreasing the anabolic activity of the
adipocyte.

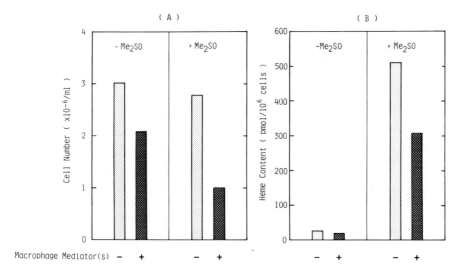

FIGURE 5. Effect of the endotoxin induced mediator from
mouse macrophage cultures on the cell growth and heme content of Friend cells. Friend cells (clone DS-19) were
incubated for 96 h in the absence or in the presence of
Me_2SO (1.5 vol %). Conditioned media (80 µl added/ml of
growth medium) from mouse peritoneal macrophage cultures
stimulated with endotoxin (5 µg/ml) were added at the
beginning of culture. Cell number (A) was counted with a
Cytograf model 6300. Heme content (B) was determined
fluorometrically. The number of trypan blue positive cells
assessed by Cytograf counting was 8-10% for all cultures.
Reproduced from Proc. Natl. Acad. Sci. 80:1717, 1983.

G. Isolation of Protein From Macrophage
Which Suppress LPL Biosynthesis

Utilizing the suppression of LPL in 3T3-Ll cells as an
assay system, we have found (15) the activity associated
with two proteins of 75,000 and 63,000 daltons in the
supernatant of thioglycolate-elicited macrophages induced
with endotoxin. The protein corresponding to 63,000 may be
a degradation product of the 75,000 since its' presence is
variable and dependent on the culture conditions. The
protein corresponding to 75,000, which we call cachectin,
has been isolated to apparent homogeneity and has many of
the properties associated with the crude macrophage
material. Further work is needed to define the complete
repetoire of biological activities associated with this
molecule.

H. Materials Which Evoke Production
of the Macrophage Factor

As described above, endotoxin is very effective at
inducing the formation of the macrophage factor which
suppresses LPL synthesis. Preliminary experiments have
revealed a number of other agents which can evoke the
macrophage factor. Table II records a partial list of the
compounds and their relative ability to promote production
of this activity in thioglycolate-elicited macrophages.
Preparations of C. parvum and zymosan, which are known to
have substantial effects on macrophages (16), are quite
effective (17). Membrane preparations of T. brucei and P.
berghei are also active (18). This finding is particularly
pleasing since the initial impetus for our studies derived
from trypanosome-infected animals. Of interest is that two
chemicals that are frequently noted to have striking effects
on macrophage function, Concanavalin A and PMA, are not
very active in promoting synthesis of the macrophage factor
that suppress the biosynthesis of LPL.

TABLE II. Effect of Materials Which Evoke Production
of Macrophage Factor Which Suppresses LPL Biosynthesis

Endotoxin	++++
C. parvum	++
Zymosan	++
Trypanosoma brucei	++
Plasmodium berghei	++
Phenbol myristatic acetate	+
Concanavalin A	+

I. Dexamethasone Inhibition of the Macrophage Factor

Preliminary experiments assessing the effect of various
agents on production of the macrophage factor have given
new insights (17). Table III lists a number of compounds
that have been evaluated for effect on either the production of the mediator by macrophages or the action of added
mediator to the 3T3-L1 cells. Indomethacin and aspirin,
agents which are known to modulate the activity of prostaglandin metabolism, have no effect on either the macrophages
or the 3T3-L1 cells. In addition, two compounds which have
been suggested for treatment of shock, naloxone and thyroid
releasing factor (TRF), are without effect on either the
production or action of the mediator. The only compound
that has significant activity is the glucocorticoid,
dexamethasone. The addition of dexamethasone to
thioglycolate-induced macrophages prior to the addition of
LPS can completely suppress the production of the factor.
Once the factor has been made, the glucocorticoid is without
effect. This observation may explain the necessity for the
early administration of glucocorticoids during the treatment of septicemic shock.

Table III. Effect of Substances on Macrophage Factor
Which Suppresses LPL Biosynthesis

	Inhibition of	
	Mediator Production	Mediator Effect
Dexamethasone 10^{-6} M	+	-
Aspirin 10^{-3} M	-	-
Indomethacin 10^{-5}	-	-
Naloxone 10^{-5} M	-	-
Thyroid Releasing Factor 10^{-7} M	-	-

II. CONCLUSION

From the studies completed to date, it appears that the
immune system can elaborate mediator(s) which can function
as hormones and alter the metabolic activity of various

tissues in the animal. Whether the cachectin factor we
have isolated effects a number of tissues, or is part of a
family of molecules, remains to be determined. These
studies should initiate insights into developing new
pharmacological agents to prevent metabolic disturbances
associated with metabolic shock or the long-term wasting
associated with chronic diseases.

ACKNOWLEDGMENTS

I would like to thank Dr. Kenneth Warren of the
Rockefeller Foundation who gave us the resources and the
time to unravel this complicated process.

REFERENCES

1. Rouzer, C.A., and Cerami, A. (1980). Mol. Biochem.
    Parasitol. 2, 31.
2. Powanda, M.C., and Canonico, P.G. (eds.) (1981). In
    "Infection" Elsevier/North Holland, 435.
3. Kawakami, M., and Cerami, A. (1981). J. Exp. Med. 154,
    631.
4. Sultzer, B.M. (1968). Nature (Lond.). 219, 1253.
5. Edelson, P.J., Zwiebel, R., and Cohn, Z.A. (1975). J.
    Exp. Med. 142, 1150.
6. Kawakami, M., Pekala, P.H., Lane, M.D., and Cerami, A.
    (1982). Proc. Natl. Acad. Sci. USA 2, 219.
7. Green, H., and Kehinde, O. (1974). Cell 1, 113.
8. Green, H., and Kehinde. O. (1975). Cell 5, 19.
9. Green, H., and Kehinde. O. (1976). Cell 7, 105.
10. Pekala, P.H., Kawakami, M., Angus, C.W., Lane, M.D.,
    and Cerami, A. (1983). Proc. Natl. Acad. Sci. USA
    80, 2743.
11. Pekala, P.H., Kawakami, M., Vine, W., Lane, M.D., and
    Cerami, A. (1983). J. Exp. Med. 157, 1360.
12. Reed, B., and Lane, M.D. (1980). Proc. Natl. Acad. Sci.
    USA 77, 285.
13. Friend, C., Priesler, H.D., and Scher, W. (1974). Cur.
    Top. Develop. Biol. 8, 81.
14. Sassa, S., Kawakami, M., and Cerami, A. (1983). Proc.
    Natl. Acad. Sci. USA 80, 1717.
15. Le Trang, N., Ikeda, I., Ludewig, R., and Cerami, A.
    (1983). Fed. Proc. 42, 1872.
16. Schorlemmer, H.V., Bitter-Suermaun, D., and Allison,
    A.C. (1977). Immunol. 32, 929.
17. Kawakami, M., Ikeda, Y., Le Trang, N., Vine, W., and
    Cerami, A. (1983). Submitted.
18. Hotez, P.J., Le Trang, N., Fairlamb, A., and Cerami, A.
    (1983). Submitted.

ACTION OF PRAZIQUANTEL AND THE BENZODIAZEPINES ON ADULT MALE SCHISTOSOMA MANSONI

Ralph A. Pax[1]
David P. Thompson[2]

Department of Zoology and Neuroscience Program
Michigan State University
East Lansing, Michigan

James L. Bennett[1]

Department of Pharmacology and Toxicology
Michigan State University
East Lansing, Michigan

I.   INTRODUCTION

Schistosomiasis is a major parasitic disease caused by a small, blood dwelling trematode (or fluke) of the genus Schistosoma. This disease is transmitted in tropical parts of the world where the vectors (various tropical snails) thrive in various bodies of water e.g., small ponds, streams and irrigation canals. Three major geographic species responsible for most of the disease are S. mansoni, S. haematobium and S. japonicum. World-wide it has been estimated that 200 million people are infected with one or more species of Schistosoma, while 1 to 1.5 billion people are at risk. In recent years, a number of methods have been designed to control this disease in the tropics. Results from various studies emphasize the use of good survey methods to detect and treat infection in combination with

---
[1]Supported by W.H.O./T.D.R. grant 790577 and N.I.H. grant AI-14993-06.
[2]Supported by N.I.H. Training Grant 5 T32 GM07392.

187

measures to improve the quality of water and reduce the presence of infected snails at heavily used watering sites, e.g., sites used for recreation, laundering and defecation.

Chemotherapy has always been considered a major ingredient in schistosomiasis control programs. The role of chemotherapy in control programs has been strengthened over the last five years due to the introduction of new antischistosomal drugs, most notable of which is a pyrazinoisoquinoline derivative called praziquantel (PZ) or Biltricide^R (1). Another compound which has intriguing pharmacologic properties, but appears to be less useful because of its side effects, is the clonazepam-like benzodiazepine Ro 11-3128 (2). In this paper we will discuss the action of these compounds on the adult male schistosome, Schistosoma mansoni.

II.   ACTION OF PRAZIQUANTEL AND RO 11-3128 ON SCHISTO-SOME MUSCLE

The effects of Ro 11-3128 and praziquantel (PZ) on the musculature of single male schistosomes was determined by connecting the parasites to an apparatus capable of measuring the mechanical activity of its musculature (3). Figure 1 (left panel) demonstrates the effects of 10^{-6}M PZ on longitudinal muscle tension of a male schistosome. Since the effect of these drugs on tension of the parasite's musculature could be easily quantified, we examined the effects of various concentrations of PZ or Ro 11-3128 on the tension of the musculature of male S. mansoni or S. japonicum. Figure 1 (middle panel) shows that PZ, at low concentrations, produced a marked effect on the tension of the musculature of the male S. mansoni or S. japonicum. This was not the case with Ro 11-3128 (Fig. 1, right panel) which was found to affect muscle tension in male S. mansoni but not male S. japonicum. This observation correlates with a report by Stohler (2), demonstrating that Ro 11-3128 could cure mice infected with S. mansoni but not with S. japonicum.

In an attempt to determine the nature of the antischistosomal action of PZ and Ro 11-3128, we examined the interaction between these drugs and putative neurotransmitters of this parasite. For example, Tomosky et al. (4) demonstrated that dopamine is one of these putative neurotransmitters which, when incubated in the presence of male schistosomes, will lengthen the parasite, i.e., a response opposite to that induced by PZ or Ro 11-3128. Thus, to determine whether dopamine would block PZ or Ro 11-3128-induced muscle tension increases in male S. mansoni we preincubated the worm in dopamine for 20 min and then added 10^{-6}M PZ or 10^{-6}M Ro 11-3128. Dopamine did not block the PZ-induced rise in tension, nor did it block the effect of Ro 11-3128. In addition to dopamine, we attempted to block the effect of PZ or Ro 11-3128 with other compounds that are known to interact with other neuroreceptive sites in $\underline{S}$. mansoni, i.e., 5-hydroxytryptamine, carbachol, spiroperidol, brom-lysergic acid diethylamide, and atropine (4,5). None of these compounds (at 10^{-4}M) blocked the PZ or Ro 11-3128-induced increase in tension in male $\underline{S}$. mansoni. We also attempted to block, without success, the PZ-induced rise with 10^{-3}M pentobarbital, a compound that lengthens and paralyzes the schistosome. The inability of neurotransmitter agonists or antagonists to block the action of PZ or Ro 11-3128 on the musculature of male $\underline{S}$. mansoni suggested to us that these drugs may be acting directly on mechanisms that regulate muscle contractility (e.g., activation of myosin kinase and/or release of Ca^{2+} ions).

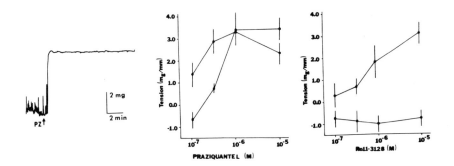

FIGURE 1.   Left: effects of 10^{-6}M PZ on longitudinal muscle tension in adult male $\underline{S}$. mansoni.   Middle: effects of various concentrations of PZ on muscle tension in $\underline{S}$. mansoni (closed circles) and $\underline{S}$. japonicum (closed squares).   Right: effects of various concentrations of Ro 11-3128 on muscle tension in $\underline{S}$. mansoni (closed circles) and $\underline{S}$. japonicum (closed squares).

To determine if inorganic ions play a vital role in mediating the action of PZ or Ro 11-3128 we performed several ion-substitution experiments.   When schistosomes were preincubated for 15 min in Ca^{2+}-free media we did not observe the PZ or Ro 11-3128-induced rise in the tension of the musculature of male schistosomes. When Ca^{2+} was added back to the Ca^{2+}-free media, containing PZ, the schistosomes would contract. Incubation of the parasites in Ca^{2+}-free media alone produced a slight rise in tension of the musculature of the parasite and a reduction in the number of spontaneous contractions. When schistosomes were preincubated for only 1 minute in Ca^{2+}-free media we noted a sharp rise in tension following addition of PZ, followed within 10 minutes, by a return to a pre-drug level of tension. This result suggests that the PZ-induced contraction can be initiated in a Ca^{2+}-free media but that a sustained increase in tension requires the presence of Ca^{2+} in the recording medium.

Since high concentrations of Mg^{2+} have been shown to attenuate biological mechanisms which depend upon Ca^{2+} (6), we studied the effects of various concentrations of Ca^{2+} and Mg^{2+} on PZ-induced contractions of the male schistosome musculature. When male schistosomes were preincubated in Hanks' balanced salt solution containing 0.4 mM Ca^{2+} and 30 mM Mg^{2+}, we noted no change in tension and a slight decrease in spontaneous contractile activity; when PZ was added we observed a transient rise in tension (Fig. 2, upper trace).

The rate of relaxation of the schistosome musculature in high Mg^{2+}, when exposed to PZ, became greater with increasing concentrations of PZ. This suggests that PZ may induce Mg^{2+} uptake by the parasite. In addition, we noted that the effect of Ro 11-3128 on the parasite's longitudinal musculature was not blocked by high Mg^{2+} (Fig. 2, lower trace).

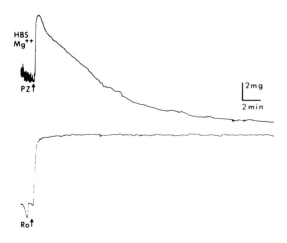

FIGURE 2.   Upper trace: effects of reducing the Ca^{2+}/Mg^{2+} ratio of the recording medium on the PZ-induced muscle tension increase in S. mansoni. Note the transient nature of the response. Lower trace: effects of reducing the Ca^{2+}/Mg^{2+} ratio on the Ro 11-3128 response.

Since Ca^{2+} and Mg^{2+} appear to play important roles in mediating the effects of PZ or Ro 11-3128 we attempted to determine if alterations in the concentration of other inorganic ions would affect the action of these drugs on the musculature of S. mansoni. We observed that decreasing or increasing the concentration of K^{+}, Na^{+}, or Cl^{-} in the media had little if any effect upon the Ro 11-3128 or PZ-induced rise in tension of the schistosome musculature.

To more accurately assess the role that inorganic ions may play in the action of PZ or Ro 11-3128 on the schistosome's musculature we studied the effects of these drugs on the influx of $^{45}Ca^{2+}$, $^{22}Na^{+}$, and $^{42}K^{+}$ into the parasite. The addition of these drugs to media containing the parasite plus radioactive cations resulted in a rapid accumulation of $^{45}Ca^{2+}$ by the male schistosome and stimulated the uptake of $^{22}Na^{+}$ but inhibited the uptake of $^{42}K^{+}$ by the parasite.

The increase in muscle tension induced by PZ can be mimicked by agents, like 60 mM K^{+}, which cause depolarization of the parasite's muscle cells. When a schistosome is preincubated in a Ca^{2+} antagonist (D-600) we noted that the high K^{+}-induced contraction was converted to a transient contraction identical to that observed when the schistosome is preincubated in high Mg^{2+} before addition of PZ. Examination of the action of PZ on the muscle cell membrane potential of the schistosome showed that the drug does not immediately depolarize the muscle cell (unlike K^{+}) even though it induces contraction immediately upon exposure. Also, the PZ-induced contraction is not blocked by the calcium antagonist D-600.

In summary, PZ initiates a rapid contraction of the parasite's muscle that is <u>not</u> dependent upon extraworm Ca^{2+}. To maintain this contraction, however, the drug does require the presence of extraworm Ca^{2+}. A reasonable explanation for the initial contraction is that PZ may 1) perturb the parasite's intramuscle storage mechanisms for Ca^{2+} and/or 2) perturb the extramuscle storage mechanisms for Ca^{2+} or interfere with the permeability of the membranes that normally restrict the rapid movement of Ca^{2+} between various cellular compartments or between the parasite and its environment. The possibility that PZ may increase the Ca^{2+} concentration within other cells was demonstrated when the drug was shown to disrupt the plasma membrane that separates the parasite from its environment.

III.   ACTION OF PRAZIQUANTEL AND RO 11-3128 ON THE PARASITE'S TEGUMENT

As with contraction, the mechanism underlying tegumental alterations in schistosomes is unknown. At concentrations of 10^{-6}M to 10^{-4}M the observed alterations were a function of time of exposure to the drug, rather than of its concentration (7-9). PZ causes vacuolization of the tegument, starting at the base of the syncytial layer. The size of the vacuoles increase with time, they begin to protrude above the surface, thus becoming visible as blebs and, finally, they burst. Vacuolization of the tegument results in tegumental lesions which then cause partial erosion of the tegument.

Recently we showed that Ro 11-3128 causes tegumental changes in <u>S. mansoni</u> morphologically identical to those caused by praziquantel, and the effect is caused only by the therapeutically active stereoisomers of the drug (9). The tegumental damage induced by Ro 11-3128 may be related to the findings of a previous study according to which this drug binds preferentially to the outer membranes of the schistosome (10). Tegumental damage is not an inherent property of antischistosomal compounds, as neither amoscanate nor oltipraz alter the tegument on in vitro incubations. It is interesting that prolonged in vivo treatment with amoscanate results in a different type of tegumental damage (11).

Since the ability to damage the tegument in vitro is not a sine qua non property of antischistosomal drugs, we assume that tegument disruption may be incidentally linked to muscle contraction. Sustained muscle contraction by itself does not inevitably lead to disruption of the parasite's tegument, as exposure of the schistosomes to 60 mM K^+, 10^{-4} M ouabain, or low temperature contract the parasite's musculature (12,13), yet they do not cause tegumental damage.

As mentioned above, increasing the Mg^{2+} concentration of the recording medium converts the sustained muscle contraction caused by PZ into a transient contraction. Recently, we demonstrated that high Mg^{2+} can also reduce the extent of PZ-induced disruption of the S. mansoni tegument (9). In light of the fact that Mg^{2+} inhibits many calcium-dependent mechanisms (14), these results suggest that the action of these drugs on both the muscle and tegument are calcium-dependent. However, while the absence of Ca^{2+} in the media markedly reduces the response of the schistosome's musculature to praziquantel (15), the tegumental damage induced by this drug is not inhibited by the absence of Ca^{2+} in the medium. Apparently, external Ca^{2+} is not required for the drug to express its action upon the tegument, but Ca^{2+} within the worm could be involved, since only 30% of the Ca^{2+} content of schistosomes is removed after a 60-min incubation in Ca^{2+}-free media containing 0.5 mM EGTA (15).

Reversal of praziquantel-induced tegumental disruption does not appear to be a general response to the presence of elevated levels of multivalent cations. Elevated levels of Ni^{2+}, La^{3+}, Co^{2+}, or Ca^{2+} all failed to attenuate the effect, even though Co^{2+} and La^{3+} do significantly reduce the muscle tension increases associated with praziquantel or elevated K^+ (12).

The tegumental disruption caused by drugs could be explained if they acted upon the cytokinetic elements of the schistosome, thereby directly or indirectly altering syncytial membrane turnover. Since colchicine (16) and cytochalasin B (17) interfere with microtubule and microfilament function of schistosomes, respectively, we analyzed the effects of these drugs on the surface of the schistosome; cytochalasin B, but not colchicine, caused tegument disruption (but not contraction of the musculature) of S. mansoni. These results indicate that microfilaments may play a role in maintaining the integrity of the parasite's tegument.

IV. OTHER BIOCHEMICAL AND PHYSIOLOGICAL EFFECTS ASSOCIATED WITH PRAZIQUANTEL'S ACTION

Praziquantel can decrease glucose uptake and the glycogen content of schistosomes. In addition, it can decrease lactate and alanine release as well as ATP content, but all of these effects take place after the drug has contracted the parasite's muscle and vacuolized its tegument. Thus, these effects are secondary to the two primary events associated with this drug. PZ is without effect on the parasite's endogenous serotonin or its uptake mechanism for this amine. PZ does not affect nucleoside incorporation into nucleic acids, bind DNA, or affect incorporation of amino acids into protein by a cell-free protein synthesizing system. PZ is also without effect on the parasite's Na^+,K^+-ATPase or Ca^{2+}-activated ATPase.

V. EFFECT OF PRAZIQUANTEL ON VERTEBRATE CARDIAC AND SMOOTH MUSCLE

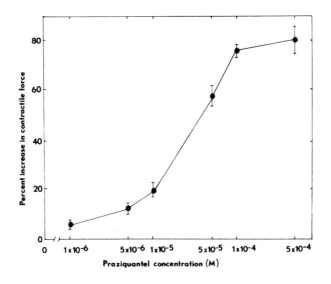

FIGURE 3. The dose-response relationship of the positive inotropic effect of praziquantel. Left atria of rat heart were stabilized for 40 min before the addition of praziquantel. Percent increase in force of contraction from stabilized value was determined at maximum inotropic effect. Each point represents the mean $\pm$ S.E.M. from at least 5 rats. The increase in force of contraction was significant ($P < .05$) between 1×10^{-6} and 5×10^{-4} M.

Using the isolated atria of the rat heart we have demonstrated that PZ produces a dose-dependent positive inotropic effect at concentrations between 10^{-6} and 10^{-4}M, with a maximum response occurring at 10^{-4}M (18) (Fig. 3).

Praziquantel increased rates of force development and relaxation, but did not alter time to peak force. The inotropic action was $[Ca^{2+}]_o$ dependent, and not blocked by 5×10^{-6}M (+)-propranolol, 5×10^{-5}M phentolamine or reserpine (5 mg/kg) pretreatment. The positive inotropic action, however, was significantly reduced in the presence of 1×10^{-7}M verapamil. Transmembrane potential recordings indicated that PZ prolonged the duration of the plateau phase without altering the maximal rate of depolarization, overshoot of the action potential or the resting membrane potential. Praziquantel $(5\times10^{-5}$M) failed to prolong the action potential duration shortened in the presence of 5×10^{-7}M verapamil (Table I). The compound did not inhibit partially purified Na^+,K^+-ATPase activity at concentrations effective in eliciting an inotropic effect. In addition, praziquantel was found to be devoid of cation ionophore properties since it was unable to translocate Ca^{2+}, Na^+ or K^+ from an aqueous into an organic phase. These findings suggest that the inotropic action of PZ seems to result from alterations in calcium flux which is mediated by a mechanism(s) other than adrenergic stimulation, Na^+,K^+-ATPase inhibition or cation ionophore translocation.

TABLE I. Effects of Praziquantel and Verapamil on Transmembrane Potential in Electrically Driven Left Atrial Preparations

Treatment	Resting Potential	Maximum Rate of Depolarization	Overshoot	Duration (Levels of Repolarization)	
				20%	50%
	mV	*V/sec*	*mV*	*msec*	*msec*
Control	75.6 ± 1.0	101.3 ± 1.4	19.6 ± 1.0	7.6 ± 0.3	21.2 ± 1.0
Praziquantel, 5×10^{5} M	74.9 ± 0.9	96.0 ± 1.1	17.1 ± 1.4	14.6 ± 0.6*	31.0 ± 0.5*
Verapamil, 5×10^{7} M	74.9 ± 1.2	100.0 ± 5.0	20.9 ± 1.0	4.0 ± 0.2*	15.9 ± 0.7*
Verapamil and praziquantel	75.8 ± 1.0	106.6 ± 7.3	21.1 ± 0.8	3.7 ± 0.3*	14.9 ± 1.0*

* P < .05.

Transmembrane potential recordings obtained first in the absence, then in the presence of praziquantel were from the same cell of 5 preparations during continuous impalement. In another set of experiments, recordings from different cells of the same preparation were obtained first in the absence of verapamil, 20 min after perfusing with verapamil and again 10 min after the addition of praziquantel. Recordings were obtained from 5 different preparations. Data represent mean ± S.E.M. P < .05.

Praziquantel $(5\times10^{-5}$M) also produced mechanical responses in guinea pig ileal muscle that were approximately 20% of those produced by muscarinic receptor stimulation (19). This effect was also dependent on extracellular calcium, and it was abolished by D-600. No evidence for a generalized and reliable contraction of mammalian smooth vascular muscle was found in isolated rabbit aortic strips tested in concentrations between 3.2×10^{-7} M and 3.2×10^{-5} M. Thus, the modulatory activity of praziquantel on calcium channels of mammalian smooth muscle is only weak (20).

VI. CONCLUSIONS

First, calcium appears to be an important common denominator in the action of praziquantel on the parasite as well as host tissue. Second, the dramatic impact of this drug on helminths is exclusively limited to the cestodes and trematodes (not nematodes), both of which share the unique morphological characteristic of having a syncytium which completely covers their internal organ system. This syncytium, along with other compartments surrounding the cestode's and trematode's muscle cells, may hold the secret as to why drugs like praziquantel are so effective against these parasites. Thus, the key to the success of praziquantel's action may be revealed when investigators begin to explore the mechanisms by which the schistosome regulates calcium within the syncytium and other compartments surrounding the parasite's musculature. At present we can only speculate about praziquantel's action and state that this drug appears to disturb, directly or indirectly, the ability of the schistosome to regulate calcium concentrations within its tissues.

REFERENCES

1. Thomas, H., and Gonnert, R. (1977). Z. Parasitenkd. 52, 117.
2. Stohler, H.R. (1977). Abstr. Congr. Chemotherapy, Sept. 18-23, Zurich, Switzerland.
3. Fetterer, R.H., Pax, R.A., and Bennett, J.L. (1977). Exp. Parasitol. 43, 286.
4. Tomosky, T., Bennett, J.L., and Bueding, E. (1974). J. Pharmacol. Exp. Ther. 190, 260.
5. Barker, L.R., Bueding, E., and Thomas, A.R. (1966). Br. J. Pharmacol. Chemother. 26, 656.
6. del Castillo, J., and Katz, B. (1954). J. Physiol. 124, 560.
7. Becker, B., Mehlhorn, P., Andrews, P., Thomas, H., and Eckert, J. (1980). Z. Parasitenkd. 63, 113.
8. Becker, B., Mehlhorn, P., Andrews, P., and Thomas, H. (1980). Z. Parasitenkd. 61, 121.
9. Bricker, C.S., Depenbusch, J.W., Bennett, J.L., and Thompson, D.P. (1983). Z. Parasitenkd. 69, 61.
10. Bennett, J.L. (1980). J. Parasitol. 66, 742.

11. Voge, M. and Bueding, E. (1980). Exp. Parasitol. 50, 251.
12. Fetterer, R.H., Pax, R.A., and Bennett, J.L. (1980). Europ. J. Pharmacol. 64, 31.
13. Fetterer, R.H., Pax, R.A., and Bennett, J.L. (1981). Parasitology 82, 97.
14. Potter, J.D., Robertson, S.P., and Johnson, J.D. (1981). Federation Proc. 40, 2653.
15. Wolde Mussie, E., VandeWaa, J., Pax, R.A., Fetterer, R.H., and Bennett, J.L. (1982). Exp. Parasitol. 53, 270.
16. Bogitsh, B.J., and Carter, O.S. (1980). Exp. Parasitol. 49, 319.
17. Wilson, R.A., and Barnes, P.E. (1974). Parasitology 68, 259.
18. Chubb, J.M., Bennett, J.L., Akera, T., and Brody, T.M. (1978). J. Pharmacol. Exp. Ther. 207, 284.
19. Jim, K., and Triggle, D.J. (1979). Can. J. Physiol. Pharmacol. 57, 1460.
20. Towart, R. (1981). Bayer AG, internal report.

SEROTONIN RECEPTORS IN TREMATODES: CHARACTERIZATION AND FUNCTION

Tag E. Mansour[1]

Department of Pharmacology
Stanford University
Stanford, California

I. INTRODUCTION

Ever since the early discovery of serotonin (5-hydroxy-tryptamine) it has been recognized that the bioamine plays an important role as a neurotransmitter in many invertebrate species. Research in my laboratory and by others during the last 25 years has accumulated evidence to indicate that serotonin and its analogs influence motility and metabolism of many parasitic flatworms. The effect of serotonin and its congeners appears to occur as a result of interaction with specific receptors which are designated here as serotonin receptors. I shall summarize here the evidence available that implicates these receptors in the regulation of motility and metabolism of these parasitic worms. The finding that these receptors are linked to a very active adenylate cyclase has provided a good opportunity to study their properties and the mechanism for their cellular control. Serotonin receptors have also been studied by their ability to bind radioligands. Binding experiments have provided an opportunity to compare the receptors from the parasite with those from the host. I shall also discuss some recent experiments done in my laboratory that explore the relationship between development of Schistosoma and the appearance of serotonin-related adenylate cyclase in the schistosomules.

[1]Supported by USPHS research grants AI 16501 and MH 23464 and a grant from the Edna McCommell Clark Foundation.

II. EFFECT OF SEROTONIN ON MOTILITY OF PARASITES

Parasitic worms have adapted their lives to specific
sites in the host. Motility appears to play an important
role in the maintenance of the parasite in the host. Coordination of the movement of parasites allow them to maintain
themselves in situ in the face of motion of host fluids such
as the gut content or bile, in the case of intestinal parasites, or the movement of blood or lymph, in the case of
some tissue parasites. Control of movement of these parasites is through a well-developed nervous system and musculature. The importance of motility in maintaining a successful
parasitic life has provided pharmacologists an impetus to use
it as a target for the development of chemotherapeutic agents.
Many neuromuscular preparations have been developed to study
the physiological and biochemical nature of its control.
There is overwhelming evidence to indicate that serotonin
is one of the bioamines that are involved in the control of
motility in parasitic flatworms. Serotonin was first reported to stimulate rhythmical movement of the liver fluke
Fasciola hepatica (1). Subsequently, several other trematodes and cestodes were shown to be stimulated by serotonin
(for references, see review, Ref. 2). A more direct evidence
that serotonin could influence the location of the parasite
in the host was reported recently in a series of experiments
by Mettrick and Cho (3). They reported that serotonin administration parenterally or by mouth caused migration of the
tapeworm Hymenolepis diminuta in the intestine.
Serotonin has been shown to be present in many parasitic
worms, both trematodes and cestodes (4-6). The parasites
that have been studied so far appear to depend on the host
for their supply of serotonin. This is because the enzyme
that is responsible for the synthesis of 5-hydroxytryptophan
from tryptophan is not present in these species (4,7,8). A
good source of serotonin to many of these parasites is the
blood platelets, in the case of the liver flukes and the
blood flukes, since it is known that they feed on the host's
blood.

III. SEROTONIN AND REGULATION OF METABOLISM IN PARASITES

Parasites in general do not appear to be responsive to
mammalian hormones (2,9). Catecholamines are known to stimulate the carbohydrate and lipid metabolism in mammals by
increasing glycogenolysis, glycolysis and lipolysis. On the

other hand, the carbohydrate metabolism of parasitic worms
does not respond to epinephrine or to norepinephrine. Serotonin has an effect on the carbohydrate metabolism of flatworms similar to that of epinephrine in the host. We have
reported in our laboratory that serotonin added to cultures
of the liver fluke Fasciola hepatica increased glycolysis and
glycogenolysis (10). The indoleamine activates three enzymes
that are involved in the regulation of carbohydrate metabolism: glycogen phosphorylase, phosphofructokinase, and adenylate cyclase (11, 12). The effect of serotonin can occur
in other parasitic flatworms such as schistosomes and the
tapeworm Hymenolepis diminuta (14-18).

IV.   EFFECT OF CYCLIC AMP AND NEUROTRANSMITTER AMINES ON DEVELOPMENT OF EUKARYOTIC CELLS

The function of cyclic AMP as a cellular regulator has
been conserved in a diverse variety of prokaryotic and
eukaryotic cells. The effect of cyclic AMP in promoting
glycolysis and energy change has been reported in a wide
variety of organisms. In bacteria, cyclic AMP exerts this
effect through catabolite repression and may be involved in
transcriptional regulation (19). In higher animal cells,
cyclic AMP acts as a second messenger coupling hormone
binding at the outer membrane surface to a variety of intracellular processes (20). In the unicellular eukaryotic cells
such as Neurospora and slime molds, the cyclic nucleotide
has been implicated in metabolic and behavioral processes
(21,22).

Neurotransmitters such as norepinephrine, serotonin, dopamine, and acetylcholine may be involved in the regulation of
differentiation and morphogenesis (23). Cyclic AMP was
reported to cause a change in the morphology of fibroblasts,
astrocytes, and neurons (24-27). The studies of Buznikov
and his colleagues suggest the involvement of neurotransmitters in the early development of metazoan organisms such as
the sea urchin embryo (28,29). The effects of these neurotransmitters may be mediated through cyclic nucleotides.
While the sensitivity of the sea urchin adenylate cyclase to
these neurotransmitters has not yet been established, the
enzyme in many other invertebrates is sensitive to these
neurotransmitters (30-33).

V. SEROTONIN-ACTIVATED ADENYLATE CYCLASE
AND DEVELOPMENT OF SCHISTOSOMA MANSONI

In view of the possible participation of serotonin and
cyclic AMP in the developmental process of eukaryotes, we
investigated the possibility that adenylate cyclase varies at
different developmental stages (16,17). Our experiments were
done on adult schistosomes from experimentally infected mice,
on cercariae (free-living stages), and on schistosomules.
Adult schistosomes have a very active adenylate cyclase,
almost all in the plasma membrane particles. On the other
hand, the activity of the enzyme in cercariae is very low.
Figure 1 shows that total adenylate cyclase in the adults,
expressed as total activity in the presence of saturating concentrations of NaF, is ten times that in the cercariae.
Figure 2 illustrates the responsivity of adenylate cyclase to
serotonin in cercariae and adults. It is clear from these
results that serotonin in the presence of GTP caused almost
no activation of the cercarial enzyme, whereas it markedly
stimulated adult adenylate cyclase. We then questioned how
rapidly adenylate cyclase develops from low to high responsiveness to serotonin. We therefore studied the enzyme
activity in the early stages of development from cercariae to
adults, the schistosomules. These organisms were cultured
at 36° in a 5% CO_2 atmosphere according to the procedure of
Basch (34). Figure 3 illustrates the changes in the activity
of the schistosomules during the first ten days of development in vitro. It can be seen that the most significant
change in total adenylate cyclase activity was on the second
and fourth days. Concomitant with such increase in total
enzyme activity, there was also a significant increase in
sensitivity of the enzyme to serotonin activation during the
same period of development. Adult parasites which are cultured in vitro or obtained from the infected animal can be
seen to have even greater adenylate cyclase activity represented as total or serotonin-stimulated adenylate cyclase
activity. It is concluded that as the parasite develops
to maturity it gains more adenylate cyclase that is sensitive
to serotonin activation. The development of serotonin-sensi-
tive cyclase comes at a time when the schistosomule is well-
established in the mammalian host, where it encounters
serotonin.

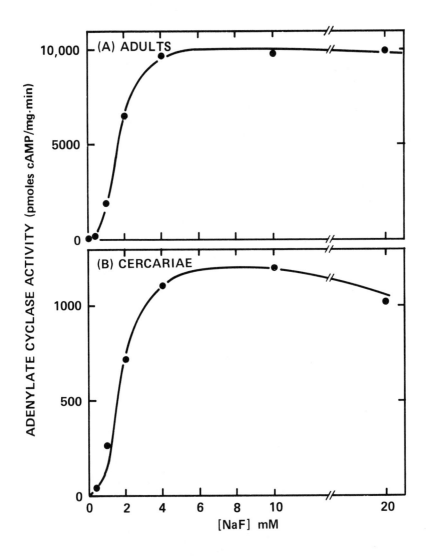

FIGURE 1. Activity of adenylate cyclase in adults and
cercariae of Schistotoma mansoni in the presence of different
concentrations of NaF. Maximal enzyme activity can be seen
in the presence of saturating concentrations of NaF. (Data
from Kasschau and Mansour, 1982, by courtesy of Molecular and
Biochemical Parasitology.)

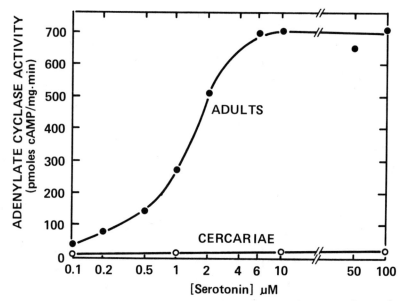

FIGURE 2. Serotonin activation of adenylate cyclase from adult (●) and cercariae (○) particles. (Data from Kasschau and Mansour, 1982, by courtesy of Nature.)

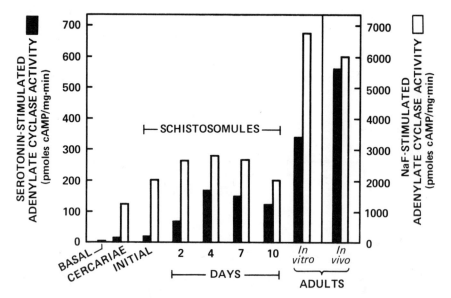

FIGURE 3. Activation of adenylate cyclase by serotonin and GTP (left ordinate) and by NaF (right ordinate) at different stages of development. (Data from Kasschau and Mansour, 1982, by courtesy of Nature.)

VI.   SEROTONIN RECEPTORS IN FASCIOLA

Serotonin-activated adenylate cyclase in Fasciola hepatica is being studied in our laboratory as a representative
of parasitic flatworms (35, 36). The membranous enzyme contains the following components: (a) the receptor that binds
the hormone; (b) the regulatory component of the cyclase
system (GTP/F⁻) is a membranous protein that binds GTP which
has the function of communicating the hormonal message from
the receptor to the cyclase catalytic component. Responsivity of the cyclase to serotonin depends on binding of GTP to
this protein (36). NaF (35) and aluminum (37) appear to
activate the cyclase through an action on this protein. (c)
the catalytic component of the cyclase is the enzyme that
catalyzes the cyclase reaction; (d) the cyclic AMP-dependent
protein kinase (38) which catalyzes the phosphorylation of
different regulatory proteins, such as glycogen phosphorylase
kinase and phosphofructokinase.

We have studied the specificity of the serotonin receptors by examining the effect of different serotonin agonists
and antagonists on adenylate cyclase activity in membrane
particles (35) and on the specific binding of ^{3}H-LSD to the
receptors (39). Among the indolealkylamines, serotonin
appears to be the best analog to activate the adenylate
cyclase. D-lysergic acid diethylamide acts as a partial
agonist; it mimics the effect of the full agonists but does
not do so maximally and antagonizes when the system is activated by a full agonist. LSD in fact has a greater affinity
to the receptors than serotonin itself, with half-maximal
activation at 46 nM compared to 2.1 µM for serotonin.
2-Bromo LSD acts as a potent antagonist of serotonin activation. The effect of LSD is stereospecific since D-LSD is
much more potent that L-LSD, both as an activator and as an
inhibitor of serotonin. The antagonism of either LSD or 2-
bromo LSD is competitive with respect to serotonin. Our
kinetic studies confirmed that agonists and antagonists
interact at the same site, the serotonin receptor (35).

Because of the greater affinity of LSD to the receptors,
it was used to study direct binding properties of different
analogs to the receptors (39). Specific binding of radioactively labeled LSD has all the characteristics of binding
to physiological receptors: specificity, stereospecificity,
and saturability. We studied the effectiveness of different
serotonin agonists and antagonists in displacing ^{3}H-LSD
binding. The concentration of each compound which caused 50%
inhibition of specific binding of ^{3}H-LSD was determined.
Data for different derivatives using the adenylate cyclase

assay procedure corresponds well with data obtained by the
radioligand binding method. The relative affinities of a
series of serotonin antagonists to the fluke receptors were
LSD = 2-bromo LSD > methiothepin > cyproheptidine = metergo-
line > mianserin = serotonin > spiroperidol > ketanserin (39).
This data was compared with binding data on serotonin receptors in the mammalian brain using the same serotonin agonists
and antagonists as reported by Peroutka et al. (40). According to these authors, the brain has two types of receptors
which respond to different sets of agonists and antagonists
of serotonin. They were designated $5-HT_1$ and $5-HT_2$ receptors. We observed major differences between binding properties of the fluke receptors and both mammalian receptors.
For example, in the mammalian system, of the compounds tested
serotonin has the highest affinity for the $5-HT_1$ receptors
while spiroperidol and ketanserin have the highest affinity
for the $5-HT_2$ receptors. The results indicate that the
flukes have serotonin receptors that are different from
those in the mammalian brain.

VII.   CONCLUSIONS

It is evident from the above discussion that serotonin
receptors regulate motility and carbohydrate metabolism in
several species of flatworms. The receptors are linked to a
very active adenylate cyclase. Cyclic AMP may be acting as
the second messenger for serotonin in the regulation of carbohydrate metabolism. The different components of the serotonin-activated adenylate cyclase in the parasite are the
same as those that have been previously described for the
host. Binding characteristics of the receptors from Fasciola
as well as the effect of different agonists and antagonists
to influence adenylate cyclase indicate that these receptors
are different from those that have been described in the host.
Serotonin-activated adenylate cyclase in Schistosoma mansoni
is activated early in the life of the schistosomule. It is
possible that the availability of cyclic AMP through serotonin activation in these parasites may be a prelude to the
development processes that take place in the parasite. Serotonin receptors offer a new site that is amenable to pharmacological manipulation in a strategy for the development of
new chemotherapeutic agents against these parasites.

REFERENCES

1. Mansour, T.E., Br. J. Pharmacol. **12**: 406 (1957).
2. Mansour, T.E., Science, **205**: 462 (1979).
3. Mettrick, D.F., and Cho, C..H., Can. J. Pharmacol. **54**: 281 (1981).
4. Mansour, T.E., Adv. Pharmacol. **3**: 129 (1964).
5. Chou, T.-C. T., Bennett, J., and Bueding, E., J. Parasitol. **58**: 1098 (1972).
6. Lee, M.B., Bueding, E., and Schiffler, E.L., J. Parasitol. **64**: 257 (1978).
7. Mansour, T.E., and Stone, D.B., Biochem. Pharmacol. **19**: 1137 (1970).
8. Bennett, J.L., and Bueding, E., Mol. Pharmacol. **9**: 311 (1973).
9. Hutton, J.C., Schofield, P.J., and McManus, W.R., Comp. Biochem. Physiol. **42**: 49 (1972).
10. Mansour, T.E., J. Pharmacol. Exp. Ther. **126**: 212 (1959).
11. Mansour, T.E., Pharmacol. Rev. **11**: 465 (1959).
12. Mansour, T.E., and Mansour, J.M., J. Biol. Chem. **237**: 629 (1962).
13. Mansour, T.E., Sutherland, E.W., Rall, T.W., and Bueding, E., J. Biol. Chem. 235: 466 (1960).
14. Hillman, G.R., Olsen, N.J., and Senft, A.W., J. Pharmacol. Exp. Ther. **188**: 529 (1974).
15. Bueding, E., and Fisher, J., J. Parasitol. **68**: 208 (1982).
16. Kasschau, M.R., and Mansour, T.E., Mol. Biochem. Parasitol. **5**: 107 (1982).
17. Kasschau, M.R., and Mansour, T.E., Nature **296**: 66 (1982).
18. Mettrick, D.F., Rahman, M.S., and Podesta, R.B., Mol. Biochem. Parasitol. **4**: 217 (1981).
19. Rickenberg, H.V., Annu. Rev. Microbiol. **28**: 353 (1974).
20. Sutherland, E.W., and Robison, G.A., Pharmacol. Rev. **18**: 145 (1966).
21. Gerisch, G., and Wick, U., Biochem. Biophys. Res. Commun. **65**: 364 (1975).
22. Pall, M.L., Microbiol. Rev. **45**: 462 (1981).
23. McMahan, D., Science **185**: 1012 (1974).
24. Hsie, A.W., and Puck, T.T., Proc. Natl. Acad. Sci. USA **68**: 358 (1971).
25. Shapiro, D.L., Nature **241**: 203 (1973).
26. Roisen, F.J., Murphy, R.A., Pichichero, M.E., and Braden, W.G., Science **175**: 73 (1972).

27. Kirkland, W., and Burton, P.R., Nature (New Biol.) **240**: 205 (1972).
28. Buznikov, G.A., Chudakova, I.V., Berdysheva, L.V., and Vyazmina, N.M., J. Embryol. Exp. Morphol. **20**: 119 (1968).
29. Buznikov, G.A., Kost, A.N., Kucherova, N.F., Mndzhoyan, A.L., Suvarov, M.N., and Berdysheva, L.V., J. Embryol. Exp. Morphol. **23**: 549 (1970).
30. Cedar, H., and Schwartz, J.H., J. Gen. Physiol. **60**: 570 (1972).
31. Nathanson, J.A., Science **203**: 65 (1978).
32. Nathanson, J.A., and Greengard, P., Proc. Natl. Acad. Sci. USA **71**: 797 (1974).
33. Gentleman, S., and Mansour, T.E., Life Sci. **20**: 687 (1977).
34. Basch, P.F., J. Parasitol. **67**: 179 (1981).
35. Northup, J.K., and Mansour, T.E., Mol. Pharmacol. **14**: 804 (1978).
36. Northup, J.K., and Mansour, T.E., Mol. Pharmacol. **14**: 820 (1978).
37. Mansour, J.M., Ehrlich, A., and Mansour, T.E., Biochem. Biophys. Res. Commun. **112**: 911 (1983).
38. Gentleman, S., Abrahams, S.L., and Mansour, T.E., Mol. Pharmacol. **12**: 59 (1976).
39. McNall, S., and Mansour, T.E., Fed. Proc. **42**: 1876 (1983).
40. Peroutka, S.J., Lebovitz, R.M., and Snyder, S.H., Science **212**: 827 (1981).

IV PROSTAGLANDINS AND LEUKOTRIENES

PROSTACYCLIN

S. Moncada
J.R. Vane

Wellcome Research Laboratories
Langley Court, Beckenham, Kent BR3 3BS, U.K.

I. INTRODUCTION

Our discovery of prostacyclin in 1976 (1) has led to intense research not only on products of arachidonic acid (AA) metabolism but also in the fields of thrombosis and hemostasis. We have proposed the concept that a balance betwen the formation of prostacyclin by the vessel wall and of thromboxane A_2 (TXA_2) by platelets is important for the control of hemostasis (2,3,4). At the present time, prostacyclin is being used as a research tool to reinvestigate fundamental areas of cardiovascular research such as platelet-vessel wall interactions, the origin of atherosclerosis and the mechanism of action of different anti-platelet drugs. The possible use of prostacyclin in different clinical conditions is also being extensively studied and it is likely that prostacyclin will be the basis for the chemical development of more powerful anti-platelet agents than those known at present.

In this brief review we will concentrate on the formation and synthesis of prostacyclin, the possible dietary manipulation of the prostacyclin/thromboxane axis and the therapeutic potential of prostacyclin. For more extensive reviews see Vane (2), Moncada (3) and Moncada and Vane (4).

II. THE FORMATION AND PROPERTIES OF PROSTACYCLIN

Prostacyclin (see Fig. 1) is the main product of arachidonic acid in all vascular tissues so far tested, including those of man. The ability of the large vessel wall to synthesise prostacyclin is greatest at the intimal surface and progressively decreases toward the adventitia (5). Culture of cells from vessel walls also shows that endothelial cells are the most active producers of prostacyclin (6,7).

Prostacyclin relaxes isolated vascular strips and is a strong hypotensive agent through vasodilation of all vascular beds studied, including the pulmonary and cerebral circulations. Several authors have suggested that prostacyclin generation participates in or accounts for functional hyperemia (8).

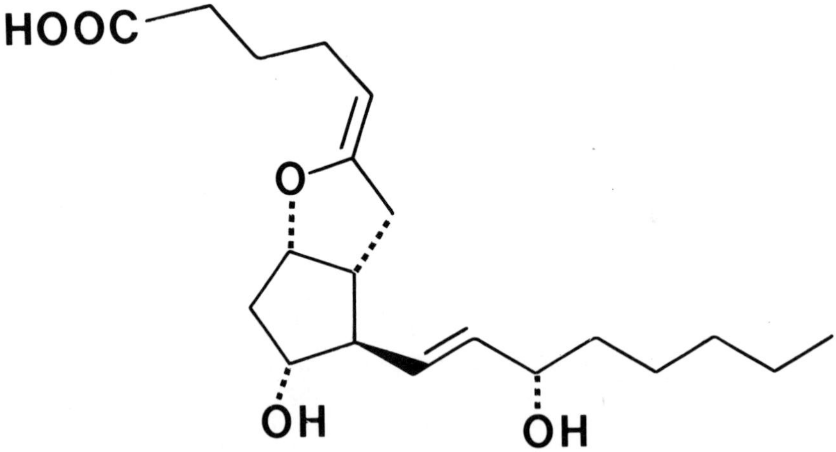

Prostacyclin (PGI$_2$)—Epoprostenol

FIGURE 1

Prostacyclin is the most potent endogenous inhibitor of platelet aggregation yet discovered. This effect is short-lasting in vivo, disappearing within 30 minutes of cessation of intravenous administration. Prostacyclin disperses platelet aggregates in vitro (1,9) and in the circulation of man (10). Moreover, it inhibits thrombus formation in models using the carotid artery of the rabbit (9) and the coronary artery of the dog (11), protects against sudden death (thought to be due to platelet clumping) induced by intravenous arachidonic acid in rabbits (12) and inhibits platelet aggregation in pial venules of the mouse when applied locally (13).

Prostacyclin inhibits platelet aggregation by stimulating adenylate cyclase, leading to an increase in cAMP levels in the platelets (14,15). In this respect prostacyclin is much more potent than either PGE$_1$ or PGD$_2$ and its effect is longer-lasting. In contrast to TXA_2, prostacyclin enhances Ca^{++} sequestration in platelet membranes (16). Moreover, inhibitory effects on platelet phospholipase (17,18) and platelet cyclo-oxygenase (19) have been described. All these effects are related to its ability to increase cAMP in platelets. Prostacyclin, by inhibiting several steps in the activation of the arachidonic acid metabolic cascade, exerts an overall control of platelet aggregability.

Prostacyclin increases cAMP levels in cells other than platelets, raising the possibility that in these cells a balance with the thromboxane system exerts a similar homeostatic control of cell behaviour to that observed in platelets. Thus, the prostacyclin/TXA_2 system may have wider biological significance in cell regulation. An example is that prostacyclin inhibits white cell adherence to the vessel wall (20,21), to nylon fibres and to endothelial monolayers in vitro (22). Prostacyclin increases cAMP in the endothelial cell itself, suggesting a negative feedback control for prostacyclin production by the endothelium (23-25).

One of the functional characteristics of the intact vascular endothelium is its non-reactivity to platelets: clearly, prostacyclin generation could contribute to this thromboresistance. Moreover, prostacyclin inhibits platelet aggregation (platelet-platelet interaction) at much lower concentrations than those needed to inhibit adhesion (platelet-collagen interaction) (26). Thus, prostacyclin may allow platelets to stick to vascular tissue and to participate in the repair of a damaged vessel wall while at the same time preventing or limiting thrombus formation.

III. DIETARY MANIPULATION OF THE
THROMBOXANE A_2:PROSTACYCLIN RATIO

Eicosapentaenoic acid (EPA) is a polyunsaturated fatty acid like AA but has a higher degree of unsaturation. It gives rise to PGs of the "3" series and, when incubated with vascular tissue, leads to the release of an anti-aggregating substance (27). Synthetic Δ^{17}-prostacyclin (PGI_3) is as potent an anti-aggregating agent as prostacyclin (27). In contrast, TXA_3 has a weaker pro-aggregating activity than TXA_2 (27,28). Phospholipids in the membranes of cells, such as platelets, from Greenland Eskimos, contain 8% EPA compared with 0.5% in Danes (29). Similarly, the AA in phospholipids of Eskimos is approximately one-third of that in Danes. These differences may explain why Eskimos have a low incidence of acute myocardial infarction, low blood cholesterol levels and an increased tendency to bleed (29). This prolonged bleeding time is related to a reduction in ex-vivo platelet aggregability (30). The plasma concentrations of cholesterol, triglyceride, low and very low-density lipoprotein are low in Eskimos, whereas the concentrations of high-density lipoprotein are high (31).

EPA inhibits in vitro aggregation of platelets stimulated by ADP, collagen, AA and a synthetic analogue of PGH_2 (27). Also, EPA inhibits aggregation in aspirin- and imidazole-treated platelets (32) and thrombin-induced aggregation (33). It is clear, therefore, that both PG-dependent and PG-independent pathways of platelet aggregation are inhibited by EPA in vitro. In vivo, however, EPA is incorporated into platelet phospholipids, to some extent replacing AA and exerting its antithrombotic effect either by competing with the remaining AA for cyclo-oxygenase and lipoxygenase (34,35) or by being converted to the less pro-aggregatory PGH_3 and TXA_3 (27). Studying seven Caucasians who had been on a mackerel diet for 1 week, Seiss and colleagues (36) showed a reduced sensitivity of platelets to collagen, associated with a reduced ability to produce TXB_2, which was dependent on the ratio of EPA:AA in platelet phospholipids. ADP-induced aggregation was significantly reduced in some subjects and platelet aggregation to exogenously added AA was unchanged, indicating normal cyclo-oxygenase activity. Similarly, Sanders and colleagues (37) showed a significant increase (40%) in bleeding time in volunteers who had taken cod liver oil (equivalent to 1.8 g EPA) daily for 6 weeks. This was accompanied by a decrease in AA and an increase in EPA in the platelet phospholipids.

Under normal peroxide levels EPA is a poor substrate for the cyclo-oxygenase, but increasing peroxide tone in an incubate containing purified cyclo-oxygenase considerably increases the conversion of EPA (34). Incubation of platelet-rich plasma with EPA does not induce the generation of a thromboxane-like material; indeed it prevents the formation of TXA_2 induced by AA or by collagen (27). Conversely, in human umbilical vasculature, Dyerberg and Jorgensen (32) demonstrated that EPA did not influence the conversion of AA to prostacyclin but gave rise to additional synthesis of prostacyclin-like material. Aortic microsomes readily convert PGH_3 to Δ^{17}-6-oxo-$PGF_{1\alpha}$ (38), but formation of this metabolite of Δ^{17}-prostacyclin from exogenous or endogenous EPA in vivo has yet to be confirmed.

Fish oil feeding increased the amount of C20:5 (n=3) fatty acids present in the heart and liver of cats and the platelets of dogs (39,40). Brain infarct volume and the neurological deficit after experimentally-induced cerebral ischemia were less in cats fed fish oil than in a corresponding control group (39). In dogs fed fish oil, thrombosis and subsequent infarct size (3% compared with 25% in a control group) induced by electrical stimulation were reduced, with less than 30% ectopic beats after 19 hours compared with 80% in the control group (40).

The prolonged bleeding time in Eskimos is reduced after aspirin ingestion (30), suggesting a decreased TX synthesizing capacity coupled with a normal or possibly increased production of prostacyclin. Feeding spontaneously hypertensive male weanling rats a diet containing fish oil as the main source of fat resulted in significantly lower blood pressure 22 weeks after the diet was started compared with rats fed corn oil (41). More recently, a study on supplementation of the diet of 8 male volunteers with 40 ml of cod liver oil daily showed after 25 days an increased bleeding time, reduced platelet aggregation, reduced TXA_2 generation during aggregation and a lowered blood pressure associated with a reduction in the hypertensive response to noradrenaline infusions (42). In separate experiments, these authors also showed the conversion of eicosapentaenoic acid into Δ^{17}-6-keto $PGF_{1\alpha}$ by human umbilical artery strips and rabbit renal cortex microsomes.

IV. PROSTACYCLIN AND ATHEROSCLEROSIS

Lipid peroxides, such as 15-hydroperoxy arachidonic acid (15-HPAA), are potent and selective inhibitors of prostacyclin generation by vessel wall microsomes or by fresh vascular tissue (43,44,45,46). There are high concentrations of lipid peroxides in advanced atherosclerotic lesions (47). Lipid peroxidation induced by free radical formation occurs in vitamin E deficiency, the ageing process and perhaps also in hyperlipidemia accompanying atherosclerosis (48). Accumulation of lipid peroxides in atheromatous plaques could predispose to thrombus formation by inhibiting generation of prostacyclin by the vessel wall without reducing TXA_2 production by platelets. Moreover, platelet aggregation is induced by 15-HPAA and this aggregation is not inhibited by adenosine or PGE_1 (49). Human atheromatous plaques do not produce prostacyclin (50,51). In normal rabbits the production of prostacyclin by the luminal surface of the aorta is abolished by de-endothelialisation and slowly recovers with re-endothelialisation over a period of about 70 days. However, the recovery of prostacyclin formation did not occur in rabbits made moderately hypercholesterolemic by diet (52). These results suggest that it would be worth exploring whether attempts to reduce lipid peroxide formation by inhibiting peroxidation influence the development of atherosclerosis and arterial thrombosis. Vitamin E acts as an antioxidant and perhaps its empirical use in arterial disease in the past (53-55) had, in fact, a biochemical rationale. For discussion of the implication of prostacyclin and TXA_2 in diseases other than atherosclerosis see reference Moncada and Vane (56).

V. CLINICAL APPLICATIONS OF PROSTACYCLIN

Prostacyclin is now produced as a stable freeze-dried preparation (Epoprostenol) suitable for human use. Intravenous infusion of prostacyclin in healthy volunteers leads to a dose-related inhibition of platelet aggregation, dispersal of circulating platelet aggregates, arteriolar vasodilation, increases in skin temperature, facial flushing and sometimes headache (for reviews see 2,3). Infusion of prostacyclin into patients susceptible to migraine or cluster headache induces, in most cases, a headache different from those usually experienced (57).

Extracorporeal circulation of blood brings it into contact with artificial surfaces which cannot generate prostacyclin. In the course of such procedures thrombocytopenia and loss of platelet hemostatic function occur and make an important contribution to the bleeding problems following charcoal hemoperfusion and prolonged cardiopulmonary bypass in man. Formation of microemboli during cardiopulmonary bypass may also contribute to the cerebral complications which sometimes follow this procedure. Platelet damage and thrombocytopenia were prevented by prostacyclin both in animal models of extracorporeal circulation (2,3) and in man.

In patients with fulminant hepatic failure undergoing charcoal hemoperfusion (58) prostacyclin infusion prevented the fall in platelet count and elevation of β-thromboglobulin seen in the control patients. Gimson and his colleagues (59) have made almost 200 charcoal hemoperfusions on a daily basis using prostacyclin for platelet protection in the treatment of 76 patients with fulminant hepatic failure. High survival rates (65%) were obtained in the 31 patients who had been referred early and in whom the serial hemoperfusions were started whilst the signs of grade III encephalopathy were still apparent (not rousable but may or may not respond to painful stimuli). The authors thought that early treatment was probably the major factor in the improved survival rate, a reflection of the better biocompatibility of the system because prostacyclin was used, allowing the patients to be treated at an earlier stage. In the group treated later, with Grade IV encephalopathy already present, 20% survived, so that the overall survival rate from the 76 patients was 38%. These results (especially those treated early) compare favourably with a survival rate of 15% in patients under standard intensive care measures.

Several double blind clinical trials of prostacyclin in cardiopulmonary bypass have been published (60-66). The treatment groups showed a preservation of platelet number and function, with a reduction in the blood loss in the first 18 hours after operation. In the trial by Longmore and colleagues (65) the blood loss was halved. In that by Walker and co-workers (64) filters were used and the formation of platelet aggregates on the filters from the placebo group contrasted strikingly with the lack of platelet adhesion to those from patients treated with prostacyclin. The heparin-sparing effect of prostacyclin was confirmed and the vasodilator effects were not troublesome; indeed, Nobak and colleagues (66) suggest that these effects may be utilised in controlling intra-bypass hypertension. Clearly, the use of prostacyclin or an analogue should allow improvements in the methodology of extracorporeal circulations.

Therapeutic assessment of prostacyclin is still in its infancy with many trials in progress. The results are, therefore, still preliminary, but nevertheless they point the way to conditions in which prostacyclin therapy may be useful. In open trials, infusions of prostacyclin for 3-4 days were of benefit to patients with peripheral vascular disease both through relief of ischemic pain and improved ulcer healing (67-72). Placebo controlled blind trials are now in progress and the results of the first to be analysed (73) are encouraging. In the 13 patients infused intravenously for 4 days with placebo, 3 showed reduction in rest pain at 5 days, 2 at 1 month and 1 at 6 months. After 6 months, 3 had died and 5 others had received surgical intervention. Of those 15 patients who were infused with prostacyclin for 4 days (average 7 ng/kg/min i.v.), at 5 days, all had reduction in rest pain. At 1 month, 9 still showed a substantial improvement, which was also evident in 7 patients at 6 months. By this time, two other patients in the group had received surgical intervention and one had died. Gryglewski and colleagues (74) infused prostacyclin into 14 patients with sudden blockage of the central retinal vein. In 8 of these patients, the prostacyclin infusion was followed by amelioration of the disturbance in visual activity, as well as disappearance of optic nerve edema, hemorrhages and tortuosity of the retinal blood vessels.

Prostacyclin also induces long-lasting improvements in Raynaud's phenomenon. Intravenous infusion of the drug for 72 hours produced striking reductions in the frequency, duration and severity of the disease in 21 of 24 patients. The improvement lasted for a mean of 9-10 weeks and in 3 patients, subjective improvement was still reported 6 months after the infusion. Pain relief was a striking feature, presumably associated with the increased blood flow as indicated by increased temperature of the hands and fingers (75). Belch and co-workers (76) have also reported successful treatment in 4 out of 5 patients and a double-blind clinical trial (77) has now confirmed these results in Raynaud's phenomenon. There was an overall improvement still present at 6 weeks in 6 of 7 patients receiving prostacyclin, but only in 1 of 7 receiving placebo. The prostacyclin patients had a significant fall in the number and duration of attacks over the 6 week period post-infusion, whereas there was no change in the placebo group.

Improvements following prostacyclin infusion have now been described in 10 patients with ischemic stroke (78). Patients with transient ischemic attacks and hemorrhagic stroke were excluded.

Prostacyclin has been successfully used in a few cases of pulmonary hypertension and is more effective than PGE_1 (79-81). Single case studies have suggested that prostacyclin may be useful in the treatment of patent ductus arteriosus (82) and pre-eclamptic toxemia (83).

Beneficial effects of intravenous infusion of prostacyclin were obtained in 9 patients with severe congestive heart failure refractory to digitalis and diuretics (84). Mean pulmonary and systemic pressures and vascular resistances were reduced and heart rate, cardiac index and stroke index were all increased during the infusion, with facial flushing as the only side effect.

Bergman and colleagues (85) gave an intravenous infusion of prostacyclin to patients with coronary artery disease with no deleterious effects. Heart rate and cardiac index were increased and mean blood pressure, systemic and pulmonary resistance all fell. Mean atrial pacing time to angina rose from 142 to 241 seconds. They concluded that acute administration of prostacyclin was beneficial in angina, having effects similar to those of the short-acting nitrates. In 5 patients with coronary artery disease, prostacyclin was safely infused directly into diseased coronary arteries (86) and there was a beneficial effect of intravenous prostacyclin infusions in patients with unstable angina (72). However, prostacyclin had no effect on the number, severity and duration of ischemic episodes in 8 of 9 patients with variant angina, although consistent relief was seen in the ninth patient (87).

A prostacyclin deficiency has been reported in thrombotic thrombocytopenic purpura (TTP) (88). Infusion of prostacyclin into two patients with TTP did not produce an increase in circulating platelet count (88,89). However, FitzGerald and colleagues (90) have reported an increase in platelet count and an improvement in the neurological status of one such patient during 18 days of prostacyclin infusion. They were sufficiently encouraged to conclude that the controlled evaluation of prostacyclin in TTP was warranted.

Infusion of prostacyclin protects transplanted kidneys from hyperimmune rejection in dogs (91) and is also protective in patients with chronic renal transplant rejection (92).

Clearly, there are many clinical conditions which may respond to prostacyclin treatment and its place (or that of chemically stable analogues) in therapeutics will be defined in the next few years. Some of these conditions are pre-eclamptic toxemia (93), hemolytic uremic syndrome (94), peptic ulceration (95), the thrombotic complications associated with transplant rejection (91), the prevention of tumour metastasis (96) and the treatment of pulmonary embolism (97).

REFERENCES

1. Moncada S, Gryglewski RJ, Bunting S, Vane JR. Nature (Lond) 1976;263:663-665.
2. Vane, J.R. J. Endocrin. 1982; 95:3P-43P.
3. Moncada S. Br. J. Pharmacol. 1982; 76:3-31.
4. Moncada S, Vane JR. Pharm Rev 1979;30:293-331.
5. Moncada S, Herman AG, Higgs EA, Vane J.R. Thromb Res 1977; 11:323-344.
6. Weksler BB, Marcus AJ, Jaffe EA. Proc Nat Acad Sci USA 1977;74:3922-3926.
7. MacIntyre DE, Pearson JD, Gordon JL. Nature (Lond) 1978;271:549-551.

8. Whittle, B.J.R.   In: Gastro-intestinal Mucosal Blood Flow. Fielding LP ed.   Edinburgh, London, Churchill Livingstone, 1980; 180-191.
9. Ubatuba FB, Moncada S, Vane JR.   Thromb Diath Haemorrh 1979;41:425-434.
10. Szczeklik A, Gryglewski RJ, Nizankowski R, Musial J, Pieton R, Mruk J. Pharmac Res Commun 1978; 10:545-556.
11. Aiken JW, Gorman RR, Shebuski RJ. Prostaglandins 1979; 17:483-494.
12. Bayer B-L, Blass KE, Forster W. Br J Pharmacol 1979; 66:10-12.
13. Rosenblum WI, El Sabban F. Stroke 1979; 10:399-401.
14. Gorman RR, Bunting S, Miller OV. Prostaglandins 1977;13:377-388.
15. Tateson JE, Moncada S, Vane JR.   Prostaglandins 1977;13:389-399.
16. Kaser-Glanzmann R, Jakabova M, George J, Luscher E. Biochim Biophys Acta 1977;466:429-440.
17. Lapetina EG, Schmitges CJ, Chandrabose K, Cuatrecasas P. Biochim Biophys Res Commun. 1977;76:828-835.
18. Minkes M, Stanford M, Chi M, Roth G, Raz A, Needleman P, Majerus P. J Clin Invest 1977;59:449-454.
19. Malmsten C, Granstrom E, Samuelsson B. Biochem Biophys Res Commun 1976;68:569-576.
20. Higgs GA, Moncada S, Vane JR.   J Physiol (Lond) 1978;280:55-56P.
21. Higgs GA. In: Herman AG, Vanhoutte PM, Denolin H & Goossens A eds., Cardiovascular Pharmacology of the Prostaglandins, New York: Raven Press 1982; 315-325.
22. Boxer LA, Allen JM, Schmidt M, Yoder M, Baehner RL. J Lab Clin Med 1980;95:672-678.
23. Hopkins NK, Gorman RR. J Clin Invest 1981;67:540-546.
24. Schafer AI, Gimbrone MA Jr, Handin RI. Biochem Biophys Res Commun 1980;96:1640-1647.
25. Brotherton AFA, Hoak JC. Proc Natl Acad Sci USA 1982; 79:495-499.
26. Higgs EA, Moncada S, Vane JR, Caen JP, Michel H, Tobelem G. Prostaglandins 1978; 16:17-22.
27. Gryglewski RJ, Salmon JA, Ubatuba FB, Weatherly BC, Moncada S, Vane, JR. Prostaglandins, 1979; 18: 453-478.
28. Raz A, Minkes MS, Needleman P. Biochim. biophys. Acta., 1977; 488: 305-311.
29. Dyerberg J, Bang HO, Stoffersen E, Moncada, S, Vane JR. Lancet, 1978; ii:117-119.
30. Dyerberg J, Bang HO. Lancet, 1979; ii: 433-435.
31. Bang HO, Dyerberg J. Acta. Med. Scand. 1972; 192: 85-94.
32. Dyerberg J, Jorgensen KA. Artery, 1980; 8: 12-17.
33. Jakubowski JA, Ardlie NG. Thromb. Res., 1979; 16:205-217.

34. Culp BR, Titus BG, Lands WEM. Prostaglandins Med. 1979; 3: 269-278.
35. Needleman P, Raz A, Minkes MS, Ferrendelli JA, Sprecher H. Proc. Nat. Acad. Sci. USA, 1979; 76:944-948.
36. Seiss W, Roth P, Scherer B, Kurzmann I, Bohlig B, Weber PC. Lancet, 1980; i:441-444.
37. Sanders TAB, Naismith DJ, Haines AP, Vickers M. Lancet 1980; i: 1189.
38. Smith DR, Weatherley BC, Salmon JA, Ubatuba FB, Gryglewski RJ, Moncada S. Prostaglandins 1979; 18:423-438.
39. Black RL, Culp B, Madison D, Randall OS, Lands WEM. Prostaglandins Med., 1979; 3: 257-268.
40. Culp BR, Lands WEM, Lucchesi BR, Pitt B, Romson J. Prostaglandins 1980; 20: 1021-1031.
41. Schoene NW, Fiore D. Progress in Lipid Research, 1981; 20: 569-570.
42. Lorenz R, Spengler U, Fischer S, Duhn J, Weber PC. Circulation, 1983; 67: 504-511.
43. Gryglewski RJ, Bunting S, Moncada S, Flower RJ, Vane JR. Prostaglandins 1976;12:685-713.
44. Moncada S, Gryglewski RJ, Bunting S, Vane JR. Prostaglandins 1976;12:715-733.
45. Bunting S, Gryglewski R, Moncada S, Vane JR. Prostaglandins 1976;12:897-913.
46. Salmon JA, Smith DR, Flower RJ, Moncada S, Vane JR. Biochim Biophys Acta 1978;523:250-262.
47. Glavind J, Hartmann S, Clemmesen J, Jessen KE, Dam H. Acta Pathol Microbiol Scand 1952; 30:1-6.
48. Slater TF. Free Radical Mechanisms in Tissue Injury. Pion. Ltd., London, 1972.
49. Mickel HS, Horbar J. Lipids 1974;9:68-71.
50. Angelo VD, Villa S, Mysliwiec M, Donati MB, De Gaetano G. Thromb Diath Haemorrh 1978;39:535-536.
51. Sinzinger H, Feigl W, Silberbauer K. Lancet 1979;ii:469.
52. Eldor A, Falcone DJ, Hajjar DP, Minick CR, Weksler BB. Am J Pathol. 1982; 107:186.
53. Boyd AM, Marks J. Angiology 1963;14:198-208.
54. Haeger K. Vasc Dis 1968;5:199-213.
55. Marks J. Vitamins and Hormones 1962;20:573-598.
56. Moncada S, Vane JR. Harvard Medical School Bicentennial Celebration Proceedings, in press.
57. Peatfield RC, Gawel MJ, Clifford Rose F. Headache 1981; 21:190-195.
58. Gimson AES, Hughes RD, Mellon PJ, Woods HF, Langley PG, Canalese J, Williams R, Weston MJ. Lancet 1980; i:173-175.
59. Gimson AES, Braude S, Mellon PJ, Canalese J, Williams R. Lancet 1982; ii:681-683.

60. Bennett JG, Longmore DB, O'Grady J. In: Lewis PJ, O'Grady J, Eds. Clinical Pharmacology of Prostacyclin. New York, Raven Press. 1981:201-208.
61. Bunting S, O'Grady J, Fabiani J-N, Terrier E, Moncada S, Vane JR, Dubost Ch. In: Lewis PJ, O'Grady J, Eds. Clinical Pharmacology of Prostacyclin. New York, Raven Press. 1981:181-193.
62. Chelly J, Tricot A, Garcia A, Boucherie J-C, Fabiani J-N, Passelecq J, Dubost Ch. In: Lewis PJ, O'Grady J, eds. Clinical Pharmacology of Prostacyclin. New York, Raven Press. 1981:209.
63. Radegran K, Egberg N, Papaconstantinou C. Scand J Thoracic Cardiovasc Surg. 1981; 15:263-268.
64. Walker ID, Davidson JF, Faichney A, Wheatley D, Davidson K. In: Lewis PJ, O'Grady J, eds. Clinical Pharmacology of Prostacyclin. New York, Raven Press. 1981:195-199.
65. Longmore DB, Bennett JG, Hoyle PM, Smith MA, Gregory A, Osivand T, Jones WA. Lancet 1981;i:800-804.
66. Nobak CR, Tinker JH, Kaye MP, Holcomb GR, Pluth JR. Circulation 1980; 62 (Suppl. 3):1242.
67. Negus D. In: Hormones and Vascular Disease. Pitman Medical. 1981; 181-189.
68. Olsson AG Lancet 1980; ii:1076.
69. Pardy BJ, Lewis JD, Eastcott HHG. Surgery 1980; 88:826-832.
70. Soreide O, Segadahl L, Trippestad A, Engedal H. Scand J Thoracic Cardiovasc Surg 1982; 16:71-73.
71. Szczeklik A, Nizanowski R, Skawinski S, Szczeklik J, Gluszko P, Gryglewski RJ. Lancet 1979;i:1111-1114.
72. Szczeklik A, Gryglewski RJ. In: Lewis PJ, O'Grady J, eds. Clinical Pharmacology of Prostacyclin, New York:Raven Press, 1981;159-167.
73. Belch JJF, McKay A, McArdle B, Lieberman P, Pollock JG, Lowe GDO, Forbes CD, Prentice CRM. Lancet 1983; i:315.
74. Gryglewski RJ. In: Samuelsson B, Paoletti R and Ramwell P. eds. Advances in Prostaglandin, Thromboxane and Leukotriene Research, New York:Raven Press, 1983; 11, 457-461.
75. Dowd PM, Martin MFR, Cooke ED, Bowcock SA, Jones R, Dieppe PA, Kirby JDT. Br J Dermatol. 1982; 106:81-89.
76. Belch JJF, Newman P, Drury JK, Capell H, Leiberman P, James WB, Forbes CD, Prentice CRM. Thromb Haem 1981; 45:255-256.
77. Belch JJF, Newman P, Drury JK, McKenzie F, Capell H, Leiberman P, Forbes CD, Prentice CRM. Lancet 1983; i:313.
78. Gryglewski RJ, Nowak S, Kostka-Trabka E, Bieron K, Dembinska-Kiec A, Blaszczyk B, Kusmiderski J, Markowska E, Szmatola S. Pharm Res Commun. 1982; 14:879-908.
79. Watkins WD, Peterson MB, Crone RK, Shannon DC, Levine L. Lancet 1980;i:1083.

80. Rubin LJ, Groves BM, Reeves JT, Frosolono M, Handel F, Cato AE. Circulation 1982; 66 (2) Part 1:334.
81. Szczeklik J, Szczeklik A, Nizankowski R. Lancet 1980;ii:1076.
82. Lock JE, Olley PM, Coceani F, Swyer PR, Rowe RD. Lancet 1979; i:1343.
83. Fidler J, Bennett MJ, de Swiet M, Ellis C, Lewis PJ. Lancet 1980; ii:31-32.
84. Yui Y, Nakajima H, Kawai C, Murakami T. Am J Cardiol 1982; 50:320-324.
85. Bergman G, Daly R, Atkinson L, Rothman M, Richardson PJ, Jackson G, Jewitt DE. Lancet 1981;i:569-572.
86. Hall RJC, Dewar HA. Lancet 1981;i:949.
87. Chierchia S, Patrono C, Crea F, Ciabattoni G, de Caterina R, Cinotti GA, Distante A, Maseri A. Circulation 1982; 65:470-477.
88. Hensby CN, Lewis PJ, Hilgard P, Mufti GJ, Hows J, Webster J. Lancet 1979; ii:748.
89. Budd GT, Bukowski RM, Lucas FV, Cato AE, Cocchetto DM. Lancet 1980;ii:915.
90. FitzGerald GA, Roberts LJ II, Maas D, Brash AR, Oates JA. In: Lewis PJ, O'Grady J, eds. Clinical Pharmacology of Prostacyclin, New York:Raven Press, 1981;81.
91. Mundy AR, Bewick M, Moncada S, Vane JR. Prostaglandins 1980;19:595-603.
92. Leithner C, Sinzinger H, Schwarz M. Prostaglandins 1981; 22:783-788.
93. Fidler J, Ellis C, Bennett MJ, de Swiet M, Lewis PJ. In: Lewis PJ, O'Grady J, eds. Clinical Pharmacology of Prostacyclin, New York:Raven Press, 1981;141-143.
94. Webster J, Borysiewicz LK, Rees AJ, Lewis PJ. In: Lewis PJ, O'Grady J, eds. Clinical Pharmacology of Prostacyclin, New York:Raven Press, 1981;77-80.
95. Whittle BJR, Kauffman GL, Moncada S. Nature 1981; 292:472-474.
96. Honn KV, Cicone B, Skoff A. Science 1981;212:1270-1272.
97. Utsunomiya T, Krausz MM, Valeri CR, Shepro D, Hechtman HB. Surgery 1980;88:25-30.

STRUCTURAL AND FUNCTIONAL DIVERSITY
OF THE LEUKOTRIENE MEDIATORS

Edward J. Goetzl
Daniel W. Goldman
Donald G. Payan

Howard Hughes Medical Institute Laboratories
and Division of Allergy and Immunology
University of California
San Francisco, California

The initial recognition of the involvement of leukotrienes and other lipoxygenase products of arachidonic acid as mediators of hypersensitivity reactions (1-3) stimulated a wide range of investigations of their roles as mediators of physiological responses. Results of studies over the past several years have demonstrated that many types of cells other than leukocytes have the capacity to generate and respond to lipoxygenase products of arachidonic acid. Examples of the broad effects of lipoxygenase products include the initiation of secretion by pulmonary airways, pancreatic islets, and intestines, and the stimulation of migration and other non-contractile functions of smooth muscle cells (4). The characteristic ability of these endogenous lipoxygenase products to influence functional activities of the cells in which they are produced has indicated the applicability of the term autocoids. Further, the dramatic suppression of function of some cells by structurally distinct inhibitors of lipoxygenation has suggested that some of the metabolites also may be critical prerequisites for cellular activation by heterologous stimuli. Much additional information is needed to elucidate definitively the physiological and pathological contributions of the lipoxygenase products of arachidonic acid. A comprehensive understanding of the roles of lipoxygenase

products is critical to the success of the development
of specific inhibitors of generation and antagonists
that are relevant to human physiology and disease.

I. GENERATION OF LEUKOTRIENES AND OTHER PRODUCTS OF THE LIPOXYGENATION OF ARACHIDONIC ACID

Most of the knowledge of lipoxygenation of arachidonic
acid is based on the isolation and characterization of metabolites of exogenous arachidonic acid that were extracted
from suspensions of cells stimulated with unspecific agonists. Sensitive and specific radioimmunoassays now permit
the quantification of metabolites at approximately 1/100 the
level needed for assessment by optical density of the same
compounds after resolution by high performance liquid chromatography (HPLC). Both methods have revealed the same
major products for cells, such as mast cells, macrophages,
and basophils, that generate large quantities of mediators
for export to the extra-cellular fluid. For each of these
sources, the 5-lipoxygenation of arachidonic acid yields 5-
hydroperoxy-eicosatetraenoic acid (5-OOHETE), which is converted to 5-hydroxy-eicosatetraenoic acid (5-HETE) or to
5,6-epoxy-eicosatetraenoic acid or leukotriene A_4 (LTA_4)
(3). LTA_4 is transformed by enzymatic hydration to 5(S),
12(R)-di-hydroxy-eicosa-6,14-cis-8,10-trans-tetraenoic acid
(LTB_4) and non-enzymatically to several other 5,12-di-HETEs
or is coupled to glutathione to form 5-hydroxy-6-S-gluta-
thionyl-eicosatetraenoic acid (LTC_4). LTC_4 is subjected to
sequential peptidolysis to yield 5-hydroxy-6-S-cysteinyl-
glycyl-eicosatetraenoic acid (LTD_4) and 5-hydroxy-6-S-
cysteinyl-eicosatetraenoic acid (LTE_4). The same cells also
generate different amounts of mono-HETEs and di-HETEs from
the 15-lipoxygenase and other lipoxygenase pathways.
    The rate of extra-cellular appearance of the lipoxy-
genase products is rapid and the quantity of each is a function both of the specific cells and the stimulus. Macrophages and mast cells, for example, generate predominantly
LTC_4 and LTB_4, of the complex mediators, whereas basophils
generate largely LTD_4 and LTB_4 (5-7). A few types of mast
cells, such as dog cutaneous mastocytoma cells, also produce
a small quantity of LTD_4, which presumably is derived from
the larger amounts of LTC_4. The quantities, but not the
relative amounts, of the lipoxygenase products of each type
of cell is dependent on the stimulus. Usually, ionophores
elicit a greater generation of lipoxygenase products than
preferential specific stimuli of any type of cell. Some

mast cell stimuli, such as 15-HETE, are selective for lipoxygenation and fail to evoke the release of histamine (8).
Other stimuli, such as compound 48/80, release histamine
from mast cells, but do not stimulate the generation of
leukotrienes.

In other cells, such as PMN leukocytes, the quantities
of products released are one-tenth or less of those released
from mast cells and macrophages. In the absence of exogenous arachidonic acid, specific stimuli often fail to elicit
the generation by PMN leukocytes of quantities of products
sufficient for detection by standard HPLC techniques. While
it is tempting to speculate that such stimuli may not release arachidonic acid or that contaminating cells may participate by supplying substrate, the insensitivity of conventional assays may be the basis for the negative results.
To examine this possibility, replicate 1 ml suspensions of 3
x 10^7 human neutrophils of greater than 98% purity in Hanks'
solution without protein were incubated for 1-20 min at 37°C
without or with 1 μM ionophore A23187 (CaI A23187) or 1 μM
chemotactic peptide N-formyl-methionyl-leucyl-phenylalanine
(fMLP). Portions of each supernate were removed for radioimmunoassay (RIA) determinations of LTB_4 and LTC_4, and the
remainder of each suspension was extracted for HPLC determination of the leukotrienes as described (5). By RIA, LTB_4
and LTC_4 were found in all supernates and the quantities
were increased both by fMLP and CaI A23187 (Table I). In
contrast, only the 20 min CaI A23187-stimulated suspension
had a detectable amount of LTC_4 by HPLC analysis. The HPLC
analysis of LTB_4 detected approximately 50% of that found by
RIA for neutrophils exposed to CaI A23187, but revealed only
marginal amounts or none for neutrophils incubated with fMLP
or buffer alone. The quantities of LTB_4 generated by neutrophils in buffer alone or exposed to CaI A23187 far
exceeded those of LTC_4, whereas the quantities of the two
mediators generated by neutrophils stimulated with fMLP were
similar (Table I). Thus, with fewer neutrophils the conventional HPLC assay would detect LTB_4 only with CaI A23187
stimulation and no LTC_4. RIAs are a more sensitive technique
and a more rapid method for studies of the effects of complex
variables on the generation of leukotrienes.

TABLE I

GENERATION OF LEUKOTRIENES BY HUMAN NEUTROPHILS

STIMULUS	INCUBATION INTERVAL (min at 37°C)	LTB_4[a] (pmoles, mean)		LTC_4[a] (pmoles, mean)	
		RIA[c]	HPLC[b]	RIA	HPLC[b]
Buffer	1	0.7	–	1.1	–
	5	3.6	–	1.3	–
	20	8.2	–	1.7	–
CaI[d]	1	145	83	7.5	–
A23187	5	710	326	64	–
(1 μM)	20	238	109	152	12.6
fMLP[e]	1	7.2	–	3.7	–
(1 μM)	5	18	11	12	–
	20	47	22	55	–

– = Not detectable.

a = Each value is the mean of two determinations for one experiment.

b = These values are uncorrected for losses during extraction and subsequent processing for high performance liquid chromatography (HPLC).

c = Radioimmunoassay.

d = Ionophore A23187.

e = N-formyl-methionyl-leucyl-phenylalanine.

II. EFFECTS OF LEUKOTRIENES ON HUMAN PMN LEUKOCYTE AND LYMPHOCYTE FUNCTION

The earliest studies of the activities of leukotrienes showed that LTC_4, LTD_4, and LTE_4 had potent vasoactive and smooth muscle contractile functions, but lacked activity for leukocytes (1-3), while LTB_4 was a potent chemotactic factor for PMN leukocytes (9). In addition to exhibiting chemotactic activity, LTB_4 also increased random migration (chemokinesis), enhanced adherence, stimulated aggregation, augmented the expression of C3b receptors, and initiated limited degranulation of PMN leukocytes (1) (Fig. 1). The only effect of LTC_4 and other C-6 peptide leukotrienes on PMN leukocytes was increased adherence, as assessed by affinity for Sephadex G-25 (10). The increased adherence of PMN leukocytes evoked by LTC_4 and LTD_4 was largely prevented by

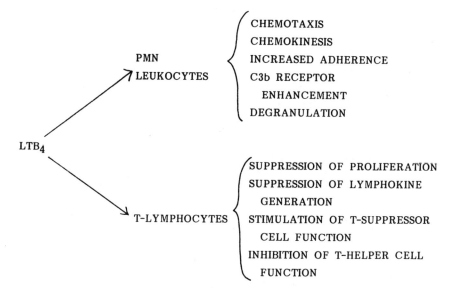

FIGURE 1.   EFFECTS OF LTB$_4$ ON HUMAN LEUKOCYTE FUNCTION

indomethacin and was associated with increased production of thromboxane B$_2$. The latter findings suggested that the effect of LTC$_4$ and LTD$_4$, but not of LTB$_4$, on PMN leukocytes is mediated by stimulation of the cyclo-oxygenation of arachidonic acid and the generation of thromboxane A$_2$, which is known to increase PMN leukocyte adherence.

Human T-lymphocyte proliferative and synthetic responses to mitogens are suppressed directly by LTB$_4$ (11). The overall suppression observed with mixed T-lymphocytes is the net effect of several activities of LTB$_4$ (Fig. 1). At concentrations that suppress mixed T-lymphocyte function, LTB$_4$ inhibits T-helper cell proliferation and stimulates T-suppressor cell proliferation. Thus the immunosuppressive effect of LTB$_4$ is the result of bidirectional modulation of the principal functional subsets of T-lymphocytes. LTB$_4$ also has the capacity to augment the expression of natural cytotoxic cell activity by a thromboxane-dependent mechanism (12). The complex immunological effects of LTB$_4$ are only now beginning to be unraveled by utilizing more specific assays and purified subpopulations of lymphocytes.

III.   LEUKOCYTE RECEPTORS FOR LTB$_4$

The complexity of the LTB$_4$ structural determinants of
chemotactic activity and the inhibition of LTB$_4$-induced
chemotaxis by less active isomers and derivatives of LTB$_4$
suggested that human neutrophils possess receptors specific
for LTB$_4$ (1).   Two different methods for the assessment of
binding of [^{3}H]LTB$_4$ (specific activity = 39 ± 19 Ci/mmole;
mean ± S.D., n = 5) to purified human neutrophils demonstrated 26,000–40,000 receptors per N with a dissociation
constant (Kd) of 1.08–1.39 x 10^{-8}M (13).   The specificity of
the receptors was confirmed by the results of studies of
competitive inhibition of the binding of [^{3}H]LTB$_4$, which
showed that isomers of LTB$_4$, but not peptide chemotactic
factors, bound to LTB$_4$ receptors at chemotactic concentrations (13).

Analyses were also performed of the binding of [^{3}H]LTB$_4$
to subcellular fractions of neutrophils disrupted by nitrogen cavitation in calcium-free buffer at 4°C.   Three fractions recovered from a sucrose gradient contained a mean of
approximately 12%, 20%, and 7% of the membranes and 0.3%,
5%, and 28% of the granules, respectively, as assessed by
quantifying enzymatic markers for each of the cellular components.   The binding of [^{3}H]LTB$_4$ by the same fractions was
4%, 36%, and 5% of that of intact neutrophils, respectively,
while the corresponding binding of the chemotactic peptide
[^{3}H] N-formyl-methionyl-leucyl-phenylalanine (fMLP) was 6%,
28%, and 13%.   Thus the receptors for both LTB$_4$ and fMLP are
localized predominantly in the plasma membranes of neutrophils, but more receptors for fMLP than LTB$_4$ are in the
granules.   Of even greater interest was the difference in
affinity for [^{3}H]LTB$_4$ exhibited by the three subcellular
fractions.   The respective mean Kd values were 1.2 x 10^{-9}M,
7.8 x 10^{-9}M, and 3.0 x 10^{-9}M for the two membrane fractions
and the granule fraction.   This result suggests that LTB$_4$
receptors in one plasma membrane compartment of human neutrophils exhibit a 10-fold higher affinity for LTB$_4$ than the
bulk of the receptors detected on intact neutrophils.

The demonstration of high- and low-affinity receptors
for LTB$_4$ on human neutrophils raises the possibility that
different receptors may mediate the distinct effects of LTB$_4$
on neutrophil function (Fig. 2).   Chemotaxis, which is stimulated to a half-maximal response by 3 x 10^{-9}M–10^{-8}M LTB$_4$
(1,9,13), and adherence, the half-maximal increase in which
is achieved by 3–5 x 10^{-9}M LTB$_4$ (10), are presumably both
initiated by the occupancy of the same or different high-
affinity receptors.   In contrast, a half-maximal stimulation

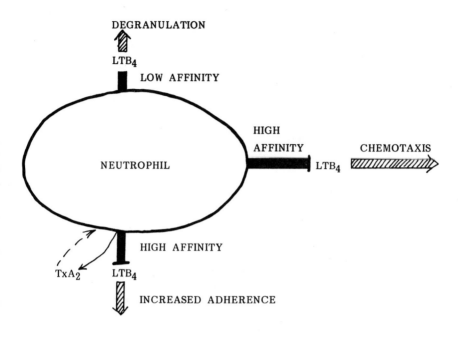

FIGURE 2. LEUKOTRIENE B_4 RECEPTORS OF HUMAN NEUTROPHILS
TxA_2 = Thromboxane A_2

of release of lysosomal enzymes from neutrophils requires
approximately $10^{-7}-10^{-6}M$ LTB_4 (9) and may be mediated by
low-affinity receptors. The possibility that each functional effect of LTB_4 is governed by a receptor with a binding affinity which is different from that of other function-
specific receptors, also suggests that the potency and net
effect of antagonists must be defined in terms of a specific
function. Similar heterogeneity may also exist among T-
lymphocyte receptors for LTB_4.

IV. CONCLUDING COMMENTS

The leukotrienes are a family of potent mediators of
hypersensitivity and inflammation. The application of sensitive and specific radioimmunoassays for leukotrienes has
revealed the generation of significant quantities of several
leukotrienes by leukocytes exposed to natural stimuli in the
absence of exogenous arachidonic acid. The C-6 peptide
leukotrienes, LTC_4 and LTD_4, are potent vasoactive and smooth
muscle contractile factors. Leukotriene B_4 and other di-

HETEs stimulate PMN leukocyte function and suppress T-lympho-cyte activities. The effects of LTB$_4$ on T-lymphocytes are subset-specific and include the activation of suppressor and cytotoxic T-cells. Receptors for LTB$_4$ on PMN leukocytes are specific, but exhibit considerable heterogeneity of binding affinity and may mediate different functional effects. The complexity of the pathways of generation and metabolism of leukotrienes, and of the leukotriene receptors suggest that carefully defined systems will be needed to test the effects of pharmacological inhibitors and antagonists.

REFERENCES

1. Goetzl, E.J. (1981). In "The Medical Clinics of North America" (B.P. Robertson, ed.), p. 809, W.B. Saunders, Philadelphia.
2. Bach, M. (1982). Annu. Rev. Microbiol. 36, 371.
3. Samuelsson, B. (1983). Science 220, 568.
4. Chakrin, L.W., and D.M. Bailey, eds. "The Chemistry and Biology of Leukotrienes and Related Substances", in press.
5. Phillips, M.J., Gold, W.M., and Goetzl, E.J. (1983) J. Immunol., in press.
6. Fels, A.O.S., Pawlowski, N.A., Kramer, E.B., King, T.K.C., Cohen, Z.A., and Scott, W.A. (1982). Proc. Natl. Acad. Sci. U.S.A. 79, 7866.
7. Jakschik, B.A., and Lee, L.H. (1980). Nature 287, 51.
8. Goetzl, E.J., Phillips, M.J., and Gold, W.M. (1983). J. Exp. Med., in press.
9. Goetzl, E.J., and Pickett, W.C. (1980). J. Immunol. 125, 1789.
10. Goetzl, E.J., Brindley, L.L., and Goldman, D.W. (1983). Immunology, in press.
11. Payan, D.G., and Goetzl, E.J. (1983). J. Immunol., in press.
12. Rola-Pleszczynski, M., Gagnon, L., and Sirois, P. (1983). Biochem. Biophys. Res. Commun., in press.
13. Goldman, D.W., and Goetzl, E.J. (1982). J. Immunol. 129, 1600.

CYTOPROTECTION WITH PROSTACYCLIN AND WITH DUAL ENZYME INHIBITORS

K.M. Mullane* and S. Moncada
Dept. of Prostaglandin Research
Wellcome Research Laboratories
Langley Court, Beckenham, Kent BR3 3BS
and
*Dept. of Pharmacology
New York Medical College
Valhalla, New York

I. PROSTACYCLIN

A. Prostacyclin and cyclic AMP

The inhibition of platelet aggregation by prostacyclin is correlated with an activation of the adenylate cyclase system, leading to a substantial rise in platelet intracellular cyclic AMP levels (1,2). Indeed, in this respect, as with its anti-aggregating activity, prostacyclin is the most potent endogenous stimulant of platelet adenylate cyclase, being more active than either PGE_1 or PGD_2. A sequential stimulation of adenylate cyclase, followed by a presumably indirect activation of phosphodiesterase has been characterized in human platelets (3). Elevated cyclic AMP levels appear to regulate platelet cytoplasmic calcium levels by stimulating calcium removed by a membrane system, probably the dense tubular system (4). Thus, prostacyclin may inhibit platelet aggregation through the cyclic AMP system by reducing cytoplasmic calcium levels, upon which platelet shape change, aggregation and the release reaction depend. In contrast, TXA_2 and PGH_2 can reduce platelet intracellular cyclic AMP levels, but only when these levels are already elevated by an adenylate cyclase stimulant such as PGE_1 (5). The induction of platelet aggregation by these compounds may not necessarily be directly linked to inhibition of adenylate cyclase, since basal levels of cyclic AMP are not lowered by TXA_2 or PGH_2. Furthermore, an adenylate cyclase inhibitor (SQ22536), which can lower basal concentrations of cyclic AMP as well as reduce those stimulated by PGE_1, fails to induce platelet aggregation (6). However, the ability of

229

TXA_2 to modulate the anti-aggregating actions of prostacyclin by attenuating its actions on intracellular cyclic AMP levels may be an important interactive mechanism between these two agents under physiological and pathophysiological conditions.

Interactions between the effects of TXA_2 and prostacyclin on the cyclic AMP system of other cells have also been reported. Thus in B16 melanoma cells, the stable epoxy-methano analogue and the thromboxane breakdown product, TXB_2, in high concentrations can reduce PGE_1-elevated intracellular cyclic AMP levels and enhanced cell proliferation, whereas prostacyclin, in high concentrations, reduced cell proliferation (7). It was proposed that tumour cell proliferation may be regulated by a balance in TXA_2 and prostacyclin production, but it is not known whether such actions could be brought about by the levels of these arachidonate metabolites produced in vivo.

Prostacyclin also increases cyclic AMP levels in cultured fibroblasts (8) and in bovine coronary arteries (9). High concentrations of prostacyclin can activate adenylate cyclase in biopsies of human gastric and duodenal mucosa (10). However, in studies with isolated parietal cells, separated from other cell types from dog gastric mucosa, low concentrations of prostacyclin and its stable analogues reduced histamine-elevated cyclic AMP levels, an action which is likely to underlie the gastric antisecretory activity of prostacyclin (11). Likewise, prostacyclin may either stimulate or inhibit cyclic AMP in rat isolated fat cells (12); thus in both cell types the levels of cyclic AMP will increase or decrease depending on the concentration of prostacyclin used, and the initial level of adenylate cyclase activation prior to treatment. Studies using cultured endothelial cells from human umbilical vein also demonstrated a potent stimulant action of prostacyclin on cyclic AMP levels in the presence of phosphodiesterase inhibition (13). It was also suggested that such elevation of cyclic AMP could act as a negative feedback control for prostacyclin biosynthesis by these cells, as previous studies had shown that in platelets cyclic AMP could inhibit the availability of endogenous arachidonate, probably by an action on the cyclo-oxygenase as well as on the phospholipase (14).

B. Prostacyclin and cytoprotection

The ability of TXA_2 or its stable analogues to promote tissue damage in the gastric mucosa (15) or myocardial tissue (16) may be correlated with its potent direct vasoconstrictor properties and with its pro-aggregating activity, resulting in platelet obstruction of microvascular beds. However, TXA_2 may also have a direct action on gastric mucosal and myocardial cellular integrity, which could contribute to its cyto-destructive properties. Thus, in cats with coronary artery occlusion, a carbocyclic thromboxane analogue significantly reduced myocardial creatine kinase activity and bound cathepsin D (an index of cellular integrity) in both the ischemic and non-ischemic areas (16). Although these findings may have resulted from its coronary vasoconstrictor action, this thromboxane analogue also can induce the release of lysosomal enzymes from large granule fractions of liver incubates. Thus, thromboxanes may exert a direct lytic action on susceptible cellular membranes, leading to the release of tissue-destructive hydrolases. In the already ischemic areas, lysosomal enzyme release would greatly augment the damage in gastric and myocardial tissue, both of which require an adequate nutrient blood flow for functional integrity. A cytolytic action of TXA_2 on other tissues and organs both in vivo and in vitro and its role in pathogenesis of cardiovascular and gastro-intestinal disease remains to be explored.

In experimental models of myocardial infarction, prostacyclin can reduce infarct size and arrhythmias while also decreasing both oxygen demand and the release of cathepsin D and creatine phosphokinase from infarcted areas (17,18). A beneficial effect of infused prostacyclin has also been reported in endotoxin shock in the dog and in the cat where it improves splanchnic blood flow and reduces the formation and release of the lysosomal hydrolase, cathepsin D (19,20). The effects of hypoxic damage in the cat isolated perfused liver are also substantially reduced by prostacyclin (21) while the release of β-glucuronidase and cathepsin D from the large granule fraction is inhibited. In an experimental assessment of prostacyclin in the harvesting of canine kidneys for transplantation, the degree of ischemic damage appeared to be reduced, since auto-transplanted kidneys pre-treated with prostacyclin had normal renal function within 48 hours, as judged by serum creatine levels (22). Furthermore, canine livers have been preserved for up to 48 hours and then successfully transplanted using a combination of refrigeration, Sacks' solution and prostacyclin (23). Prostacyclin has also been shown to protect against liver injury induced by carbon tetrachloride in rats (24).

In contrast to TXA_2, which has cytolytic activity in the gastric mucosa, myocardium and liver, prostacyclin can thus exert protective actions against experimental damage in these tissues. Whereas this effect may reflect its potent vasodilator and anti-aggregating activity, reversing the vasoconstriction and platelet plugging actions of TXA_2, other mechanisms may also play an important role in the overall protective processes of prostacyclin, as in the gastro-intestinal tract.

All these effects could be related to an effect observed recently in our laboratory. We found that the addition of prostacyclin during the separation from blood and the subsequent washing of platelets substantially improves their viability in vitro, but more importantly, whereas normal in vitro platelet survival time is about 4 to 8 h, platelets prepared with the aid of prostacyclin remain functional for more than 72 h (25). This effect was not accompanied by (although it was subsequent to) an increase in cAMP level in platelets, thus separating it from the classical anti-aggregating effect (26). Interestingly, there has been a study demonstrating a dissociation between anti-aggregating and cytoprotective effects of a prostacyclin analogue in a model of acute myocardial ischemia (27). At the moment then it is not clear whether this cytoprotective effect is related in any way to the effect on cyclic AMP or is a totally independent phenomenon. More work is necessary to elucidate this problem, however, these results suggest that some of the therapeutic effects of prostacyclin might be related to this cytoprotective effect and indicate a wider therapeutic use of prostacyclin in cell or tissue preservation in vivo and in vitro.

II.   DUAL INHIBITORS

A.   Inflammation and leukocytes

During the last 50 years, the participation of locally produced chemical substances in an inflammatory response has been demonstrated. In particular, evidence has accumulated to show that prostaglandins play a key role in the development of the signs and symptoms of inflammation (28). The discovery that aspirin-like drugs inhibit the synthesis of prostaglandins (29) and the subsequent demonstration that this action accounts for the anti-inflammatory, as well as some of the toxic, effects of aspirin and related compounds, explained the mechanism of action of this class of compounds (for review see 30).

Virtually all cells have the capacity to synthesize prostaglandins which result from the transformation of arachidonic acid by the cyclo-oxygenase enzyme. Arachidonic acid can also be metabolized by a lipoxygenase enzyme, which is the preferred pathway of metabolism in polymorphonuclear leukocytes (PMNs) (31). PMNs accumulate in an acute inflammatory lesion to ingest and remove foreign agents, bacteria, etc., and in doing so release lysosomal enzymes and other mediators. Stimulation of PMNs by chemotactic agents or bacteria induces the release of arachidonic acid and the formation of products of the 5'-lipoxygenase enzyme. One of these, called leukotriene B_4 (5,12 diHETE) (32), is a potent chemotactic agent (33) and promotes leukocyte degranulation (34). It also appears that the integrity of the lipoxygenase is critical for normal leukocyte function (35). Aspirin-like drugs generally have little or no effect on leukocyte infiltration into an inflammatory lesion (36). Moreover, while aspirin-like drugs provide symptomatic relief in chronic inflammation, reducing pain and swelling for example, they do little to ameliorate the underlying progression of the disease (37). The failure of these drugs to suppress leukocyte-mediated events may account for the permanence of the inflammatory damage.

In 1979 Higgs, Flower and Vane (38) described a new compound called BW755C, which not only inhibits the cyclo-oxygenase enzyme, like other non-steroidal anti-inflammatory agents, but also inhibits the lipoxygenase enzyme. This "dual" inhibitor represents a new class of powerful anti-inflammatory drugs which, in addition to preventing local prostaglandin generation, inhibits leukocyte infiltration into the inflammatory lesion (36). Higgs and co-workers, (36,37,39) have performed an exhaustive study whereby the abilities of a variety of anti-inflammatory drugs to suppress leukocyte infiltration, inhibit prostaglandin formation and attenuate edema formation were compared. It became apparent that doses of these agents required to reduce an inflammatory response (edema formation) also suppress leukocyte infiltration and, with the exception of BW755C, are 3-50 times greater than the dose required to inhibit prostaglandin formation.

B.   Inflammation and Myocardial Ischemia

Ischemic heart disease is the leading cause of death and disability in the western world. The concept of reducing infarct size to improve patient prognosis results from 2 major observations. First, myocellular death does not occur uniformly but in discrete areas. Oxygen deprivation first induces reversible damage in the myocytes, which becomes irreversible, giving rise to a necrotic region, if the oxygen supply continues to be compromised. A "wave-front" of cell damage moves out from the subendocardium (40) and potentially necrotic tissue can be salvaged by agents which suppress this movement. Second, full development of myocardial infarction may take several days rather than just hours since infarct expansion or extension can contribute to the final degree of damage (41).

The initiating cause of myocardial ischemia is a critical reduction in oxygen supply to the heart due to coronary atherosclerosis or vasospasm. Consequently, most attempts to limit infarct size have been directed towards either improving the oxygen supply or reducing the oxygen demands of the heart (42). However, drugs which act in this manner need to be given either before or early during the period of ischemia. This factor severely limits the usefulness of such drugs except as prophylactic treatment to reduce the chances of reinfarction.

We (43) have recently highlighted the similarities between myocardial infarction and other forms of acute inflammation induced by tissue injury. All the cardinal features of an inflammatory response can be observed. First, myocardial ischemia is accompanied by an early migration of PMNs into the ischemic area (43). Within 60 min of occlusion, scanning electron microscopy revealed leukocytes adhering to the endothelium of vessels draining the ischemic zone. In some areas the endothelium appeared "blebbed" or "blistered" due to leukocytes which migrated through the endothelial layer. Over the subsequent 5 hrs large numbers of PMNs infiltrate into the ischemic myocardium, many apparently migrating from "normal" areas of the myocardium and converging on the necrotic zone. Some small arteries were also found to be totally occluded by PMNs. A similar observation was recently made by Engler and co-workers (44), who suggested that blockade of vessels by leukocytes could account for the "no-reflow phenomenon".

Second, potentially pro-inflammatory mediators are produced by the ischemic myocardium. The release of prostaglandins and TXA_2 during myocardial ischemia has already been observed (45-47). We found that infarcted tissue converts arachidonic acid primarily to the lipoxygenase product 12-HETE, with smaller quantities of 15-HETE also formed (43). The formation of these lipoxygenase products is attributed to the invading leukocytes since the formation of 12- and 15-HETE is proportional to the degree of cell invasion, and a semi-purified preparation of peripheral leukocytes from the dog shows an identical metabolic profile when incubated with arachidonic acid. The formation of 12-HETE by infarcted myocardium is important since it indicates that migrating cells alter the metabolic profile of the tissue which they invade. 12-HETE has chemotactic activity (48) and constricts cat coronary arteries in vitro (49) - actions which may contribute to myocardial injury.

The third cardinal sign of inflammation observed in myocardial infarction is edema (50). This symptom may also be dependent on PMNs since the interaction between a chemotactic factor such as $C5_a$ or LTB_4, the PMNs and a locally produced vasodilator prostaglandin such as PGI_2 (all of which have been identified in the ischemic myocardium) leads to edema formation in rabbit skin and is attenuated in leukopenic animals (51).

The final inflammatory features observed in myocardial infarction are pain and loss of function (reduced contractility).

C. Myocardial ischemia and leukocytes

The PMNs appear to play a central role in enhancing the myocardial injury observed in our model of myocardial ischemia in the dog (43). Activation of peripheral blood PMNs has also been reported in patients with myocardial infarction (52). In vitro studies have shown that during the process of phagocytosis PMNs can release proteolytic enzymes and toxic oxygen metabolites (free radicals) such as superoxide, or hydrogen peroxide, together with metabolites of arachidonic acid, into the external tissue environment. Measuring the net formation of tyrosine (an amino acid neither synthesized nor degraded by cardiac muscle) as an index of lysosomal protease activity in the myocardium, Bolli (53) found that proteolysis correlated with leukocyte infiltration and probably reflects leukocyte-mediated digestion of the necrotic debris. The fact that inhibition of lysosomal protease activity with leupeptin, antipain, pepstatin and chymostatin totally suppressed proteolysis but did not influence infarct size suggests that other leukocyte-derived mediators, such as free radicals or arachidonic acid metabolites, are more important in exacerbating ischemia-induced myocardial injury.

Oxygen metabolites can directly alter structural components of tissues, producing degradation of glycosaminoglycans (54), proteoglycans and collagen (55). These free radicals can also cause injury and lysis of a number of different cell-types (56), including endothelial cells, and may, in turn, provide a thrombogenic surface for intravascular platelet aggregation. The release of oxygen metabolites by phagocytosing leukocytes could extend the area of myocardial necrosis by damaging further the adjoining "reversibly"-injured cells during the process of phagocytosis of "irreversibly"-injured cells.

The formation of oxygen metabolites by the ischemic myocardium itself has been proposed (57). These are formed via a xanthine-xanthine oxidase system (57) rather than the NAD(P)H oxidase system of the neutrophil (58). Hess and co-workers (59) have proposed that free radicals and protons generated during myocardial ischemia alter myocardial contractility by the uncoupling of calcium transport from ATP hydrolysis.

Oxidation of polyunsaturated fatty acids, either enzymic or auto-oxidation by oxygen metabolites, to lipid peroxides can enhance cell toxicity and has been implicated in, for example, liver cell injury (60). Lipid peroxides react with proteins to produce a loss of enzymic activity, the destruction of some labile amino acids such as cystein and lysine, polymerisation and polypeptide chain scission (60). Moreover, reincorporation of hydroperoxides of polyunsaturated fatty acids into membrane phospholipids by reacylation enzymes can change the membrane characteristics to increase the leakiness of cells. Oxidized di- and trienoic fatty acids, leukotriene B_4 and phosphatidic acid are thought to serve as endogenous calcium ionophores in cells (61,62) and could, thereby, promote mitochondrial damage and lysosomal enzyme release, as well as the liberation of fatty acids and other mediators. Thus, lipid peroxidation secondary to the release of PMN-derived mediators, can also contribute to ischemia-induced cell damage. Lipid peroxides and/or hydroxides may contribute to the pain of myocardial ischemia (angina) for they are amongst the most potent hyperalgesic substances tested (63).

Complement activation may represent the initial stimulus for PMN infiltration. Hill and Ward (64) found that coronary artery ligation led to the stimulation of a tissue protease present in the myocardium which cleaves the third component of complement into chemotactically active fragments. Pinckard's group (65,66) have localized complement fragments C_3, C_4 and C_5 in the ischemic myocardium using immunofluorescent techniques and found C_3 and C_5 located in the walls of small arteries in infarcted myocardium as well as on myocardial fibers. The interaction of the complement component C_{3b} with a specific receptor on the surface of PMN triggers phagocytosis (67). Complement-stimulated neutrophils also produce platelet-activating factor (68), another pro-inflammatory lipid mediator which induces aggregation of platelets and leukocytes (69). The depletion of complement with cobra venom factor attenuates leukocyte infiltration into the myocardium and reduces infarct size (65,70,71).

D.   Anti-inflammatory drugs and myocardial infarction

A corollary of the proposal that the acute inflammatory response exacerbates ischemia-induced myocardial injury is that agents which abrogate the inflammatory process should similarly reduce ischemic damage.   However, the   non-steroidal   anti-inflammatory   drug indomethacin actually increases infarct size rather than decreases it (72). Indomethacin is a cyclo-oxygenase inhibitor and has been shown, at certain doses, actually to increase leukocyte infiltration into an inflammatory lesion (36). Consequently indomethacin is a poor agent with which to test the hypothesis that PMNs and the inflammatory response contribute to the myocardial damage.   Since infarcted myocardium metabolizes arachidonic acid via the lipoxygenase pathway and inhibitors of the lipoxygenase enzyme reduce leukocyte infiltration, it seemed pertinent to study the effects of a lipoxygenase inhibitor.   The agent selected was BW755C, and its effects were compared with those of the cyclo-oxygenase inhibitor, indomethacin (43,73).   BW755C attenuated leukocyte infiltration into the myocardium, abolished 12-HETE formation and significantly reduced infarct size, whereas indomethacin had no effect on these parameters. Moreover, BW755C was effective even when administered after the period of occlusion, during the reperfusion phase, so its beneficial effects could not be attributed to improvements in myocardial oxygenation during the critical period of occlusion.   Depletion of circulating leukocytes by chronic treatment with hydroxyurea also reduced infarct size, with few PMNs observed in the ischemic tissue (43).

Lucchesi and co-workers have reached similar conclusions. These workers found that the ability of another non-steroidal anti-inflammatory drug, ibuprofen, to reduce infarct size correlated with inhibition of leukocyte infiltration and not with platelet accumulation (74). The ability of ibuprofen to reduce the leukocyte invasion into the heart is interesting since ibuprofen does not inhibit the lipoxygenase enzyme.   Ibuprofen may interfere with the binding of chemotactic factor(s) to the neutrophil, to prevent its activation.   In contrast ibuprofen does not inhibit leukocyte infiltration in an inflammatory model   whereby   a   carrageenin-impregnated   polyester   sponge   is implanted subcutaneously (36).   Complement appears to be an important chemotactic factor in myocardial ischemia (64-66), whereas LTB_4 may be an important chemotactic agent in the sponge model (75). Undoubtedly, there are a number of potential sites of action for anti-inflammatory agents to inhibit leukocyte function. Lucchesi and co-workers then went on to show that neutrophil depletion with specific anti-sera also reduces infarct size (76), confirming the importance of leukocytes in ischemia-induced myocardial injury.

A variety of anti-inflammatory drugs have been tested in myocardial ischemia with varying results (see Table 1).   However, many of these agents were selected for additional properties such as inhibition of platelet aggregation or of prostaglandin biosynthesis or "lysosomal stabilization" rather than prevention of leukocyte infiltration. If the ability of these anti-inflammatory agents to reduce infarct size is compared with their ability to suppress neutrophil invasion into an inflammatory lesion, there is a clear correlation between these two actions. Moreover, a variety of other drugs which suppress different aspects of the inflammatory process also reduce infarct size (Table 2).

Further experiments are now necessary to elucidate the precise relationship between white cell migration and tissue damage and, perhaps more important, the role of white cells in the process of tissue repair.   We have evidence that reduction of white cell migration reduces the development of myocardial infarction. If this approach also leads to decreased healing then the therapeutic potential of this type of intervention will be in doubt.

Table 1

Comparison of the ability of different anti-inflammatory drugs to
reduce infarct size and suppress leukocyte infiltration

Anti-inflammatory Drug	Infarct Size	Leukocyte Infiltration (into inflammatory exudate)	Reference
BW755C	↓	↓	43,73
Ibuprofen	↓	↓	74,77
Flurbiprofen	↓	↓	78,79
Indomethacin	↑	↑	36,72
Aspirin	no effect	no effect	36,80
Sulfinpyrazone	"	"	81
Zomepirac	"	?	82
Naproxen	"	no effect	36,81
Meclofenamate	"	"	36,83
Corticosteroids*	↓	↓	39,84,85

*   Only effective in doses approx. 5-fold greater than anti-
inflammatory doses

Table 2

Additional agents which supress the inflammatory response and
reduce infarct size

Mechanism	Agent	Reference
complement depletion	cobra venom factor	70,71
serine protease inhibition	trasylol (aprotinin)	86
free radical scavengers	mannitol	87
	glucose-insulin-potassium	88,89
	dimethylsulfoxide	90
	superoxide dismutase and catalase	91
neutrophil depletion	anti-neutrophil antibodies	76

REFERENCES

1. Tateson JE, Moncada S & Vane JR (1977) Prostaglandins, 13, 389-399.
2. Gorman RR, Bunting S & Miller OV (1977) Prostaglandins, 13, 377-388.
3. Alvarez R, Taylor A, Fazzari JJ & Jacobs JR (1981) Mol. Pharmacol., 20, 302-309.
4. Kaser-Glanzmann R, Jakabova M, George JN & Luscher EF (1977) Biochim. Biophys. Acta., 466, 429-440.
5. Miller OV, Johnson RA & Gorman RR (1977) Prostaglandins, 13, 599-609.
6. Salzman EW, MacIntyre DE, Steer ML & Gordon JL (1978) Thromb. Res., 13, 1089-1101.
7. Honn KV & Meyer J (1981) Biochem. Biophys. Res. Comm., 102, 1122-1129.
8. Gorman RR, Hamilton RD & Hopkins NK (1979) J. Biol. Chem., 254, 1671-1676.
9. Dembinska-Kiec A, Ruker W & Schonhofer PS (1979) Naunyn Schmiedeberg's Arch. Pharmacol., 308, 107-110.
10. Simon B & Kather H (1980) Digestion, 20, 111-114.
11. Soll AH & Whittle BJR (1981) Prostaglandins, 21, 353-365.
12. Fredholm BB, Hjemdahl P & Hammarstrom S (1980) Biochem. Pharmacol., 29, 661-663.
13. Hopkins NK & Gorman RR (1981) J. Clin. Invest., 67, 540-546.
14. Hassid A (1982) Am. J. Physiol., 243, C205-211.
15. Whittle BJR, Kauffman GL & Moncada S (1981) Nature, 292, 472-474.
16. Smith EF, Lefer AM, Aharony D, Smith JB, Magolda RL, Claremon D & Nicolaou KC (1981) Prostaglandins, 21, 443-456.
17. Ogletree ML, Lefer AM, Smith JB & Nicolaou KC (1979) Eur. J. Pharmac., 56, 95-103.
18. Ribeiro LGT, Brandon TA, Hopkins DG, Reduto LA, Taylor AA & Miller RR (1981) Am. J. Cardiol., 47, 835-840.
19. Fletcher JR & Ramwell PW (1980) Circ. Shock, 7, 299-308.
20. Lefer AM, Tabas J & Smith EF (1980) Pharmacol., 21, 206-212.
21. Araki H & Lefer AM (1980) Am. J. Physiol., 238, H176-H181.
22. Mundy AR, Bewick M, Moncada S & Vane JR (1980) Transplantation, 30, 251-255.
23. Monden M & Fortner JG (1982) Ann. Surg., 196, 38-42.
24. Guarner, F., Fremont-Smith, M., Corzo, J., Quiroga, J., Rodriguez, J.L. and Prieto, J. (1983). In: Advances in Prostaglandin, Thromboxane and Leukotriene Research, Vol. 12, ed. B. Samuelsson, R. Paoletti & P. Ramwell, Raven, Press, New York., 75-82.
25. Moncada S, Radomski M, Vargas JR (1982). Br J Pharmacol, 75,165P.

26. Blackwell GJ, Radomski M, Vargas JR, Moncada S (1982). Biochim. Biophys. Acta., 718:60-65.
27. Schror K, Ohlendorf R, Darius H (1981). J. Pharmac. Exp. Ther., 219, 243-249.
28. Moncada S and Vane JR (1979). Adv. Intern. Med., 24, 1-22.
29. Vane JR (1971). Nature (New Biol.), 231, 232-235.
30. Flower RJ (1974). Pharmacol. Rev., 26, 33-67.
31. Borgeat P and Samuelsson B (1979). J. Biol. Chem., 254, 2643-2646.
32. Borgeat P and Samuelsson B (1979). Proc. Nat. Acad. Sci. USA., 76, 2148-2152.
33. Palmer RMJ, Stepney RJ, Higgs GA and Eakins KE (1980). Prostaglandins, 20, 411-418.
34. Serhan CN, Radin A, Smolen JE, Korchak H, Samuelsson B and Weissmann G (1982). Biochem. Biophys. Res. Comm., 107, 1006-1012.
35. Hirata F, Corcoran BA, Venkatasubramarian K, Schiffman E and Axelrod J (1979). Proc. Nat. Acad. Sci. USA, 76, 2640-2643.
36. Higgs GA, Eakins KE, Mugridge KG, Moncada S and Vane, JR (1980). Eur. J. Pharmacol., 66, 81-86.
37. Higgs GA, Palmer, RMJ, Eakins KE and Moncada S (1981). Molec. Aspects Med. 4, 275-301.
38. Higgs GA, Flower RJ and Vane JR (1979). Biochem. Pharm., 28, 1959-1961.
39. Higgs GA and Mugridge KG (1982). Br. J. Pharmacol., 76, 284P.
40. Reimer KA, Lowe JE, Rasmussen MM and Jennings RB (1977). Circulation, 56, 786-794.
41. Hutchins GM and Bulkley BH (1978). Am. J. Cardiol., 41, 1127-1132.
42. Maroko PR and Braunwald E (1973). Ann. Intern. Med., 79, 720-733.
43. Mullane KM, Read N, Salmon JA and Moncada S (1983). J. Pharmacol. Exp. Ther., (in press).
44. Engler RL, Schmid-Schonbein GW and Pavelec RS (1983). Am. J. Pathol., 111, 98-111.
45. Berger HJ, Zaret BL, Speroff L, Cohen LS and Wolfson S (1976). Circ. Res. 38, 566-571.
46. Coker SJ, Parratt JR, McA Ledingham I and Zeitlin IJ (1981). Nature, 291, 323-324.
47. Sakai K, Ito T and Ogawa K (1982). J. Cardiovasc. Pharm., 4, 129-135.
48. Turner SR, Tainer JA and Lynn WS (1975). Nature, 257, 680-681.
49. Trachte GJ, Lefer AM, Aharony D and Smith JB (1979). Prostaglandins, 18, 909-914.
50. Reimer KA and Jennings RB (1979). Circulation, 60, 866-876.
51. Wedmore CV and Williams TJ (1981). Nature 289, 646-650.
52. Lauter LB, El Kharib MR, Rising JA and Robin E (1973). Ann. Intern. Med., 79, 59-62.

53. Bolli R (1982). Cardiovasc. Research Center Bulletin (July-Sept.), 1-33.
54. Greenwald RA and Moy WW (1980). Arthritis Rheum., 23, 455-463.
55. Greenwald RA and Moy WW (1979). Arthritis Rheum., 22, 251-259.
56. Fantone JC and Ward PA (1982). Am. J. Pathol., 107, 397-418.
57. McCord JM and Roy RS (1982). Can. J. Physiol. Pharmacol., 60, 1346-1352.
58. Suzuki Y and Lehrer RI (1980). J. Clin. Invest., 66, 1409-1418.
59. Hess ML, Marson NH and Okabe E (1982). Can. J. Physiol. Pharmacol., 60, 1382-1389.
60. Recknagel RO (1967). Pharmacol. Rev., 19, 145-208.
61. Serhan C, Anderson P, Goodman E, Dunham P and Weissmann G (1981). J. Biol. Chem., 256, 2736-2741.
62. Serhan C, Fridovich J, Goetzl EJ, Dunham PB and Weissmann G (1982). J. Biol. Chem., 257, 4746-4752.
63. Ferreira SH (1972). Nature (New Biol.), 240, 200-203.
64. Hill JH and Ward PA (1971). J. Exp. Med., 133, 885-900.
65. Pinckard RN, O'Rourke RA, Crawford MH, Grover FS, McManus LM, Ghidoni JJ, Storrs SB and Olson MS (1980). J. Clin. Invest. 66, 1050-1056.
66. McManus LM, Kolb WP, Crawford MH, O'Rourke RA, Grover FS and Pinckard RN (1983). Lab. Invest., 48, 436-447.
67. Griffin FM, Jr and Silverstein SC (1974). J. Exp. Med., 139, 323-336.
68. Cusack NJ (1980). Nature, 285, 193-195.
69. Benveniste J, Jouvin E, Pirotzky E, Arnoux B, Mencia-Huerta JM, Roubin R and Vargaftig BB (1981). Int. Archs. Allergy Appl. Immun., 66 (Suppl. I), 121-126.
70. Maroko PR, Carpenter CB, Chiariello M, Fishbein ML, Radvany P, Krestman JD and Hale SL (1978). J. Clin. Invest., 61, 661-670.
71. Hartmann JR, Robinson JA and Gunnar RM (1977). Am. J. Cardiol., 40, 550-555.
72. Jugdutt BI, Hutchins GM, Bulkley BH, Pitt B and Becker LC (1979). Circulation 59, 734-743.
73. Mullane KM and Moncada S (1982). Prostaglandins, 24, 255-266.
74. Romson JL, Hook BG, Rigot VH, Schork MA, Swanson DP and Lucchesi BR (1982). Circulation, 66, 1002-1011.
75. Simmons PM, Salmon JA and Moncada S (1983). Biochem. Pharm., 32, 1353-1359.
76. Romson JL, Hook BG and Kunkel SL, Abrams GD, Schork MA and Lucchesi BR (1983). Circulation, 67, 1016-1023.
77. Jugdutt BI, Hutchins GM, Bulkley BH and Becker LC (1980). Am. J. Cardiol., 46, 74-82.
78. Darsee JR, Kloner RA and Braunwald E (1981). Circulation, 63, 29-35.

79. Meacock AC and Kitchen EA (1976). Agents and Actions, 6, 320-325.
80. Bonow RO, Lipson LC, Sheehan FH, Capurro NL, Isner JM, Roberts WC, Goldstein RE and Epstein SE (1981). Am. J. Cardiol., 47, 258-264.
81. Bolli R, Goldstein RE, Davenport N and Epstein SE (1981). Am. J. Cardiol., 44, 841-847.
82. Hook BG, Romson JL, Jolly SR, Bailie MB and Lucchesi BR (1982). J. Cardiovasc. Pharm., 5, 302-308.
83. Ogletree ML and Lefer AM (1976). J. Pharmacol. Exp. Ther., 197, 582-593.
84. Libby P, Maroko PR, Bloor CM, Sobel BE and Braunwald E (1973). J. Clin. Invest., 52, 599-607.
85. Johnson AS, Scheinberg SR, Gerisch RA and Saltzstein HC (1953). Circulation, 7, 224-228.
86. Diaz PE, Fishbein MC, Davis MA, Askenazi J and Maroko PR (1977). Am. J. Cardiol., 40, 541-549.
87. Kloner RA, Reimer KA, Willerson JT and Jennings RB (1976). Proc. Soc. Exp. Biol. Med., 151, 677-683.
88. Hess ML, Okabe E, Poland J, Warner M, Stewart JR and Greenfield LJ (1983). J. Cardiovasc. Pharm., 5, 35-43.
89. Maroko PR, Libby P, Sobel BE, Bloor CM, Sybers HD, Shell WE, Covell JW and Braunwald E (1972). Circulation, 45, 1160-1175.
90. Shlafer M, Kane PF and Kirsh MM (1982). Cryobiology, 19, 61-69.
91. Shlafer M, Kane PF and Kirsh MM (1982). J. Thorac. Cardiovasc. Surg., 83, 830-839.

EICOSANOIDS AND THE ENDOTHELIUM:
STUDIES IN VIVO AND IN VITRO[1]

Babette B. Weksler
Division of Hematology-Oncology
Department of Medicine
Cornell University Medical College
New York, NY 10021

I. INTRODUCTION

The vascular endothelium has been termed nature's most
blood-compatible container, implying its suitability for
maintaining blood liquidity and for efficient repair of any
breaching injury. The functions of the endothelium reach far
beyond those of a passive container. Endothelium is an
active secretory and excretory tissue, produces hemostatic as
well as anti-thrombotic substances, provides a selective
permeability and filtration system, regulates normal
leukocyte exodus from the blood, modulates vascular tone, and
has immunologic function. Keeping the circulating blood
liquid is now known to be an active process in which the
endothelium plays many roles. For example, endothelium
releases Von Willebrand factor, necessary for normal platelet
function (1), and specifically binds several coagulation
factors including factors IX, X and thrombin (2,3). Through
such localized thrombin-mediated activation of plasma protein
C involving an endothelial cell cofactor, thrombomodulin,
coagulation factors Va and VIIIa are inactivated (4). In
addition, endothelium produces and releases plasminogen
activator which initiates the fibrinolytic process (5). The
plasma surface membrane of endothelium is coated with heparan
sulphate, an anticoagulant, and contains ecto-enzymes which
break down adenine nucleotides to adenosine, inactivate
kinins and convert angiotensin I to II (6). Finally,
endothelium produces the antiaggregatory prostaglandin
prostacyclin (PGI_2) (7,8), which inhibits platelet shape
change, secretion and aggregation and prevents the binding of
Von Willebrand factor and fibrinogen to receptors on the
platelet surface membrane (9,10).

Prostacyclin production thus represents only one of
several antithrombotic properties of the vascular endo-

[1]Supported by grants from a NIH SCOR in Thrombosis (HL
18828), Research Center in Cerebrovascular Disease (5PO
NS03346) and by a Faculty Research Award from the American
Cancer Society.

thelium. However, this powerful autocoid - for PGI_2
is probably not a circulating hormone, but a locally active
substance (11-13) - has a major role in normal hemostasis and
blood flow. This chapter will review the present state of
knowledge about control of PGI_2 synthesis in the vascular
endothelium, and the interaction of endothelium with other
arachidonic acid metabolites.

II. SYNTHESIS OF PGI BY VASCULAR ENDOTHELIUM

When PGI_2 was first identified as the main enzymatic
product of arachidonic acid metabolism in aortic homogenates,
it was soon recognized that vascular endothelial cells
on a tissue mass basis, synthesized the largest amount of
this PGI_2. Endothelium from rabbit aorta, which represents
1% by weight of the aortic wall, synthesized 40% of the PGI_2;
the medial smooth muscle layer another 40%, and the
adventitia a smaller amount (14). Most PGI_2 which reaches
the vascular lumen is derived from the endothelium and not
from smooth muscle layers. In tissue denuded of endothelium,
PGI_2 production diminishes acutely and returns toward the
normal range only with the development of a vascular
neointima consisting of migrated smooth muscle cells, or with
reendothelialization (15,16). PGI_2 is the main product of
arachidonic acid metabolism in endothelium derived from human
umbilical vein, pulmonary artery and vein and aorta; bovine
aorta, pulmonary artery and capillaries (cerebral, adrenal,
retinal, or cardiac); rat aorta and porcine aorta. The
spectrum of tissues producing PGI_2 has recently been
summarized (17).

PGI_2 synthesis by endothelium grown in tissue culture
requires stimulation; all the PGI_2 produced is promptly
released from the cells; none remains intracellular. While
PGI_2 is usually produced from endogenous arachidonate, it has
been clearly shown that stimulated platelets in close
contiguity to endothelial cells donate released endoperoxide
for conversion by the endothelial cells to PGI_2 (18). This
"endoperoxide steal" phenomenon is enhanced by inhibition of
platelet thromboxane synthetase (19).

Factors controlling the synthesis of PGI_2 by endothelial
cells in tissue culture include growth state, availability of
substrate, type of stimulus, and the tonicity, ionic
composition and protein components in the medium. Agents
which stimulate PGI_2 synthesis in endothelium are listed in
Table 1.

Table I. Stimuli for PGI_2 Synthesis

Physical:	Hypoxia, hypotonicity, change in shear stress, Temperature
Chemical:	Arachidonic acid, prostaglandin endoperoxides Angiotensin II, histamine, bradykinin Thrombin, trypsin, ADP, ATP High density lipoprotein
Pharmacologic:	Nitroglycerin, dipyridamole, hydralazine, heparin, furosemide, calcium ionophores

These agents activate endothelial cell phospholipase A_2 which releases endogenous arachidonate for immediate enzymatic conversion to PGI_2 and to a lesser extent, other prostaglandins. Only a small percent of the total intra-cellular arachidonate content is available for PGI_2 synthesis. In contrast, exogenous arachidonate is not efficiently used for PGI_2 synthesis, with less than 1% of substrate being converted even at optimal arachidonate concentration (10-20 μM in buffer systems) (18). Exogenous endoperoxide, however, is 80% or more converted to PGI_2. The growth state of the tissue culture is an important determinant of PGI_2 synthetic capacity, which varies with species. In human cells, maximal PGI_2 synthesis occurs at a preconfluent stage, especially if thrombin is used as the stimulus. It can be shown that thrombin receptors are present in greater number in log phase as opposed to confluent cultures (20). The behavior of bovine aortic endothelium provides an opposite example. Bovine aortic endothelial cells produce more PGI the longer they remain in a confluent state (21).

III. CONTROL OF PGI_2 BIOSYNTHESIS BY ENDOTHELIUM

Vascular endothelium requires preformed arachidonate for PGI_2 synthesis, and appears to lack the capacity to transform linoleic acid to arachidonic acid (22,23), since it lacks elongation and desaturation enzymes necessary for this step (human fibroblasts and smooth muscle cells, however, can convert linoleic to arachidonic acid). Incubation of endothelial cells with linoleate results in an inhibition of PGI_2 synthesis and a decrease in cellular arachidonate content, suggesting that linoleic acid can block arachidonate accumulation and utilization by endothelium. Similarly,

eicosapentaenoic acid produces decreased endothelial PGI_2
production, without a compensatory increase in PGI_3
formation; eicosapentaenoic acid is a poor substrate for
endothelial cyclooxygenase and inhibits the function of this
enzyme, as it does in platelets (24).

The regulation of phospholipase activity in the vascular
endothelium has been less well studied. Vasoactive hormones
and amines, serine proteases and mechanical factors which
stimulate prostaglandin synthesis from endogenous
arachidonate all activate phospholipase A_2 via surface
receptor-mediated mechanisms (25). These stimuli can be
shown to release cellular arachidonate if cyclooxygenase is
blocked and a binding substance such as albumin is present in
the medium. This activation is calcium dependent, and can be
enhanced by calcium ionophores and inhibited by EDTA or TMB-8
(8,N,N-diethylamine)-octyl-3,4,5-trimethyoxy benzoate), an
antagonist of cytoplasmic free calcium ion (26). This
activation is only weakly calmodulin dependent and is not
easily blocked by trifluoroperazine (Weksler, unpublished
observations). Because PGI_2 itself strongly stimulates
adenylate cyclase, and cyclic AMP regulates cytosolic Ca^{++}
concentration, the possibility that PGI_2 may regulate its own
synthesis by inducing high cAMP concentrations in endothelial
cells producing PGI_2 has been explored (27). High
endothelial cell cAMP phosphodiesterase activity requires the
presence of a phosphodiesterase inhibitor in order for PGI_2
to raise cAMP levels. In the presence of the
phosphodiesterase inhibitor, isobutylmethylxanthine (MIX),
PGI_2 synthesis induced with thrombin or the ionophore A23187
was blocked and arachidonate release partially inhibited but
PGH_2-induced PGI_2 production was unaffected (28,27).
However, when endothelial cell cAMP was raised by exposing
cells to forskolin, a strong direct stimulus of adenylate
cyclase, PGI_2 production was not inhibited although cAMP
levels rose higher than in the presence of PGI_2-MIX (29).
Thus, PGI_2 synthesis is not controlled directly by
endothelial levels of cAMP. The inhibition of PGI_2
production observed in the presence of phosphodiesterase
inhibitors represents a different effect, probably
phospholipase inhibition. The partial inhibition of PGI_2
synthesis by the combination of isoproterenol and MIX or
isoproternol and propranolol most likely also represents
blocking of arachidonate release (30).

Exposure of endothelium to arachidonate at first
activates, and then rapidly inactivates, endothelial
cyclooxygenase because of peroxidative attack by products of

this reaction (29). It has been recently demonstrated that
"protection" of the cyclooxygenase by a reversible inhibitor
(such as ibuprofen) during exposure of endothelial cells to
arachidonate will prevent the inactivation of cyclooxygenase;
the exogenous arachidonate is acylated into cellular
phospholipids and becomes available for eicosanoid synthesis
when the cyclooxygenase inhibitor is subsequently removed
(29). Prostacyclin synthetase, in contrast, is not
inactivated by exposure of cells to arachidonate or to
endoperoxides, and continues to produce PGI_2 during repeated
exposure to endoperoxide. While PGI_2 synthetase in intact
cells appears resistant to inactivation by its products,
isolated PGI_2 synthetase can be inactivated by peroxidation
(31,32). Similar findings have been obtained when
arachidonate metabolism was studied in intact rabbit aortas
perfused in situ: cyclooxygenase was preferentially
inactivated during perfusion with arachidonate whereas
prostacyclin synthetase activity, evaluated by PGI_2
production upon perfusing with endoperoxides, was maintained
(33). Lipid peroxides, in particular 15-hydroperoxy-
arachidonic acid (15-HPAA) and 12-HPAA, are specific
inhibitors of PGI_2 synthesis at concentrations which do not
affect cyclooxygenase (10-100 µM) (34), and may also inhibit
arachidonate release from phospholipid (35).

These recent studies may help to explain the inhibitory
effects of low density lipoproteins (LDL) on endothelial cell
PGI_2 production (36), as low density lipoproteins are easily
peroxidized and thus may serve as inhibitors of endothelial
cyclooxygenase. In contrast, high density lipoproteins (HDL)
have been shown to enhance PGI_2 synthesis during cell
culture, without having an immediate stimulatory effect on
PGI_2 production (37). The HDL appear to serve as a source of
arachidonate -- rat HDL which are unusually rich in
arachidonate content, had a greater effect than porcine or
human HDL on bovine endothelial cells. HDL may also displace
LDL from endothelial membrane receptors. All these actions
of HDL would tend to augment both the synthesis of enzymes
in the prostaglandin pathway and PGI_2 synthesis itself.
Additionally, endothelial cells can "process" LDL and degrade
it so that the LDL are taken up by tissue macrophages by a
salvage mechanism, via the acetyl LDL receptor (38).

IV. INHIBITION OF PGI_2 SYNTHESIS
Despite earlier controversy, it has become clear that
endothelial cell cyclooxygenase in intact cells in vitro or
in blood vessels is as sensitive to inhibition by aspirin and
non-steroidal anti-inflammatory agents as is the platelet

enzyme (39). The ID_{50} for aspirin in vitro is less than 3 µM. Because protein synthesis by endothelial cells rapidly replaces inactivated cyclooxygenase, the recovery of cellular capacity to synthesize PGI_2 begins within a few hours, and is complete by 24-36 hours (39,40). Cyclooxygenase inhibition by other non-steroidal anti-inflammatory agents is of briefer duration, as many agents appear to block cyclooxygenase by a competitive, reversible mechanism. Ibuprofen, for example, must be present in the medium to block PGI_2 production by cultured monolayers (40a). Sulfinpyrazone is 100 times weaker an inhibitor of endothelial cell PGI_2 synthesis than is aspirin (41).

Since large clinical trials using aspirin to prevent recurrent myocardial infarction or stroke have shown only modest to no benefit, despite the documented platelet-inhibitory effect of the drug, attention has recently been focused on the possibility that vascular PGI_2 inhibition accompanied platelet inhibition by the aspirin used. This has led to examination of how vascular production of PGI_2 was affected by usual clinical doses of aspirin. Preston demonstrated that 150-300 mg oral aspirin profoundly inhibited ex-vivo PGI_2 synthesis by biopsies of normal veins for at least 8 hours (42). These findings were confirmed and extended by Hanley et al (43) who showed that 160 mg of aspirin taken by patients pre-operatively inhibited PGI_2 production by vein removed during saphenous vein surgery, and that partial inhibition continued at least 48 hours. In studies aimed at determining the minimal dose of aspirin which selectively inhibited platelet thromboxane formation, Patrignani et al (44) observed that 20-30 mg of aspirin daily inhibited platelet TXA_2 by 95% but did not inhibit urinary 6-keto PGF_{1a}, the main metabolite of renal PGI_2 synthesis. Correlating steady state aspirin dosage of 20-2600 mg/day with the urinary production of 2,3-dinor-6-keto-PGF_{1a}, the main metabolite of vascular PGI_2, Fitzgerald et al (45), showed that inhibition of 2,3-dinor production did not exceed 80-85%, even with high doses of aspirin every six hours. Further studies have been carried out in atherosclerotic subjects by Weksler et al (46). A single dose of 40-325 mg aspirin was administered 12 hours before coronary artery bypass graft surgery, and platelet function, platelet TXA_2 production and vascular PGI_2 production by segments of aorta and saphenous vein at the time of surgery were measured. TXA_2 production was partially inhibited (67%) by 40 mg aspirin and 95% inhibited by 80 mg aspirin, whereas inhibition of PGI_2 production by vascular tissue was less impaired: aortic PGI_2 production was inhibited 38% after 80 mg aspirin and 80% after 325 mg. Saphenous vein PGI_2 production was not inhibited after 80 mg aspirin but was 80% inhibited after 325 mg. Recently, these studies were extended to similar patients who took 20 mg of aspirin daily for the 7 days prior to their surgery (47). While serum TXB_2 fell by 85% and platelet aggregation was inhibited, aortic and venous PGI_2 were also partially inhibited after the course of aspirin compared to controls. The extent of PGI_2 inhibition depended upon the interval from the last dose of aspirin: when this was 24 hours, vascular PGI_2 fell by 48-52%; when the interval since the last aspirin dose was only 3 hours, PGI_2 fell by 70% in both aorta and vein. These studies and others (48), confirm the cumulative effect of even low dose aspirin on vascular cyclooxygenase, as well as on platelet cyclooxygenase. They also suggest a rapid restoration of vascular PGI_2 synthesis after aspirin. However, studies of urinary excretion of 2,3-dinor-6-keto PGF_{1a} in subjects treated with 20-2600 mg aspirin daily showed that recovery of vascular PGI_2 metabolite excretion after aspirin was discontinued was rather slow, requiring several days (45).

V. OTHER EICOSANOID PRODUCTS OF ENDOTHELIUM

In tissue culture, the main eicosanoid synthesized by endothelial cells is PGI_2, although smaller amounts (10% of total) of PGE_2, PGF_{2a}, and hydroxyacids are produced, especially when endogenous arachidonate serves as substrate. Dedifferentiation in culture, as occurs with porcine endothelial cells which lose the capacity to produce Von Willebrand factor, is accompanied by a shift from PGI_2 to PGE_2 production (49). Thromboxane A_2 production by endothelium has been documented in several systems: bovine endothelial cells in tissue culture and bovine aortic endothelium in intact vascular segments (50), rabbit intrapulmonary arterial rings (but not rabbit mesenteric or celiac arteries), (51) umbilical vessel rings and umbilical vein segments (52). In the latter system, thromboxane synthesis was favored at unphysiologically high concentrations of exogenous arachidonate. Ratios of PGI_2:TXA production in cultured endothelial cells ranged from 5-10:1 and in vascular segments were 100:1. Perfused lung releases many prostaglandins, thromboxane and leukotrienes: it is not clear which cells produce which eicosanoids as alveolar macrophages and lung interstitial cells have broad eicosanoid-synthesizing capacities. Lipoxygenase activity in endothelium appears to be very low. The hydroxyacid 12-HETE was identified in rabbit aortic rings, but not in human endothelial cells (53). Leukotrienes are produced in very

low amounts in cultured endothelium, although a recent report
indicated that chopped preparations of vascular tissue from
pig, rabbit, rat and dog can synthesize leukotrienes (54).

VI. ENHANCEMENT OF ENDOTHELIAL PGI_2 PRODUCTION

Certain vasodilator drugs stimulate PGI_2 production by
vascular endothelium in culture, whereas other vasodilators
enhance the biologic effect of PGI_2 or inhibit platelet
function directly. Nitroglycerin has been shown to increase
PGI_2 production by unstimulated endothelial cells (55), and
by vascular strips (56). The effect is rapid and is produced
by concentrations of nitroglycerin corresponding to those
achievable in clinical usage; these concentrations are less
than those required for a direct inhibitory effect upon
platelet function. Dipyridamole also has a modest
stimulatory effect, and also enhances the biologic effect of
PGI_2 through its phosphodiesterase inhibitory activity (57).
Nitroprusside, although a potent vasodilator, does not affect
PGI_2 production by cultured human endothelial cells.
However, the inhibitory effect of PGI_2 on platelet
aggregation is enhanced by nitroprusside in a synergistic
fashion (58).

Heparin produces relaxation of the dog coronary artery
strip and increased coronary flow in the isolated perfused
guinea pig heart by a mechanism which is aspirin-inhibitable
(59). In the heart, heparin perfusion produces an increase
in flow and in PGI_2 production (Eldor, unpublished
observations). Bolus heparin administered to human subjects
with coronary artery disease produces a prompt rise in
coronary flow accompanied by an increase in plasma PGI_2; both
enhancement of coronary flow and the increase in PGI_2 do not
occur in patients pre-treated with aspirin (60).

VII. AGE AND DISEASE-RELATED CHANGES IN ENDOTHELIAL PGI_2 PRODUCTION

Age-related differences in vascular PGI_2 production have
been described in animals and inferentially in humans. PGI_2
production is greater in fetal than in maternal vessels (61).
Aortic intimas from six month old pigs spontaneously produced
similar amounts of PGI_2 as intimas from mature (2-4 year old)
pigs, but in the presence of exogenous arachidonate the
initmal strips from the young animals synthesized twice as
much PGI_2 as strips from old animals. The fatty acid content
and composition of the intimas were the same for the two age
groups (62). It could be speculated that accumulation of

inhibitors of PGI_2 synthesis such as hydroperoxy fatty acids accumulate with age and limit PGI_2 production. The observation that bleeding time in humans shortens with age and is less affected by aspirin ingestion in older subjects (63) has been interpreted to indicate that vascular PGI_2 production may decrease with increasing age. However, our own direct measurements of PGI_2 production by segments of human aorta, both basal and stimulated with arachidonate, show no increase but rather a slight increase with age over the age range of 40-80 years (Weksler, unpublished observations). These observations, however, were made on full-thickness arterial segments and not on endothelium only, which may respond differently.

Several case reports in which atheromatous plaques were assayed for PGI_2 activity have indicated that vascular prostacyclin activity is decreased in the atherosclerotic lesion concomitant with a decrease in fibrinolytic activity (64). One report suggested that even a fatty streak lesion showed the same decrease in PGI_2 production (about 35%) as a complicated atheromatous plaque (66). On the other hand, we have studied aortic biopsies from patients with atherosclerosis who were having coronary artery surgery; aortic atherosclerosis was minimal to moderate (intimal-medial ratios of 5-25%; little cholesterol deposition or cellular infiltration) (46). Within the range of atherosclerosis observed, there was no correlation between PGI_2 production and the amount of atherosclerotic change determined morphologically. In rabbits made hypercholesterolemic for 5 months, aortic mesenteric artery rings, as well as perfused heart preparations, showed decreased PGI_2 synthetic capacity which was explained as the possible result of increased exposure to lipid peroxides (65). Similar findings were reported in rats made diabetic with streptozotocin (67), and in vascular tissue of infants of diabetic mothers (68). Many of these studies utilized vascular rings, so that it is not possible to distinguish endothelial from smooth muscle contributions to the PGI_2 production. In several conditions associated with thrombosis, vascular tissue has been found to produce increased amounts of PGI_2. Animals given high dose estrogen-progesterone combinations, spontaneously hypertensive rats (which are stroke-prone), and rabbits fed a high cholesterol-high fat diet all showed increased vascular prostacyclin (69).

Speculation about disturbed PGI_2 synthesis has been advanced in several other disease states. In the

hemolytic-uremic syndrome, some patients' plasma fail to
elicit PGI_2 production from normal vascular tissue or
cultured endothelial cells and it has been postulated that a
deficiency of a stimulatory plasma factor is responsible for
the syndrome. In women who have a circulating "lupus"
anticoagulant, with a history of multiple thrombotic episodes
and multiple miscarriages, the presence of a plasma inhibitor
of PGI_2 production has been documented; this presumably is an
antibody directed against phospholipid which inhibits
phospholipase activity, as lupus anticoagulants are
antibodies with anti-phospholipid specificity (70).
Conversely, in uremic patients, who manifest bleeding
tendencies and poor platelet function, a plasma factor has
been found which stimulates the release of PGI_2 from cultured
endothelial cells (71). In Bartter's syndrome, there is
evidence that the defective platelet function and hypotension
may be related to high levels of circulating PGI_2 or a
metabolite (72). Since recent studies have indicated that
normally plasma levels of PGI_2 are almost undetectible and
(11-13) certainly are several orders of magnitude lower than
that needed to affect platelet function or vascular tone,
these earlier studies warrant repeating with measurement of
steady state urinary excretion of 2,3-dinor-6-keto PGF_{1a}, the
major metabolite of plasma PGI_2.

VIII. OTHER ENDOTHELIAL EFFECTS ON VASCULAR WALL FUNCTION
INVOLVING ARACHIDONIC METABOLISM

The relaxation of isolated arteries induced by
vasoactive mediators such as acetylcholine, ATP, bradykinin,
thrombin, and arachidonic acid is dependent upon the presence
of endothelium in human, canine and rabbit vessels (73).
However, except for relaxation induced by arachidonate, the
mechanism of the vascular response does not appear to involve
prostacyclin. Prostacyclin relaxes de-endothelialized
vascular strips directly, and its action is not affected by
cyclooxygenase or lipoxygenase inhibitors. Acetylcholine
relaxes arteries from humans, dogs or rabbits via the
endothelial-dependent production of a factor which is not a
prostaglandin (no inhibition by cyclooxygenase or PGI_2
synthetase inhibitors), but is derived from arachidonic acid,
possibly via lipoxygenase (75). Variable inhibitory effects
of different lipoxygenase inhibitors on production of the
relaxing factor in different species have made its
characterization difficult. Bradykinin relaxes canine and
human arteries by a mechanism which also requires endothelium
and which is partially blocked by mepacrine and by ETYA,
inhibitors respectively of phospholipase A_2 and of

cyclooxygenase/lipoxygenase (76). This suggests that the relaxing factor is a fatty acid derivative of unknown type, possibly a hydroxyacid. Thrombin also causes relaxation of canine femoral arteries and veins by pathway requiring the presence of endothelium. It should be recalled that endothelium avidly binds thrombin. However, this type of relaxation is not inhibited by indomethacin, mepacrine, ETYA or HPETE and therefore does not appear to involve any known metabolites of arachidonate. Tachyphylaxis to the effect of thrombin was observed; relaxation responses were not restored by arachidonate but could be restored by acetylcholine. ATP produced a similar relaxation response unmodified by inhibitors of arachidonate metabolism.

IX. SUMMARY

Vascular endothelium has multiple anti-thrombotic and hemostatic functions, many of which involve eicosanoids, in particular, prostacyclin. It is now recognized that arachidonate metabolism by endothelium may differ from that in deeper layers of the vessel wall, and may affect both blood cell behavior and vascular smooth muscle function. Methods now under development will permit evaluation of the biochemical interactions between the endothelium and adjacent tissues and thus allow their pharmacological control.

REFERENCES

1. Jaffe, E.A., Hoyer, L.W., and Nachman, R.L. (1974). Proc. Nat. Acad. Sci. 71:1906.
2. Awbrey, B.J., Hoak, J.C., and Owen, W.G. (1979). J. Biol. Chem. 254:4092.
3. Stern, D., Drillings, M., and Nossel, H.L. (1983). Clin. Res. 31:485A.
4. Esmon, C.T., and Owen, W.G. (1981). P. N. A. S. 78:2249.
5. Levin, E.G., and Loskutoff, D.J. (1979). Thrombosis Research, 15:869.
6. Johnson, A.R. (1980). J. Clin. Invest. 65:841.
7. Moncada, S., Gryglewski, R., Bunting, S., and Vane, J.R. (1976a). Nature 263:663.
8. Weksler, B.B., Marcus, A.J., and Jaffe, E.A. (1977). Proc. Nat. Acad. Sci. 74:3922.
9. Hawiger, J., Parkinson, S., and Timmons, S. (1980). Nature 283:195.
10. Fujimoto, T., O'hara, S., and Hawiger, J. (1982). J. Clin. Invest. 69:1212.
11. Haslam, R.J., and McClenaghan, M.D. (1981). Nature 292:364.

12. Siess, W., and Dray, F. (1982). J. Lab. Clin. Med. 99:388.
13. Fitzgerald, G.A., Brash, A.R., Falardeau, and P. Oates, J.A. (1981). J. Clin. Invest. 68:1272.
14. Moncada, S., Herman, H.G., Higgs, E.A., and Vane, J.R., (1977). Thrombosis Research 11:323.
15. Eldor, A., Falcone, D.J., Hajjar, D.P., et al. (1981). J. Clin. Invest. 67:735.
16. Goldsmith, J.C., Jafvert, C.T., Lollar, P., Owen, W.G., and Hoak, J.C. (1981). Lab. Invest. 45:191.
17. Dusting, G.J., Moncada, S., and Vane, J.R. (1982). In "Advances in Prostaglandin, Thromboxane and Leukotriene Research" (J.A. Oates, ed.), Vol. 10, p. 59, Raven Press, N.Y.
18. Marcus, A.J., Weksler, B.B., and Jaffe, E.A. (1979). J. Biol. Chem. 253:7138.
19. Needleman, P., Wyche, A., and Raz, A. (1979). J. C. I. 63:345.
20. Shuman, M.A., Isaacs, J.D., Maerowitz, T., Savion, N. et al. (1981). Ann. N.Y. Acad. Sci. 370:57.
21. Eldor, A., Vlodavsky, I., Hyam, E., and Atzmon, R. et al. (1983). J. Cell Physiol. 114:179.
22. Spector, A.A., Hoak, J.C., Fry, G.L., Denning, G.M., et al. (1980). J. Clin. Invest. 65:1003.
23. Spector, A., Kaduce, T., Haok, D.C., Fry, G. (1981). J. Clin. Invest. 68:1003.
24. Whitaker, M.O., Wyche, A., Fitzpatrick, F., Sprecher, H., et al. (1979). Proc. Natl. Acad. Sci. 76:5919.
25. Alhenc-Gelas, F., Tsai, S., Callahan, K., Campbell, W., et al. (1982). Prostaglandins 24:723.
26. Brotherton, A.F.A., MacFarland, D.E., and Hoak, J.C. (1982) Thrombosis Research 28:637.
27. Hopkins, N.K., and Gorman, R.G. (1981). J. Clin. Invest. 67:540.
28. Brotherton, A.F.A. and Hoak, J. (1982a). Proc. Natl. Acad. Sci. USA 79:495.
29. Brotherton, A.F.A. and Hoak, J. (1982b). Circulation 66 (Supp II):178.
30. Adler, B., Gimbrone, M., Schafer, A., and Handin, R. (1981). Blood 58:514.
31. Turk, J., Wyche, A., and Needleman, P. (1980). BBRC 94:1628.
32. Weiss, S.J., Turk, J., and Needleman, P. (1981). Blood 53:1191.
33. Kent, R.S., Diedrich, S.L., and Whorton, A.R. (1982). Fed. Proc. 41:1642.
34. Moncada, S., Gryglewski, R.J., Bunting, S., and Vane, J.R. (1979b). Prostaglandins 12:715.

35. Hong, S.L., Carty, T., and Deykin, D. (1980). J. Biol. Chem. 255:9538.
36. Nordoy, A., Svensson, B., Wiebe, D., and Hoak, J.C. (1978). Circ. Res. 43:527.
37. Fleisher, L.N., Tall, A.R., Witte, L.D., Miller, R.W., et al. (1981). Circulation 64 (Suppl. IV):216.
38. Henriksen, T., Mahoney, E.M., Steinberg, D. (1981). Proc. Natl. Acad. Sci. (USA) 78:6499.
39. Jaffe, E.A., and Weksler, B.B. (1979). J. Clin. Invest. 63:532.
40. Czervionke, R.L., Smith, J.B., Fry, G.L., Hoak, J.C., et al. (1979). J. Clin. Invest. 63:1089.
40a. Parks, W.M., Hoak, J.C., Cervionke, R. (1981). J. Pharm. Exp. Ther. 219:415.
41. Gordon, J.L., and Pearson, J.D. (1978). Br. J. Pharmacol. 64:481.
42. Preston, F.E., Whipps, S., Jackson, C.A., French, A.J., et al. (1981) N. Engl. J. Med. 304:76.
43. Hanley, S.P., Cockbill, S.R., Bevan, J., Heptinsall, S. (1981). Lancet I:969.
44. Patrignani, P., Filabozzi, P., and Patrono, C. (1982). J. Clin. Invest. 69:1366.
45. Fitzgerald, G.A., Oates, J.A., Hawiger, J., Maas, R.L., et al. (1983). J. Clin. Invest. 71:676.
46. Weksler, B.B., Pett, S.B., Richter, R.C., Stelzer, P., et al. (1983a). N. Eng. J. Med. 308:800.
47. Weksler, B.B., Tack-Goldman, K., Karwande, S.V., and Gay, W.A., Jr. (1983b). Clin. Res. 31:486a.
48. Preston, F.E., Greaves, M., Jackson, C.A. and Stoddard, C.J. (1982). Thromb. Res. 27:447.
49. Ager, A., Pearson, J.D., and Gordon, J.L. (1979). Biochemical Soc. Trans. 7:1065.
50. Ingerman-Wojenski, C., Silver, M.J., Smith, J.B., and Macarak, E. (1981). J. Clin. Invest. 67:1292.
51. Salzman, P.M., Salmon, J.A., and Moncada, S. (1980). J. Pharm. Exp. Therap. 215:240.
52. Mehta, P., Mehta, J., Crews, F., Roy, L., et al. (1982). Prostaglandins 24:743.
53. Greenwald, J.C., Biandine, J.R., Wong, L.K. (1979). Nature 281:588.
54. Piper, P.J., Letts, L.G., Galton, S.A. (1983). Prostaglandins 25:591.
55. Levin, R.I., Jaffe, E.A., Weksler, B.B., Tack-Goldman, K. (1981). J. Clin. Invest. 67:762.
56. Schror, K., Grodzinska, L., Darius, H. (1981). Thromb Res. 23:59
57. Blass, K.E., Block, H.U., Forster, W., and Ponicke, K. (1980). Br. J. Pharmac. 68:71.

58. Levin, R.I., Weksler, B.B., Jaffe, E.A. (1982) Circulation 66:1299.
59. Eldor, A., Allan, G., Weksler, B.B. (1980). Thromb. Res. 19:719.
60. Wallis, J., Moses, J.W., Borer, J.S., Weksler, B.B., et al. (1982). Circulation 66 (Suppl II):263.
61. Terragno, N.A., Terragno, A. (1979). Fed. Proc. 38:75.
62. Kent, R.S., Kitchell, B.B., Shand, D.G., Whorton, A.R. (1981). Prostaglandins 21:483.
63. Jorgensen, K.A., Olesen, A.S., Dyerberg, J., and Stoffersen, E. (1979). Lancet II:302.
64. Sinzinger, H., Silberbauer, K., Winter, M., and Auerswald, W. Experientia 35(6):785.
65. Gryglewski, R.J., Dembinska-Kiec, A., Zmuda, A., and Gryglewska, T. (1978). Atherosclerosis 31:385.
66. Sinzinger, H., Silberbauer, K., Feigl, W., Wagner, O. et al. (1977) Thrombos. Haemost. 42:803.
67. Harrison, H.E., Reece, A.H. Johnson, M. (1978). Life Sciences 23:351.
68. Stuart, M.J., Sunderji, S.G., Allen, J.B. (1981). J. Lab. Clin. Med. 98:412.
69. Galli, C., Agradi, E., Petroni, A., Tremoli, E. (1981). Lipids 16:165.
70. Carreras, L.O., Machin, S.J., Deman, R., Defreyn, G. et al. (1981). Lancet I:244.
71. Defreyn, G., Vergara Dauden, M., Machin, S.J., and Vermylen, J. (1980). Thromb. Res. 19:695.
72. Gullner, H.G., Bartter, F.C., Cerletti, C., Smith, J.B. et al. (1979). Lancet II:767.
73. Furchgott, R.F., Zawadzki, J.V. (1980). Nature 288:373.
74. DeMey, J.G., Claeys, M., Vanhoutte, P.M. (1982). J. Pharmacol. Exp. Therapeut. 222:166.
75. Chand, N., Altura, B.M. (1981) Science 213:1376.
76. Cherry, P.D., Furchgott, R.F., Zawadzki, J.V. and Jothianandan, D. (1982). Proc. Natl. Acad. Sci. (USA) 79:2106.

V   BIOCHEMICAL BASIS
OF THE
ACTION OF TOXIC SUBSTANCES

MONOCLONAL ANTIBODY DIRECTED PHENOTYPING, RADIOIMMUNOASSAY,
AND PURIFICATION OF CYTOCHROMES P-450 THAT METABOLIZE
DRUGS AND CARCINOGENS

H. V. Gelboin, S.S. Park, B.J. Song, T. Fujino,
D. Robinson, and F. Friedman

Laboratory of Molecular Carcinogenesis
National Cancer Institute
NIH, Bethesda, Maryland   20205

I.   INTRODUCTION

The mixed-function oxidases containing cytochromes P-450
are the primary enzyme systems responsible for the metabolism
of a variety of xenobiotics including drugs, carcinogens, and
pesticides (1-3).   In addition, the cytochromes P-450 also
metabolize numerous classes of endogenous compounds such as
steroids, fatty acids, and prostaglandins (4).   With respect
to xenobiotics, including drugs and carcinogens, the cytochromes P-450 are the enzymatic interface between these environmental chemicals and higher organisms including humans.
The results of cytochrome P-450 catalyzed metabolism may be
either beneficial or hazardous to the organism.   Thus the
P-450's catalyze reactions that lead to detoxified metabolites that are safely excreted, as well as reactions that
convert the xenobiotics to their toxic, mutagenic, or carcinogenic forms.   For example, the microsomal cytochromes
P-450 convert benzo(a)pyrene in vitro to an active form that
is covalently bound to DNA (5).   The microsomal cytochromes
P-450 are the active component of the "S-9" fraction which is
extensively used for mutagen activation in the Ames mutagen
assay (6).   Thus, a very large preponderence of environmental
chemicals and drugs are either detoxified and/or activated by
the cytochrome P-450 system.

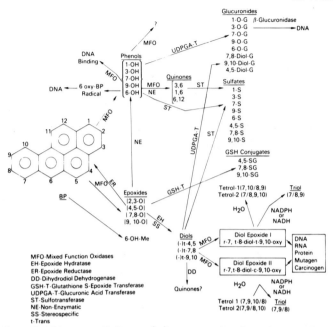

FIGURE 1. Pathways of Benzo(a)pyrene Activation and
Metabolism

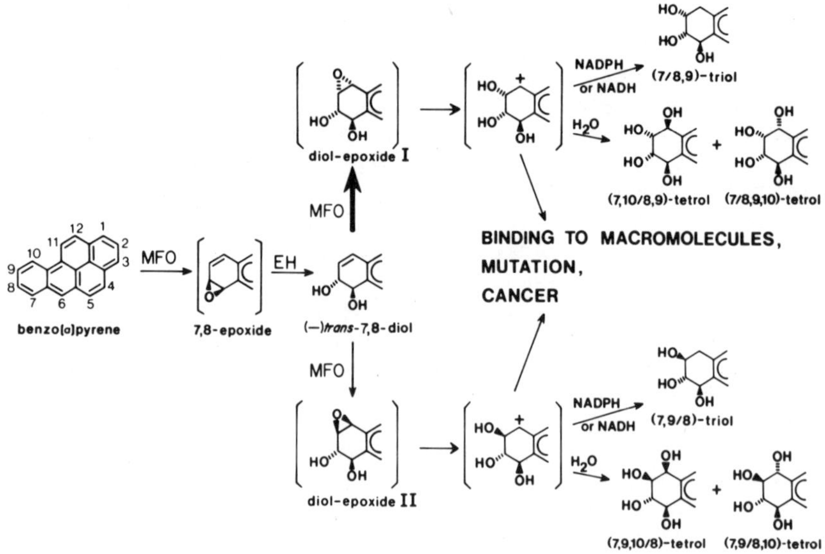

FIGURE 2. Activation Pathway of Benzo(a)pyrene to Diol
Epoxides

The Metabolic Activation and Detoxification of Benzo(a)pyrene (BP)

Figure 1 is a summary of our current knowledge of BP metabolism (1). BP is converted by the mixed-function oxidases to four unstable epoxide intermediates and five phenols, the 1,3,6,7 and 9 phenols. The phenols arise largely through epoxide re-arrangement but can also be formed by direct oxygenation. The epoxides are also enzymatically hydrated to three dihydrodiols by epoxide hydratase. We have shown that these two reactions are highly stereospecific and result in the production of three optically active trans dihydrodiols, the (-)-trans-7,-8, the 9,-10, and the 4,-5- dihydrodiol. The phenols also can be converted to three quinones. All of these oxygenated intermediates are further metabolized to water-soluble products by conjugation with either glutathione, sulfate, or glucuronic acid. Almost all of these metabolites are detoxification products and exhibit little or no mutagenic, DNA-binding, or carcinogenic activity. The free phenols however do show some toxicity to cells in culture, but in vivo are found as non-toxic conjugated forms. Figure 2 shows the major pathway of activation of BP is by oxygenation by the mixed function oxidases to the 7, 8-epoxide which is stereospecifically converted to one of four possible isomers, the (-)-trans-7, 8-diol. This product in turn is further metabolized by the mixed-function oxidases to predominantly one of eight possible isomers, a 7,8-diol-9,10-epoxide which we have termed diol epoxide I. About 10% of the biologically formed (-)-trans-7,8-diol is also converted to a different isomeric 7,8-diol-9,10-epoxide which we term diol epoxide II. The diol epoxides are very unstable and are rapidly converted to specific tetrols in the presence of water or to triols in the presence of NADPH. We were able to characterize the unstable diol epoxide by isolating and characterizing the respective tetrol hydrolysis and triol reduction products. Each diol epoxide forms two unique tetrols and a unique triol which we separated by HPLC and characterized by mass spectrometry and the formation of acetonide derivatives (7,8). The numbers on each side of the slash indicate which hydroxyl groups are on the same side of the ring. We also measured the mutagenic activity of all the unconjugated metabolites of benzo(a)pyrene in the Ames assay and a mutagen detecting mammalian cell system in vitro. We found the diol epoxide I to be a super mutagen with as as much as 100-to 1000-fold greater activity than the other metabolites. (see review-reference 1 and 8). The phenols, diols and quinones exhibit very low or insignificant levels of mutagenic activity. Subsequent studies (9) showed that the major form of BP bound to DNA was the same as the compound

TABLE 1

BP Metabolites Formed by Purified Cytochromes P-450 from Liver
of 3-MC, and PB-treated rats

BP metabolites formed	Sp. act.(pmol/min/nmol P-450)				Ratios of Metabolites (%) 3MC:PB
	MC-P-450	%	PB-P-450	%	
Unknown II	115	(2)	11	(5)	2:5
9,10-Diol	112	(2)	25	(10)	2:10
4,5-Diol	228	(4)	21	(9)	4:9
7,8-Diol	410	(8)	10	(4)	8:4
Fraction 1	165	(3)	27	(11)	3:11
9-OH-BP	548	(10)	7	(3)	10:3
7-OH-BP	362	(7)	2	(1)	7:1
1-OH-BP	92	(2)	15	(6)	7:6
3-OH-BP	1503	(27)	15	(6)	27:6
1,6-Quinone	568	(11)	4	(2)	11:2
3,6-Quinone	639	(12)	4	(2)	12:2
6,12-Quinone	158	(3)	4	(2)	3:2
Unknown	493	(10)	111	(44)	1:4

TABLE 2.   Stereospecificity of Diol Epoxide I and Diol
            Epoxide II Formation from (-)-trans-7,8-diol
            by Various Forms of Cytochrome P-450

Metabolites of (-)-trans-7,8-diol	Activity (pmol/min/nmol P-450)					
	LM_2	LM_4 (BNF)	LM_4 (PB)	LM_1	LM_{3b}	LM_7
Diol epoxide I	5.7	117.5	178.8	28.9	7.8	13.5
Diol epoxide II	6.5	10.7	15.7	17.8	4.0	42.8
Ratio I/II	0.9	11.0	11.4	1.6	2.0	0.3

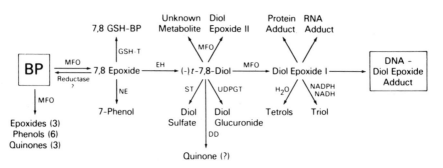

FIGURE 3.   Alternative Pathways of BP to Diol Epoxide I
             Formation

we characterized as diol epoxide I with super-mutagen
activity. Figure 3 is a summary of the activation pathway
from BP to the diol epoxide I which covalently binds to
DNA. It also shows all the possible alternative pathways
that the benzopyrene molecule can traverse. These are all
largely detoxification pathways.

Cytochrome P-450 Regio- and Stereoselectivity

At this state of our studies we were confronted with the
problem of understanding the factors that govern alternate
routes of metabolism. We have found that the different
forms of cytochrome P-450 exhibit both substrate and product
positional selectivity as well as stereoselectivity (1). We
used a high-pressure liquid chromatography system to analyze
the amount of benzo(a) pyrene metabolites formed in a reconstituted microsomal mixed-function oxidase systems containing
different cytochromes P-450 (1,10). We separated and identified ten metabolites of BP which included three diols: the
9,10-, 4,5-, and 7,8-dihydrodiols; four phenols, 9-, 7-,1-,
and 3-hydroxybenzo(a)pyrene and three quinones: the 1,6-.
3,6-, and 6,12-quinones. Table 1 shows that the ratio of
metabolites formed by the MC-induced P-450 and the PB-induced
P-450 of rat liver differ greatly. For example, the 9,10-and
4,5-diols are preferentially formed by the PB-P-450 while the
7,9-diol is preferentially formed by the MC-P-450. Similar
differences exist with the phenols formed. Table 2 shows
that with BP(-)trans-7,8-diol as substrate, six different
purified rabbit liver cytochromes P-450 form relatively
different amounts of diol epoxides I and II. The ratios of
diol epoxide I to diol epoxide II range from 0.3 to 11.3.
Thus, different P-450s prefer to oxygenate the 7,8-diol on
different sides of the plane of this BP metabolite. These
studies indicated that each cytochrome P-450 exhibits a
positional specificity as well as a stereoselectivity in
respect to both substrate utilization and product formation.
Benzo(a)pyrene metabolism can be viewed as a prototype for
other carcinogens and for drugs. Thus, the form and amount
of the different cytochromes P-450 in a tissue may regulate
the balance between activation and detoxification pathways
of carcinogens and drugs and may determine tissue or individual susceptibility to drug sensitivity or to the carcinogenic
activity of chemicals.

With BP we soon realized that analysis of metabolite
levels in either in vivo or in vitro experiments could not
easily or precisely measure individual differences in active
metabolite formation since metabolic flux was altered by a
number of factors which could not adequately be controlled.
These include the multiplicity of cytochromes P-450, their

TABLE 3

CLASSES OF MONOCLONAL ANTIBODIES
TO DIFFERENT CYTOCHROMES P-450

P-450	Species	Inducer	Code	RIA	Immuno-Prec.	Enzyme Inhib.
LM_2	Rabbit	PB	1-26-11	+	+	+
			1-31-1	+	+	-
			1-31-4	+	-	-
LM_4	Rabbit	BNF	1-1-8	+	+	+ -
			1-4-3	+	-	-
MC	Rat	MC	1-7-1	+	+	+
			1-36-1	+	+	-
			1-43-1	+	-	-
PB	Rat	PB	2-66-3	+	+	-
			2-8-1-2	+	+	-
			1-48-9	+	-	-

heterogenous distribution in different tissues, endogenous
or exogenous inducer levels, local substrate and cofactor
levels, as well as competing metabolic pathways.

Monoclonal Antibodies to Cytochromes P-450

Numerous studies on cytochrome P-450 including enzyme
purification, kinetic, genetic, inhibitor, and immunological
studies have shown a multiplicity of basal and inducible
P-450s (11). Enzyme multiplicity and overlapping stereo-
and regioselectivity for different substrates and products
have limited the determination of P-450 phenotype in tissues
or individuals. Thus, the precise role of P-450s in the
metabolism or activation of specific xenobiotics and in
individual variation in drug and carcinogen responsiveness
has not been defined. We thought that a useful approach to
this problem could be made with monoclonal antibodies to
specific types of cytochromes P-450. Monoclonal antibodies
(MAbs) formed by potentially immortal hybridomas are pure
and precise probes for specific antigenic sites on enzyme
proteins (12, 13). Monoclonals that interefere with enzyme
activity can identify and target proteins functioning in
specific reactions. In the last three years we have prepared
and characterized panels of MAbs to four different types
of cytochrome P-450. These are a phenobarbital induced
P-450 (PB-P-450 LM2), and a 7,8-benzoflavone-induced P-450

(BNF-P-450 LM4), both from rabbit liver, and a 3-methyl-
cholanthrene (MC)-induced P-450 (MC-P-450) and a PB-induced
P-450 from rat liver. We have obtained in each case several
panels of different types of monoclonal antibodies to each
cytochrome P-450. One class binds the P-450 as measured by
radioimmunioassay (RIA), immuno-precipitates the P-450,
and inhibits P-450 enzyme activity. The other two classes
of monoclonal antibodies either bind only or bind and
precipitate the P-450 but do not inhibit enzyme activity
(14-17).

Inhibition of Cytochrome P-450 AHH and ECD Catalytic Activity by MAb 1-7-1

MAb 1-7-1 is a monoclonal that is specific for MC-P-450
in RIA binding, immuno-precipitation and enzyme inhibition.
We measured the inhibitory effects of the MAb 1-7-1 on two
enzyme activities catalyzed by cytochromes P-450, the aryl
hydrocarbon hydroxylase (AHH) which measures the oxidation
of benzo(a)pyrene to phenols and ethylcoumarin deethylase
(ECD) which measures the de-ethylation of this drug. The
MAb 1-7-1 is highly specific for the purified MC-P-450 rat
liver, inhibiting both of the latter activities by 92%. MAb
1-7-1 does not inhibit the activity of three other purified
P-450's tested. Table 4 also shows that the MAb 1-7-1 can
be useful in determining what proportion of enzyme activity
of a tissue is catalyzed by the class of P-450 which is
bound and inhibited by the MAb. Table 4 shows that both the
AHH and ECD activity of microsomes from control and PB induced
rats are entirely insensitive to inhibition by MAb 1-7-1.
Thus, both AHH and ECD in these microsomes are a function of
P-450s other than the type inhibited by MAb 1-7-1. With
microsomes from MC-treated rats, 70% of the activity of
both AHH and ECD is inhibited by MAb 1-7-1. Thus 70% of the
AHH and ECD activity in MC-microsomes is contributed by a
P-450 recognized by MAb 1-7-1. Thus 70% of both AHH and ECD
are catalyzed by either the identical P-450 or two P-450s
sharing a common antigenic site. The former is the more
plausible explanation since both activities are inhibited to
the same extent by MAb-1-7-1.

Phenotyping Tissue Content of Antigenically Distinct Cytochromes P-450 Responsible for Drug and Carcinogen Reactions

The same approach described above can be used to identify
the type of cytochrome P-450 responsible for any specific
drug or carcinogen reaction. Table 5, shows the liver AHH
and ECD of four different species and two strains of mice

TABLE 4. MAb 1-7-1 INHIBITION OF P-450 AND MICROSOMAL AHH AND ECD

Enzyme Source	AHH			ECD		
	Control	1-7-1	% Inhibition	Control	1-7-1	% Inhibition
Purified Cyt. P-450*						
P-450-MC	1177	97	92	110	9	92
Microsomes**						
MC-	11704	2872	75	5280	1556	71
PB-	600	615	0	1266	1164	8
Control	367	384	0	815	953	0

*pmol/min/nmol; **pmol/min/mg

TABLE 5. MAb 1-7-1 INHIBITION OF HEPATIC AHH AND ECD OF DIFFERENT SPECIES AND STRAINS

Species	Induction	AHH (pmol/min/mg)			ECD (nmol/min/mg)		
		Control	1-7-1	% Inhibition	Control	1-7-1	% Inhibition
Rat Sprague-Dawley	none	367	384	0	.82	.95	0
	PB	600	615	0	1.27	1.16	8
	MC	11704	2872	75	5.28	1.56	71
Mouse C57BL/6	none	88	87	1	6.4	5.6	12
	PB	128	125	2	7.0	5.8	17
	MC	5716	699	88	21.9	13.2	39
Mouse DBA/2	none	70	0	0	4.0	3.5	11
	PB	51	94	0	4.7	3.6	25
	MC	501	486	3	16.9	18.9	0
Guinea Pig NIH Outbred	none	282	209	0	2.0	2.1	0
	PB	703	722	0	2.9	3.0	0
	MC	1642	804	47	5.3	6.2	0
Hamster Golden Syrian	none	100	136	25	8.7	9.1	0
	PB	192	219	0	18.0	17.0	5
	MC	387	204	51	22.1	23.7	0

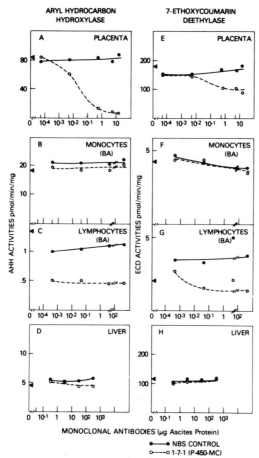

FIGURE 4.   Effect of Monoclonal Antibody 1-7-1 on the AHH
            and ECD Activities of Different Human Tissues

exposed to different inducers. The liver enzymes in rats are
highly induced for both AHH and ECD by MC and induced to a
lesser extent by PB. The MAb sensitive P-450 contributes
75% of the total activity of rat liver MC microsomes but
contributes none of the AHH or ECD activity of either the rat
liver control or PB microsomes. With the highly inducible
C57 strain mouse, 87% of liver AHH activity but only 39% of
ECD activity is contributed by the 1-7-1 sensitive P-450.
Thus, sixty percent of ECD depends on a P-450 that is different than the MAb 1-7-1 sensitive P-450. With DBA mice there
is far less induction by MC than in the C57 strain. The data
clearly show that the P-450 induced by MC in the DBA mice is
different than that induced in the C57 strain. Thus, the

inducible enzyme in the DBA mice is completely insensitive to
inhibition by MAb 1-7-1. In either control or induced guinea
pigs and hamsters none of the ECD is sensitive to MAb 1-7-1.
Thus all of the ECD in these species is catalyzed by a P-450
other than that sensitive to MAb 1-7-1. Like in rats, but
to a lesser extent, the MC induced form of AHH in guinea pigs
and hamsters is inhibited by MAb 1-7-1. Twenty five percent
of the control guinea pig AHH is due to MAb 1-7-1 sensitive
P-450. In other studies we found that we could measure the
contribution made by antigenically defined cytochromes P-450
to the metabolism of specific drugs in different tissues.

Analysis of P-450 Type in Human Tissue

We are interested in understanding the basis for individual variability of drug and carcinogen metabolism in humans.
Figure 4 shows the effects of MAb 1-7-1 on the control and
hydrocarbon inducible AHH and ECD of several human tissues
(18). Both AHH and ECD are elevated in the placenta of women
that smoke cigarettes (1-3). In non-smokers ECD is present
but at generally lower levels than in smokers, while AHH is
not detectable in the placenta of nonsmokers. The upper
section shows that at saturating levels of MAb 1-7-1 more
than 90% of AHH is inhibited whereas the ECD is inhibited
about 40%. In both normal and hydrocarbon-induced monocytes
none of the AHH or ECD activity is inhibited by the MAb
1-7-1 indicating that the P-450 responsible for this activity
in monocytes is different than the MAb 1-7-1 sensitive P-450
in placenta. With both control and induced lymphocytes,
about 50% of the AHH and ECD are inhibited by MAb 1-7-1
demonstrating that there are forms of P-450 sharing a common
antigenic site in both the control as well as in the induced
lymphocytes. Thus, a type of P-450 in induced lymphocytes is
also present in the basal control cells. Previous reports
have shown the presence and inducibility of AHH in human
lymphocytes (1), and genetic and lung cancer population
studies have suggested a trimodal distribution of AHH inducibility and a relationship to lung cancer (19, 20). However,
the latter studies have not been confirmed in twin studies
and studies in lung cancer patients (21). Thus, the status
of the theory that AHH inducibility is related to cancer is
uncertain. Our finding of two different forms of P-450
responsible for lymphocyte AHH and ECD may help to resolve
this issue. Normal human liver behaved like the monocytes
in that both the AHH and ECD activity were not inhibited by
the 1-7-1 and thus are catalyzed by a cytochrome P-450
antigenically distinct from the MAb 1-7-1 sensitive P-450.

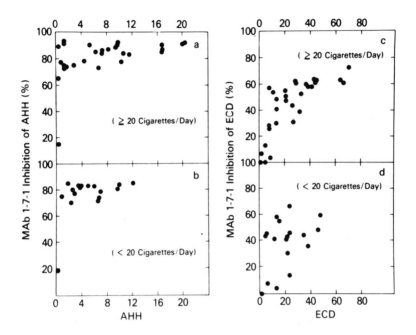

FIGURE 5.   Monoclonal Antibody 1-7-1 Inhibition of AHH
and ECD of Human Placenta from Women who
Smoke Cigarettes (Each point represents a
single placenta).

Figure 5 shows a population study of the effects of MAb
1-7-1 in both AHH and ECD of women who smoked cigarettes
(22). Each dot represents a placenta from a single individual
and shows that in both heavy and moderate smokers more than
80% the AHH is catalyzed by a type of P-450 containing an
antigenic site sensitive to MAb 1-7-1. With ECD, however,
there is a wide range of inhibition indicating the presence
of a second P-450 type which does not contain the antigenic
site sensitive to MAb 1-7-1. Thus, the ECD is catalyzed by
two types of P-450, one insensitive and one sensitive to MAb
1-7-1. Figure 6 shows the effect of 1-7-1 on the ECD of
non-smokers and smokers. With the exception of one individual
the ECD in non-smokers was inhibited by less than 20% by the
MAb 1-7-1. In twelve of the non-smoker individuals there was
no inhibition of the ECD by the MAb 1-7-1. With smokers
there was a positive relationship between the level of ECD

and its inhibition by MAb 1-7-1. Thus, our studies indicate
that there are two forms of P-450 responsible for placental
ECD. The MAb 1-7-1 can measure the amount of P-450 catalyzed
enzyme activity contributed by both the inducible and non-
inducible forms.

Monoclonal Antibody Directed Radioimmunoassay

In addition to analyzing tissues for the amount of cytochromes P-450 contributing to different xenobiotic reactions,
we have been developing methods for a competitive radioimmunoassay which would measure directly the cytochrome P-450
protein. With this type of assay it should be possible to
quantitatively determine the amount of cytochromes P-450
present in a tissue containing the antigenic site recognized
by specific monoclonal antibodies. This type of assay would
be able to detect P-450s independent of their catalytic
activity and would be useful with P-450 forms that are
unstable and that easily lose their enzymatic activity.
Figure 6 is an example of a competitive radioimmunoassay.
In this assay, the wells are coated with a standard preparation of microsomes from MC-treated rats or coated with purified MC-P-450. The ^{35}S-labelled MAb 1-7-1 is mixed with
the tissue containing an unknown amount of cytochrome P-450
antigen which titrates the MAb 1-7-1. The amount of MAb
1-7-1 remaining is measured by its binding to the well coated
with the known antigen. Figure 6 shows that serum albumin
or cytochrome C do not compete for ^{35}S-labelled MAb 1-7-1.
The MC induced rat liver microsomes compete most effectively
for antibody while the control and PB microsomes contain
less than one fiftieth of the MAb 1-7-1 recognized cytochrome
P-450 antigen. With this type of assay the monoclonal
antibody need not be of the enzyme inhibiting type but
simply one that binds the cytochrome P-450. This may be
useful in detecting P-450's that are labile with respect to
enzyme activity or P-450's present in exceedingly low concentrations in a tissue such as placenta or lymphocytes.

Monoclonal Antibody Directed Immunopurification of Cytochromes P-450

In another important application of the monoclonal antibodies we have found that a specific monoclonal antibody
covalently linked to Sepharose can be a useful immunoadsorbant
for the purification of individual cytochromes P-450. Figure
7 shows an SDS gel analyses of detergent-treated microsomes
from MC-treated, PB-treated and control rats. These microsomes were added to the Sepharose linked MAb 1-7-1. The right

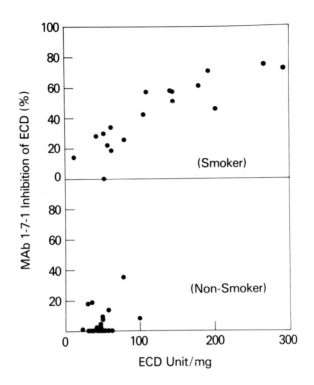

FIGURE 6.   Monoclonal Antibody 1-7-1 Inhibition of Placental
            ECD from Smokers and Non-Smokers. (Each point
            represents a single placenta)

side of the gel shows the Coomassie blue stained proteins
present in microsomes from control, PB and MC-treated rats
and the second three rows are the microsomal proteins that
did not bind to the Sepharose linked MAb 1-7-1. The left
side of the gel shows a single band of a P-450 present in
the microsomes from MC-treated rats which was bound by and
then eluted from the Sepharose linked MAb 1-7-1. Thus, the
Sepharose linked MAb 1-7-1 can selectively remove an antigenically distinct type of cytochrome P-450. No such protein
was found in either the control or the PB-microsomes. The
previously shown semi-quantitiative RIA data, however,
indicated the presence of a large amount of a MAb 1-7-1
binding P-450 in MC-microsomes but also a low level of this
type of P-450 in control and PB microsomes. The RIA indicated

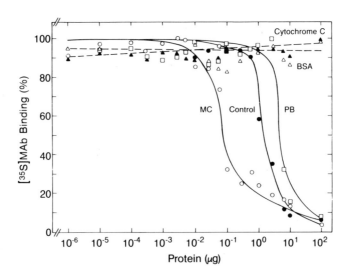

FIGURE 7.   Competitive Radioimmunoassay for MAb 1-7-1 specific
Cytochromes P-450 in the Liver Microsomes of
Control, PB-and MC-treated Rats.

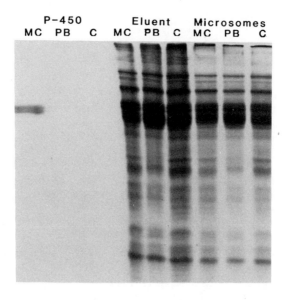

FIGURE 8.   Gel Electrophoresis of Proteins from solubilized
Rat Liver Microsomes and Protein bound and eluted
from Sepharose Bound MAb 1-7-1.

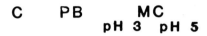

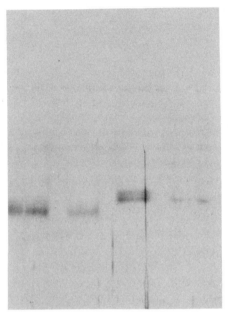

FIGURE 9.   Liver Microsomal Proteins from Control,
            Phenobarbital and MC-treated Rats That
            Bind and Elute from Sepharose bound MAb
            1-7-1.

that this protein was present at levels about one-fiftieth of
that in MC microsomes. We then examined the gels with a much
more sensitive silver staining method. Figure 8 shows the
Sepharose 1-7-1 bound P-450s present in MC, PB and control
microsomes. Two double bands of cytochromes P-450 of MW
54,000 and 52,000 from MC microsomes are recognized by the
MAb 1-7-1. We also observed MAb 1-7-1 binding cytochromes
P-450 at far lower concentrations in preparations from both
the control and the PB microsomes. The MAb 1-7-1 bound
cytochromes P-450s from both control and PB microsomes,
however, have a MW of 50,000 and migrate differently than
the MAb 1-7-1 bound P-450s from MC microsomes. Thus, the
MAb 1-7-1 recognizes the same epitope on two different

P-450's having different molecular weights. We expect that
this methodology will add much to our potential for isolating
and characterizing the multiplicity of cytochromes P-450.
The data also clearly indicate that the MC-induced P-450s
recognized by 1-7-1 are not present in control or PB rat
liver. The cytochromes P-450 are the enzyme interface between
higher organisms and environmental chemicals, drugs, and
many endogenous metabolites. Biochemical individuality in
responsiveness to these agents is complex and relates to both
environmental and genetic factors. The monoclonal antibodies
should be generally useful in determining the amount of a
specific cytochromes P-450 type, especially where a multiplicity of enzyme forms exist. The monoclonal antibody
directed characterization of tissue phenotype for cytochromes
P-450 may be useful in defining the enzymatic basis for
biochemical individuality. A library of monoclonal antibodies
to the different cytochromes P-450, may serve to prepare an
atlas of specific P-450s in different species, strains,
tissues, and individuals. These MAbs may be useful for
studying genetic control, phylogenetic evolution and the
changing distribution of cytochromes P-450 during fetal and
sexual development and after exposure to different inducers
and in different nutritional states. The monoclonal antibodies may thus be useful in understanding the role of
cytochromes P-450 in individual differences in responsiveness
to drugs and toxic agents and susceptibility to carcinogens.

ACKNOWLEDGMENT

    We wish to thank Holly Miller and Donna West for
excellent technical assistance.

REFERENCES

1. Gelboin, H. V., Physiol. Rev. 60:1107-1165 (1980).
2. Conney, A. H., Pharmacol. Rev. 19:317-366 (1967).
3. Conney, A. H., Burns, J. J., Science, 178:576-586,
    (1972).
4. Sato, R., Kato, R. (eds.)," Microsomes, Drug Oxidations,
    and Drug Toxicity". Japan Scientific Societies Press,
    (1982).
5. Gelboin, H. V., Cancer Res. 29:1272-1276, (1969).

6. Ames, B. N., Durston, W. E., Yamasaki, E., & Lee, F. D.,
    Proc. Natl. Acad. Sci. USA 79:281-2285, (1973).
7. Yang, S. K., McCourt, D. W., Roller, P. P., & Gelboin,
    H. V., Proc. Natl. Acad. Sci. USA 73:2594-2598, (1976).
8. Huberman, E., Sachs, L., Yang, S. K., & Gelboin, H. V.,
    Proc. Natl. Acad. Sci. USA 73:607-611, (1976).
9. Weinstein, I. B., Jeffrey, A., Jennette, K., Blobstein,
    H., Harvey, R., Harris, C., Autrup, H., Kasai, H., and
    Nakanishi, K., Science 193: 592-595, (1976).
10. Gozukara, E. M., Guengerich, F. P., Miller, H., and
    Gelboin, H. V., Carcinogenesis, 3:129-133, (1982).
11. Lu, A. Y. H., & West, S. B., Pharmacol. Rev. 31:277-295,
    (1980).
12. Kohler, G., & Milstein, D., Nature (London) 256:495-497,
    (1975).
13. Yelton, D. E., & Scharff, M. D., Ann. Rev. Biochem.
    50:657-680, (1981).
14. Park, S. S., Fujino, T., West, D., Guengerich, F. P., &
    Gelboin, H. V., Cancer Res. 42:1798-1808, (1982).
15. Park, S. S., Persson, A. V., Coon, M. J. & Gelboin,
    H. V., FEBS Lett. 116:231-235, (1980).
16. Park, S. S., Cha, S. J., Miller, H., Persson, A. V.,
    Coon, M. J., & Gelboin, H. V., Mol. Pharmacol.
    21:248-258, (1981).
17. Boobis, A. R., Slade, M. B., Stern, C., Lewis, K. M.,
    & Davies, D. S., Life Sc. 290:1443-1448, (1981).
18. Fujino, T., Park, S. S., West, D., Gelboin, H. V.,
    Proc. Natl. Acad. Sci. USA 70:3682-3686, (1982).
19. Kellermann, G., Lyuten-Kellerman, M., Shaw, D. R.,
    Am. J. Hum. Genet. 25:327-331, (1973).
20. Kellerman, G., Shaw, C. R., Luyten-Kellerman, M.,
    N. Engl. J. Med., 289:934-937, (1973).
21. Paigen, B., Gurtoo, H. L., Minowada, J., Houten L.,
    Vincent, R., Paigen, K., Parker, N. B., Ward, E., Hayner,
    N. T., N. Engl J. Med., 297:346-350, (1977).
22. Fujino, T., Gottlieb, K., Manchester, D. K., Park, S. S.,
    West, D., Gurtoo, H. L., and Gelboin, H. V., submitted
    for publication.

METAL REGULATION AND TOXICITY IN AQUATIC ORGANISMS[1]

Kenneth D. Jenkins

Department of Biology
California State University
Long Beach, California

Brenda M. Sanders

Duke University Marine Laboratory
Beaufort, North Carolina

William G. Sunda

National Marine Fisheries Service, NOAA
Southeast Fisheries Center
Beaufort Laboratory
Beaufort, North Carolina

I. INTRODUCTION

In recent years there has been substantial interest in
the impact of elevated trace metal concentrations on aquatic
organisms. While much of this attention has focused on the
relative toxicity of various metals or the relative sensitivity of species and their life stages, increasing emphasis
has been placed on the mechanisms which underly metal
metabolism and toxicity. These studies have drawn heavily
from mammalian toxicology and biochemistry and an improved
understanding of metal chemistry in complex aqueous systems.

Supported by grants from the Ecological Division, Department of Energy and the Ocean Assessment Division, National
Ocean Services, NOAA.

The development of metal-chelate buffer systems, which
control speciation of a number of metals simultaneously, has
proven to be a particularly useful tool for examining metal
bioavailability, metabolism and toxicity in aquatic systems
(1). In this paper we will briefly review previous work
with metal buffer systems and discuss the advantages they
provide. We will also review studies in which metal buffers
are used to examine the effects of metal interactions on
algal growth and the relationships between cupric ion
activities, copper uptake and growth in crab larvae.

II. METAL SPECIATION IN AQUEOUS MEDIA: THE IMPORTANCE OF FREE METAL ION ACTIVITY

The study of interactions between metals and aquatic
organisms is complicated by the fact that metals often exist
in a number of redox states and form complexes with a
variety of inorganic and organic ligands. The degree to
which these metal species occur is determined not only by
the activity of the metal ion in question but also by
activities of other metal ions, including H^+, which compete
for binding sites (2,3). The number of metal species and
their potential variability make it difficult to establish
causal relationships between dissolved metal concentrations
and biological effects. Metal speciation, however, can be
controlled and quantified by using highly chelated trace
metal ion buffers in which the ionic activities of the
metals are determined by equilibria between free metal ions
and chelated metal. As with pH buffers, metal ion
activities in trace metal buffers can be computed from
chemical equilibrium theory (4) and thermodynamic data for
stability constants (5,6).

From studies with these buffer systems it has been
demonstrated that availability and toxicity of metals such
as Cu, Cd, Zn are related to their free ion activities. As
an example Sunda and Guillard (1) have demonstrated that
both the cellular Cu content and growth rate (divisions/day)
of estuarine algae were related to cupric ion activity
rather than total Cu in the media. Furthermore, they found
a hyperbolic relationship between cellular Cu concentrations
and cupric ion activity. Similarly, higher order hyperbolic
relationships between Cu accumulation and free cupric ion
activity have been demonstrated in a number of marine
invertebrates (7,8,9). As with Cu, Cd accumulation has been
related to free cadmium ion activity but the relationship
appears to be linear rather than hyperbolic (10,11). Metal

toxicity in marine algae (12), invertebrates (13,14) and vertebrates (15) has also been related to free metal ion activity as has Cu inhibition of glucose and amino acid uptake by marine bacteria (16,17).

As with hydrogen ions, where the free ion activity (pH) determines hydrogen availability, there are thermodynamic considerations which dictate that metal availability and toxicity should be related to free metal ion activity: The activities of metal ions are a direct function of their free energy which at equilibrium determines the extent to which metals undergo complex formation or other chemical reactions. It is these chemical reactions – for example, the binding of metals to transport proteins which result in metal accumulation and toxicity.

III. EFFECTS OF COPPER-MANGANESE INTERACTIONS ON PHYTO-
     PLANKTON

Since trace metal buffers can be used to control the free ionic activities of several metals simultaneously they provide a useful tool for examining interactions between metals. Buffers utilizing EDTA (ethylenediaminetetraacetic acid), for example, have been used to control copper and manganese free ion activities in experiments that examined the effects of interactions between copper and manganese ions on the growth of unicellular algae (3,18). Manganese is a required trace nutrient of particular importance in algal cells where it functions in the oxidation of water during photosynthesis (19). Initial matrix experiments in which both copper and manganese ions were varied suggested copper toxicity in these organisms was a consequence of copper interfering with manganese metabolism (3).

To examine the mechanisms by which copper-manganese interactions affect copper toxicity, algal growth rates and cellular manganese concentrations were followed as a function of both copper and manganese ion activity (18). These data indicated that both cellular manganese concentration and growth rate increased with manganese activity (Figs. 1,2) approaching saturation values at high manganese ion activity. Increased cupric ion activity shifted these curves to higher manganese ion activities without changing either the shape of the curve or their maximum values. These data indicated that copper acted as a competitive inhibitor of manganese uptake. Furthermore, plots of growth rate vs cellular manganese concentrations indicated that cellular manganese was the principal factor controlling growth rate in these organisms (Fig. 3). These data then support a model in which algal growth rate is related to cellular manganese concentrations which is, in turn, controlled by competition between manganese and copper. Copper, therefore, was acting as a competitive inhibitor of manganese uptake, and its toxicity was a consequence of Mn deficiency.

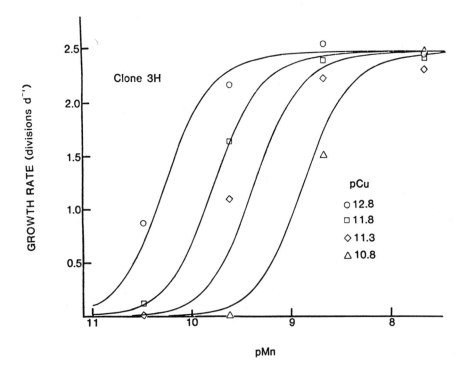

Figure 1. Growth rates of <u>Thalassiosira</u> <u>pseudonana</u> (Clone 3H) as functions of pMn at four different pCu values. pMn and pCu are negative logs of the computed free manganese and cupric ion activities and solid lines are model curves. From ref. (18).

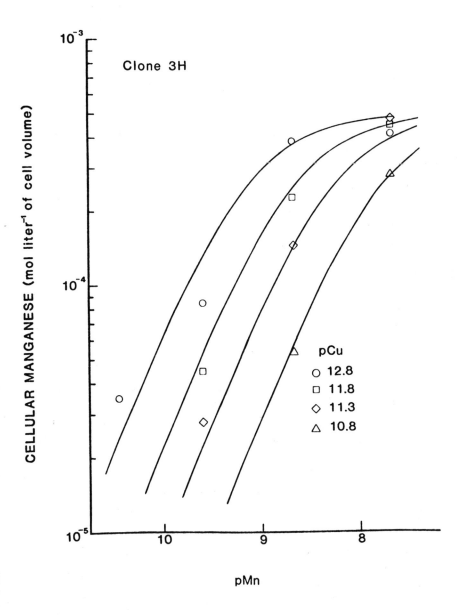

Figure 2. Cellular manganese concentrations as functions of pMn at four different pCu values. From ref. (18).

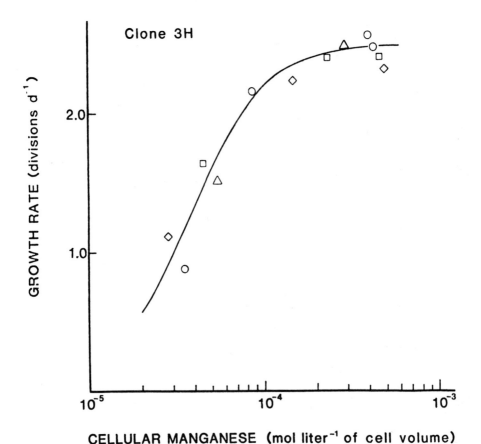

Figure 3. Growth rate as a function of cellular manganese concentrations for culture media at pCu 12.80 , 11.8⊔ , 11.3◇, and 10.8 △ . From ref. (18).

IV.   FREE CUPRIC ION ACTIVITY AFFECTS METALLOTHIONEIN AND
      GROWTH IN CRAB LARVAE

To further investigate the relationships between free metal ion activity, metal metabolism and toxicity we examined Cu uptake and subcellular distributions in crab larvae exposed to a range of free cupric ion activities (6). Metallothionein, a cysteine rich metal binding protein, serves as a major intracellular ligand for metals such as Cu, Zn, and Cd (17). Metallothioneins have been isolated

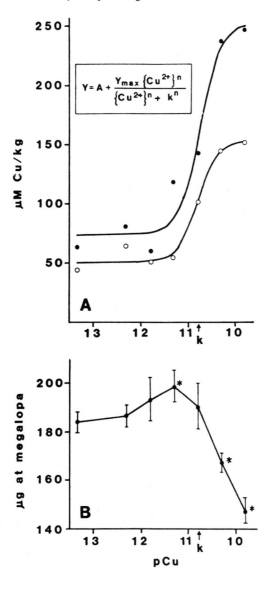

Figure 4.(A) Cytosolic distribution of copper in mud crab <u>Rhithropanopeus harrisii</u> megalopa exposed to a range of free cupric ion activities for the duration of larval development. Solid lines are derived from the inset equation. (B) Dry weights of mud crab megalopa described above. Vertical lines represent one standard error and asterisks indicate points which are significantly different by ANOVA and SNK. From ref. (9).

from vertebrates, invertebrates and higher plants and have been implicated in metal uptake, metabolism and detoxification (20,21,22,23). The primary structures of crab thioneins is homologous to mammalian thioneins and their synthesis is induced by Cu, Zn and Cd (22,23,24,25). The potential role of metallothionein in copper metabolism and toxicity therefore made the relationship between Cu-thionein accumulation, growth and cupric ion activities of particular interest.

Following Cu exposure, most of the cytosolic Cu (47–82%) was associated with metallothionein, with Cu-thionein most prominent (72–82%) at lower cupric ion activities (Fig. 4a). Copper thionein and total cytosolic Cu were independent of cupric ion activities at low exposure levels, increased at intermediate levels and approached saturation at higher levels. These relationships between cupric ion activity in the media, and Cu-thionein and cytosolic copper can be described by a second order hyperbolic equation. Although the biological significance of this relationship is as yet unclear, these data imply that crab larvae are able to regulate cytosolic copper concentrations over several orders of magnitude of cupric ion exposure.

To understand the physiological significance of these data we related free cupric ion activity to survival, duration of larval development and growth. Larval survival and duration did not change significantly over the entire range of cupric ion activities. Significant differences were observed, however, in the dry weight of larvae at megalopa: megalopa weight increased at a cupric ion activity of 5×10^{-12} M and decreased at activities beyond ca. 2×10^{-11} M (Fig. 4b). The observed increase in growth is termed hormesis, and is thought to result from transient overcorrections in the homeostatic regulation of growth in response to stress (26). At higher cupric ion activities the larvae have exceeded their capacity to compensate for stress and growth is inhibited. When Cu-thionein and growth were compared we found that larval growth was significantly reduced at cupric ion activities beyond the half-saturation constant (k) for the relationship between Cu-thionein and growth. This approach allowed us to establish a quantifiable relationship between increase in Cu-thionein, the major cytosolic Cu pool, and perturbations in larval growth.

V.   CONCLUSIONS

This paper demonstrates, with several examples using aquatic organisms, the advantages of using metal-chelate buffer systems to study the mechanisms of metal metabolism and toxicity. When used in seawater or modified growth media these buffer systems control the free ion activities of a number of metals simultaneously. This control enables the experimenter to systematically vary the free ion activity of the metal(s) of interest while maintaining the activities of the other essential metals constant. Because of the potential for metal interaction this control is particularly important to assure that changing the metal ion activity of one metal does not inadvertently alter the activities of other metals. Since it is the free metal ion activity which usually determines both biological availability and toxicity, these buffer systems are a powerful tool for the precise control of important experimental variables.

REFERENCES

1. Sunda, W., and Guillard, R.L. (1976) J. Mar. Res. 34, 511.

2. Cross, F.A., and Sunda, W.G. (1978) In "Estuarine interactions: 4th International Estuarine Research Conference" (M.L. Wiley, ed.) Academic Press, New York.

3. Sunda, W.G., Barber, R.T., and Huntsman, S.A. (1981) J. Mar. Res. 39, 567.

4. Stumm, W., and Morgan, J.J. (1981) "Aquatic Chemistry" 2nd ed. Wiley-Interscience, New York.

5. Sillen, L.G., and Martell, A.E. (1964) Stability Constants, special publication #17. The Chem. Soc. of London.

6. Smith, R.M., and Martell, A.E. (1976) Critical Stability Constants. Vol. 4. Plenum Press, New York.

7. Zamuda, C.D., and Sunda, W.G. (1982) Mar. Biol. 66, 77.

8. Crecelius, E.A., Hardy, J.T., Gibson, C.I., Schmidt, R.L., Apts, C.W., Gurtisen, J.M., and Joyce, S.P. (1982) Mar. Environ. Res. 6, 13.

9. Sanders, B.M., Jenkins, K.D., Sunda, W.G., and Costlow, J.D. (1983) in press.

10. Engel, D.W., Sunda, W.G., and Fowler, B.A. (1981) In "Biological Monitoring of Marine Pollutants" (J. Vernberg, A. Calabrese, F.P. Thurberg and W.G. Vernberg, eds.). Academic Press, New York.

11. Jenkins, K.D., Sanders, B., and P.S. Oshida (1983) MS in preparation.

12. Anderson, D.M., and Morel, F.M.M. (1978) Limnol. Oceanogr. 23(2), 283.

13. Andrew, R.W., Biesinger, K.E., and Glass, G.E. (1977) Water Res. 11, 309.

14. Sunda, W.G., Engel, D.W. and Tohuotte, R.M. (1978) Environ. Sci. Technol. 12, 409.

15. Engel, D.W., and Sunda, W.G. (1979) Mar. Biol. 50, 121.

16. Sunda, W.G., and Gillespie, P.A. (1979) J. Mar. Res. 34, 761.

17. Sunda, W.G., and Ferguson, R.L. (1983) In "Trace Metals in Sea Water" (Wong, Boyle, Bruland, Burton and Goldberg, eds.) Plenum, New York.

18. Sunda, W.G., and Huntsman, S.A. (1983) Limnol. Oceanogr. in press.

19. Wydrzynski, T., and Sauer, K. (1980) Biochem. Biophys. Acta 589, 56.

20. Kagi, J.R.R., and Nordberg, M. (eds.) (1979) Metallothionein: Proceedings of the First International Meeting on Metallothionein and Other Low Molecular Weight Metal Binding Proteins. Bukhauser Verlag, Massachusetts.

21. Kissling, N.M., and Kagi, J.H.R. (1977) FEBS Letts. 82, 247.

22. Learch, K., Amer, D., and Olafson, R.W. (1982) J. Biol. Chem. 257, 2420.

23. Rauser, W.E., and Curvetto, N.R. (1980) Nature 284, 368.

24. Overnell, J. (1982) Comp. Biochem. Physiol. 73B, 555.

25. Olafson, R.W., Kearns, A., and Sim, R.G. (1979) Comp. Biochem. Physiol. 628, 417.

26. Stebbing, A.R.D. (1981) Aquatic Tox. 1, 227.

ACTIVATION OF ADENYLATE CYCLASE BY TOXIN-CATALYZED ADP-RIBOSYLATION

Joel Moss
Martha Vaughan

National Heart, Lung, and Blood Institute
National Institutes of Health
Bethesda, Maryland

I. INTRODUCTION

Choleragen and Escherichia coli heat-labile enterotoxin
are bacterial toxins responsible, at least in part, for the
clinical syndromes of cholera and "traveler's diarrhea," respectively. The effects of the toxins result from the activation of adenylate cyclase and consequent increase in intracellular cAMP. In the disease state, the toxins produced in
the lumen of the small intestine apparently act only on
intestinal cells. Choleragen, however, can activate adenylate cyclase and increase cAMP in almost all animal cells (for
reviews of the biochemical studies of toxin, see 1-10).
    The toxins are oligomeric proteins of $\sim 84,000$ daltons
made up of one A subunit ($M_r = 29,000$) and five B ($M_r =
11,600$) subunits. The A subunit consists of two peptides,
A_1 ($M_r = 23,000$) and A_2 ($M_r = 6,000$), linked through a single
disulfide bond; it is synthesized as a single polypeptide
chain, which is then proteolytically nicked (11,12). The
separated A and B subunits of choleragen have been used to
study their different functions. Activation of adenylate
cyclase is catalyzed by the A_1 peptide after its release from
the A subunit (13). The B subunits bind to the cell surface
through specific interaction with the monosialoganglioside
$Gal\beta1 \rightarrow 3GalNAc\beta1 \rightarrow 4Gal[3 \leftarrow 2\alpha AcNeu]\beta1 \rightarrow 4Glc\beta1 \rightarrow ceramide$ (G_{M1}).
    The initial event in toxin action is binding of the B
subunit of the toxin to the cell surface, perhaps followed by
patching and capping (14,15). During its entry, the A

MECHANISM OF DRUG ACTION

subunit may be reduced to A_1 and A_2 peptides. Thiol:protein
oxidoreductase, a ubiquitous plasma membrane enzyme, can
accelerate the reduction (16). The reduced A subunit (A_1
peptide) exhibits NAD:arginine ADP-ribosyltransferase (and
NAD glycohydrolase) activity (17-19). In cultured fibroblasts (as in other cells), there is a delay between addition
of choleragen and activation of adenylate cyclase (20,21).
This is similar in length to and may reflect the time required for release of the A_1 peptide (21). Using photoacti-
vatable cross-linkers, it was demonstrated that the A_1 peptide, but not the B subunit, was inserted into the bilayer
(22-24). The substrate for the A_1 peptide is a stimulatory
GTP-binding protein (G_s) of the adenylate cyclase system (see
Section III.B.). The A_1 peptide catalyzes the transfer of
ADP-ribose from NAD to an arginine, or similar, residue in G_s
(see Section IV). ADP-ribosylation of G_s by toxin increases
the activity of the catalytic unit of the cyclase (see Section III.A.).

Another toxin, secreted by <u>Bordetella pertussis</u>, also
causes the activation of adenylate cyclase. This toxin catalyzes the ADP-ribosylation of an inhibitory GTP-binding protein (G_i) of the cyclase system; the modified G_i cannot function and thus the action of the stimulatory arm of adenylate
cyclase is unopposed (Section VI).

II. INTERACTION OF CHOLERAGEN WITH THE CELL SURFACE

Van Heyningen <u>et al</u>. (25) first showed that gangliosides
inhibited the action of choleragen on the gut; it was subsequently found that gangliosides blocked choleragen action on
many tissues (26-28). The effect of gangliosides is due to
the monosialoganglioside G_{M1}. G_{M1} formed aggregates with
toxin (29-32), interfered with choleragen binding and action
(29,31,33-39), and, when immobilized on agarose beads (40)
or as a ganglioside-cerebroside complex (41), bound toxin.
The interaction of choleragen and G_{M1} involves specifically
the B subunit of the toxin and the oligosaccharide moiety of
the ganglioside. G_{M1}-oligosaccharide inhibited the binding
of ^{125}I-choleragen to fibroblasts (42), caused a "blue-shift"
in the tryptophanyl fluorescence spectrum of toxin or its B
subunits (42), an effect similar to that observed with G_{M1}
(43,44), altered the circular dichroic spectrum of choleragen
and its B subunit (42) and led to increase in molecular
weight determined by sedimentation equilibrium (42), consistent with the multivalent structure of the B oligomer.

Several types of studies established the role of G_{M1} in the responsiveness of cells to choleragen. The effect of toxin on cells appeared to be proportional to their G_{M1} content. Treatment of cells with neuraminidase, which increases G_{M1} by converting tri- and disialogangliosides to the monosialoganglioside, increased toxin responsiveness and binding (27,39,45-49). Incorporation of exogenous G_{M1} into cells enhanced their toxin responsiveness (13,14,37,50,51). Fibroblasts that had incorporated G_{M1} but not other gangliosides responded to choleragen with an increase in cellular cAMP that was proportional to the amount of G_{M1} incorporated (52,53). As expected, fibroblasts containing G_{M1} exhibited ^{125}I-toxin binding; gangliosides G_{M2} (GalNAcβ1→4Gal[3←2αAc-Neu]β1→4Glcβ1→ceramide) and G_{M3} (AcNeuα2→3Galβ1→ 4Glcβ1→ceramide) were clearly less effective (52). Involvement of the G_{M1} oligosaccharide in toxin binding to cells was further demonstrated by the fact that choleragen blocked oxidation of the terminal galactose and the sialic acid moieties of G_{M1} by galactose oxidase and periodate, respectively (54). Toxin effectively protected G_{M1} in human fibroblasts containing endogenously synthesized ganglioside and in mouse fibroblasts that had incorporated exogenous G_{M1} from the medium (54).

III. ACTIVATION OF ADENYLATE CYCLASE BY CHOLERAGEN-CATALYZED ADP-RIBOSYLATION

A. Requirements for ADP-Ribosylation and Adenylate Cyclase Activation

Gill first reported that NAD is required for toxin activation of adenylate cyclase (55,56). It was later shown that NAD serves as an ADP-ribose donor in an ADP-ribosyltransferase reaction catalyzed by the toxin. The ADP-ribose acceptor is a regulatory component of the cyclase system, G_s (Reaction 1).

$$NAD + G_s \; \rightleftharpoons \; ADP\text{-ribose}^\cdot G_s + nicotinamide + H^{\oplus} \quad (1)$$

Activation of adenylate cyclase by choleragen requires GTP (57-67). To determine the role of GTP, the activation process in a membrane preparation was separated into three steps (67). The first step was the NAD- and toxin-dependent activation reaction, i.e., the transfer of ADP-ribose from NAD to G_s. In the second step, thermal stability of the toxin-activated cyclase was assessed. Finally, the effect of GTP on catalytic function of the activated cyclase was determined. In all steps, GTP was more effective than ITP or ATP (67).

Components in addition to GTP are required to maximize
choleragen activation of adenylate cyclase and expression of
the activated enzyme. Calmodulin (M_r = 17,000) is a heat-
stable, calcium-binding protein (68). First described as an
activator of cyclic nucleotide phosphodiesterase, it is now
known to activate a number of enzymes (68). In some instances, e.g. brain, adenylate cyclase is activated by calmodulin (61,69-74). Brain cyclase, solubilized in Triton X-100
and separated from calmodulin by DEAE-cellulose chromatography, was dependent on calmodulin for demonstration of Gpp(NH)p
or choleragen-stimulated activity (61). Several cytosolic and
membrane factors have been reported to facilitate toxin activation of adenylate cyclase (63,66,75-77). Schleifer et al.
(77) partially purified a membrane protein required to obtain
maximal ADP-ribosylation of purified G_s by choleragen. The
role of this protein, and the other factors, in the interaction of toxin, G_s, and NAD remains to be determined.

B.   Identification of Cellular Substrates for Choleragen

Cassel and Pfeuffer (78) found that in pigeon erythrocytes
choleragen ADP-ribosylated a 42,000 dalton membrane protein.
Based on the affinity of the protein for a GTP-Sepharose, it
was postulated to be the GTP-binding protein of the cyclase
system. Similarly, in pigeon erythrocytes, Gill and Meren
(79) found a 42,000 dalton substrate. In S49 cell membranes,
choleragen ADP-ribosylated, in addition to a 42,000 dalton
protein, a doublet of 52-53,000 daltons (80). Incubation of
intact S49 cells with choleragen prevented the subsequent
[^{32}P]ADP-ribosylation of both substrates in membranes (80).
Presumably both sets of proteins were modified during incubation of the cells with toxin and thus were not available for
[^{32}P]ADP-ribosylation. Thus, these proteins were cellular
substrates for choleragen. Genetic evidence that these proteins are components of the adenylate cyclase system was obtained with an S49 variant, known as AC$^-$ or cyc$^-$. These
cells lack functional G_s and did not have the 42,000 and
52-53,000 dalton toxin substrates (80). Other tissues have
42,000 or both 42,000 and 52,000 dalton substrates (78-82).

C.   Mechanism of Activation of Adenylate Cyclase by
Choleragen

Hormone-stimulated adenylate cyclase systems consist of
at least three different components (83,84). The catalytic
unit (C) converts ATP to cAMP. Specific cell surface

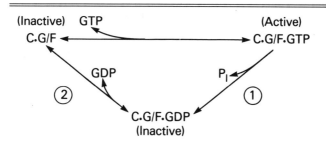

① Inhibition of Specific GTPase Would Prolong Lifetime of Active Complex.

② Accelerating Release of GDP Would Promote GTP Binding and Generation of Active Complex.

FIGURE 1. Activation of adenylate cyclase.

receptors for stimulatory ligands are coupled to C through a GTP-binding protein termed G_s; the G_s proteins appear to be heterodimers of a 35,000 and either a 42-45,000 or 52-53,000 dalton protein (85-87). Guanyl nucleotides bound to G_s influence its interaction with receptors and with C. It is believed that C is active when GTP is bound to G_s in the $G_s \cdot C$ complex (Fig. 1). The active $C \cdot G_s \cdot GTP$ species is inactivated when GTP is hydrolyzed by a specific low K_m GTPase (Fig. 1, Reaction 1) (88). Following ADP-ribosylation of G_s by choleragen, GTP hydrolysis is decreased, stabilizing the active $C \cdot G_s \cdot GTP$ complex. In addition, ADP-ribosylation of G_s promotes release of GDP from $C \cdot G_s \cdot GDP$ (Fig. 1, Reaction 2) (89,90). Burns et al. (89) showed that isoproterenol enhances the release of [3H]GDP from turkey erythrocyte membranes that had bound [3H]GTP (Fig. 1, Reaction 2). It was postulated that isoproterenol thereby promotes GTP binding and formation of $C \cdot G_s \cdot GTP$ (Fig. 1). Choleragen also caused release of [3H]GDP from membranes that had bound [3H]GTP. Similar amounts of [3H]GDP were released by toxin and by isoproterenol (89) apparently from the same guanyl nucleotide pool. To demonstrate that both were acting on G_s, erythrocyte membranes with bound [3H]GDP were incubated with or without toxin or isoproterenol, solubilized and chromatographed on a gel permeation column. The protein(s) from which [3H]GDP was released by toxin or isoproterenol cochromatographed with the 42,000 dalton toxin substrate and with the proteins that restored guanyl nucleotide sensitivity to membranes from cells

lacking functional G_s (90). Thus, choleragen may stimulate
adenylate cyclase by inhibiting the hydrolysis of GTP bound
to $C \cdot G_s$ and stabilizing the active complex. In addition,
toxin accelerates release of GDP from the inactive $C \cdot G_s \cdot GDP$
species, facilitating GTP binding and formation of the active
$C \cdot G_s \cdot GTP$ complex (89,90).

IV. ENZYMOLOGY OF CHOLERAGEN: ADP-RIBOSYLTRANSFERASE
AND NAD GLYCOHYDROLASE ACTIVITIES

To demonstrate ADP-ribosyltransferase and NAD glycohydrolase activities of choleragen in the absence of cellular components, the active A_1 peptide must be released (12,17,19).
With proteolytically nicked holotoxin or A subunits, this is
achieved by reduction of the disulfide bond linking A_1 and
A_2. The cysteine sulfhydryl is not required for catalytic
function, since after its alkylation with iodoacetate A_1
remained active (19). With toxin that is not proteolytically
nicked, trypsin is required in addition to thiol to generate
maximal activity (12).
     Choleragen catalyzes the transfer of ADP-ribose from NAD
to purified proteins (91) (Reaction 2) as well as to low
molecular weight guanidino compounds, such as arginine (Reaction 3) (18). Presumably, it is an arginine or similar guanidino residue in the protein substrate that serves as an
ADP-ribose acceptor. The ADP-ribosylation of arginine is
stereospecific; β-NAD is the substrate and α-ADP-ribose-argi-
nine is the product (92). The environment of a guanidino
moiety influences its ability to serve as an ADP-ribose acceptor; compounds with a positive charge near the guanidino
moiety (e.g., agmatine, arginine methyl ester) were more
effective acceptors than those with a negative charge (e.g.,
guanidinopropionate) (18,93).
     In the absence of an ADP-ribose acceptor, choleragen cat-
alyzes the hydrolysis of NAD to ADP-ribose and nicotinamide
(Reaction 4) (17); NAD is a much more effective substrate
than NADP, consistent with the finding that NADP cannot substitute for NAD in adenylate cyclase activation (44,55). The
ability of choleragen to catalyze NAD hydrolysis indicates
that the toxin can activate the ribosyl-nicotinamide bond in
the absence of a specific acceptor (17).

$$NAD + protein \rightleftharpoons ADP\text{-ribose-protein}$$
$$+ \ nicotinamide + H \oplus \qquad (2)$$

$$NAD + guanidino\text{-}R \rightleftharpoons ADP\text{-}ribose\text{-}guanidino\text{-}R$$
$$+ \text{ nicotinamide-H} \oplus \qquad (3)$$

$$NAD + H_2O \longrightarrow ADP\text{-}ribose + nicotinamide + H \oplus \qquad (4)$$

V. ESCHERICHIA COLI HEAT-LABILE ENTEROTOXIN: COMPARISON WITH CHOLERAGEN

Several strains of Escherichia coli produce enterotoxins that are involved in the pathogenesis of "traveler's diarrhea." One of these, termed LT (heat-labile toxin), is similar in many ways (structural, immunological, functional) to choleragen. There is considerable homology between the two toxins both in holotoxin composition (one A and five B subunits) and subunit size (for review, see 10,94-99).

A. Interaction with Cell Surface

The nature of the specific cell surface binding site(s) for LT is still in question. There is considerable evidence that the toxin, like choleragen, interacts with G_{M1}. In addition, however, LT may also bind to a site not recognized by choleragen that has the properties of a glycoprotein (100). G_{M1} can block the action of LT (33,35); the affinity of LT for G_{M1} was slightly less than that of choleragen (33). Transformed mouse fibroblasts that had incorporated G_{M1} but not G_{M2} or G_{M3} responded to LT with an increase in cellular cAMP (101). These cells responded to choleragen only after they had incorporated exogenous G_{M1} (52). ^{125}I-LT bound to rat C6 glioma cells deficient in G_{M1} that had incorporated G_{M1} but not other gangliosides (102). Choleragen inhibited binding of labeled LT to C6 glioma cells that had incorporated G_{M1}.
Like choleragen, LT appeared to interact specifically with the oligosaccharide moiety of G_{M1}. G_{M1}-oligosaccharide altered the physical properties of LT and its B subunits (LT_B) (102). The tryptophanyl fluorescence spectra of LT and LT_B were "blue-shifted" by G_{M1}-oligosaccharide but not by other oligosaccharides (102). A similar effect was observed with choleragen. The tryptophanyl fluorescence spectra of LT and LT_B differed, however, from those of choleragen and choleragenoid, respectively (102). The concentrations of G_{M1}-oligosaccharide that "blue-shifted" the tryptophanyl fluorescence spectra of LT and choleragen were similar (102). These studies as well as the data on the interaction of LT

with G_{M1}-deficient cells incubated with the ganglioside support the conclusion that there is specific binding of G_{M1}
oligosaccharide to the B subunit of LT and G_{M1} may be the
site of LT binding on the cell surface. A number of studies,
however, are consistent with the proposal that LT and choleragen do not have identical receptors (33,34,100). In
rabbit small intestine, LT_B blocked the activity of LT and
choleragen, whereas choleragenoid inhibited choleragen, but
not LT, action (100). In addition, isolated epithelial cells
or brush border membranes bound ten times more LT than choleragen (100). Binding sites for choleragen appeared to be
G_{M1}, but LT-binding sites, which were inactivated by periodate and stable to boiling, had properties of a glycoprotein
(100). An unidentified LT-binding material was solubilized
by proteolysis of delipidated membranes (100). In dog intestine in contrast to rabbit, choleragenoid blocked the action
of LT (103); in this species the two toxins may use the same
binding sites, presumably ganglioside G_{M1}.

B. ADP-Ribosyltransferase Activity

Like choleragen, LT activates adenylate cyclase in a reaction that requires NAD (104,105). With [^{32}P]NAD and GTP,
LT catalyzes the [^{32}P]ADP-ribosylation of a 42,000 dalton
protein in fat cells that is identical to the choleragen substrate (104). Other membrane proteins may also be LT substrates; in rat liver, an 11,000 dalton protein is ADP-ribosylated (106). Its relationship to LT action is unknown.
The A subunit of LT is analogous to choleragen A. In
contrast to some commercial preparations of choleragen, LT as
isolated in several laboratories appears to have an A subunit
that has not been proteolytically nicked (102). During incubation with a protease such as trypsin, peptides corresponding to choleragen A_1 and A_2 are generated (102). The NAD:
arginine ADP-ribosyltransferase activity of nicked LT, like
that of choleragen, was dependent on thiol (102,107). The
specific activity of maximally activated LT approximated that
of choleragen (102).
In addition to the ADP-ribosylation of its membrane substrate, LT catalyzes the transfer of ADP-ribose from NAD to
numerous purified proteins and to guanidino compounds such
as arginine (Reactions 2 and 3) (107,108); in the absence of
an amino acid acceptor, LT hydrolyzes NAD to ADP-ribose and
nicotinamide (Reaction 4) (102,107). The β-NAD-dependent
ADP-ribosylation of arginine by LT is stereospecific and
yields α-ADP-ribose-L-arginine (108,109). As with choleragen, a negative charge near the guanidino moiety appeared to

decrease its ability to serve as an ADP-ribose acceptor (107,
108). Other amino acids, such as lysine, histidine, and serine are inactive (107). Among the purified proteins tested,
polyarginine and histone were excellent substrates (109).
The proteins that served as ADP-ribose acceptors in the LT-
catalyzed reaction were not identical to those modified by
choleragen.

VI. PERTUSSIS TOXIN (ISLET-ACTIVATING PROTEIN)

Pertussis toxin, secreted by <u>Bordetella pertussis,</u> is an
oligomeric protein of 117,000 daltons composed of five different kinds of subunits; their molecular weights are: S_1,
28,000; S_2, 23,000; S_3, 22,000; S_4, 11,700; S_5, 9,300 (110).
In the holotoxin, two S_4 subunits are present as heterodimers with S_2 and S_3; the structure of the toxin molecule
can be represented as $S_1(S_2S_4)(S_5)(S_3S_4)$ (110). Two functional domains can be separated and studied independently
(110). S_1 catalyzes the ADP-ribosylation of G_i, a regulatory
protein in the adenylate cyclase system, and also exhibits
NAD glycohydrolase activity (110). $(S_2S_4)(S_5)(S_3S_4)$ is involved in toxin binding to the cell surface. The nature of
the binding site is unknown, but its structure may be analogous in some way to the haptoglobin affinity matrix that can
bind $(S_2S_4)(S_5)(S_3S_4)$ (110).

Pertussis toxin was isolated based on its ability to
enhance the secretion of insulin from pancreatic islets and
was referred to as islet-activating protein (111-113). It
was subsequently found that the toxin acts on the adenylate
cyclase system, altering its activity and responsiveness to
both inhibitory and stimulatory ligands (113-116). Incubation of rat heart cells with pertussis toxin increased their
response to activators of the cyclase and decreased the response to inhibitors (114). These effects apparently result
from the toxin-catalyzed ADP-ribosylation of G_i, a guanyl
nucleotide-binding protein that is involved in translating
agonist occupancy of an inhibitory receptor into decreased
activity of the catalytic unit (117). The subunit of G_i that
is ADP-ribosylated has a molecular weight of ~ 41,000 (117-
122). Incubation of NG108-15 (neuroblastoma x glioma hybrid)
cells with pertussis toxin decreased inhibitory agonist binding by the membranes and decreased the effect of guanyl nucleotide on agonist binding, but had no effect on antagonist
binding (123). It appears that ADP-ribosylation of the
41,000 dalton subunit of G_i results in a loss of its activity
(120,124); it may interfere with the ability of G_i to interact

normally with inhibitory receptors so that receptors are
effectively "uncoupled," preventing, for example, opiate stimulation of GTPase and inhibition of adenylate cyclase (120).

ACKNOWLEDGMENT

We thank Mrs. D. Marie Sherwood for expert secretarial
assistance.

REFERENCES

1. Finkelstein, R. A., *CRC Crit. Rev. Microbiol.* 2:553
    (1973).
2. Bennett, V., and Cuatrecasas, P., *in* "The Specificity
    and Action of Animal, Bacterial and Plant Toxins.
    Receptors and Recognition" (P. Cuatrecasas, ed.),
    Series B, vol. 1, p. 1. Chapman and Hall, London,
    1976.
3. Gill, D. M., *Adv. Cyclic Nucl. Res.* 8:85 (1977).
4. van Heyningen, S., *Biol. Rev.* 52:509 (1977).
5. Moss, J., and Vaughan, M., *Annu. Rev. Biochem.* 48:581
    (1979).
6. Fishman, P. H., *in* "Secretory Diarrhea" (M. Field, J. S.
    Fordtran, and S. G. Schultz, eds.), p. 85. American
    Physiological Society, Bethesda, Maryland (1980).
7. Moss, J., and Vaughan, M., *Mol. Cell. Biochem.* 37:75
    (1981).
8. Holmgren, J., *Nature (London)* 292:413 (1981).
9. van Heyningen, S., *Bioscience Reports* 2:135 (1982).
10. Moss, J., and Vaughan, M., *in* "Handbook of Natural
    Toxins" Vol. 11 "Bacterial Toxins" (A. T. Tu, W. H.
    Habig, and M. C. Hardegree, eds.), Marcel Dekker, Inc.,
    New York, in press.
11. Gill, D. M., and Rappaport, R. S., *J. Infect. Dis. 139*:
    674 (1979).
12. Mekalanos, J. J., Collier, R. J., and Romig, W. R.,
    J. Biol. Chem. 254:5855 (1979).
13. Gill, D. M., and King, C. A., *J. Biol. Chem.* 250:6424
    (1975).
14. Révész, T., and Greaves, M., *Nature (London)* 257:103
    (1975).
15. Craig, S. W., and Cuatrecasas, P., *Proc. Natl. Acad.
    Sci. U. S. A.* 72:3844 (1975).

16. Moss, J., Stanley, S. J., Morin, J. E., and Dixon, J. E., *J. Biol. Chem. 255*:11085 (1980).
17. Moss, J., Manganiello, V. C., and Vaughan, M., *Proc. Natl. Acad. Sci. U. S. A. 73*:4424 (1976).
18. Moss, J., and Vaughan, M., *J. Biol. Chem. 252*:2455 (1977).
19. Moss, J., Stanley, S. J., and Lin, M. C., *J. Biol. Chem. 254*:11993 (1979).
20. Kimberg, D. V., Field, M., Johnson, J., Henderson, A., and Gershon, E., *J. Clin. Invest. 50*:1218 (1971).
21. Kassis, S., Hagmann, J., Fishman, P. H., Chang, P. P., and Moss, J., *J. Biol. Chem. 257*:12148 (1982).
22. Wisnieski, B. J., and Bramhall, J. S., *Biochem. Biophys. Res. Commun. 87*:308 (1979).
23. Wisnieski, B. J., Shiflett, M. A., Mekalanos, J., and Bramhall, J. S., *J. Supramol. Struct. 10*:191 (1979).
24. Wisnieski, B. J., and Bramhall, J. S., *Nature (London) 289*:319 (1981).
25. van Heyningen, W. E., Carpenter, C. C. J., Pierce, N. F., and Greenough, W. B., III, *J. Infect. Dis. 124*:415 (1971).
26. Wolff, J., Temple, R., and Cook, G. H., *Proc. Natl. Acad. Sci. U. S. A. 70*:2741 (1973).
27. Haksar, A., Maudsley, D. V., and Péron, F. G., *Biochim. Biophys. Acta 381*:308 (1975).
28. Wolff, J., and Cook, G. H., *Biochim. Biophys. Acta 413*:283 (1975).
29. Holmgren, J., Lönnroth, I., and Svennerholm, L., *Infect. Immun. 8*:208 (1973).
30. Holmgren, J., Månsson, J.-E., and Svennerholm, L., *Med. Biol. 52*:229 (1974).
31. Staerk, J., Ronneberger, H. J., Wiegandt, H., and Ziegler, W., *Eur. J. Biochem. 48*:103 (1974).
32. Wiegandt, H., Ziegler, W., Staerk, J., Kranz, T., Ronneberger, H. J., Zilg, H., Karlsson, K-A., and Samuelsson, B. E., *Hoppe-Seyler's Z. Physiol. Chem. 357*:1637 (1976).
33. Holmgren, J., *Infect. Immun. 8*:851 (1973).
34. Pierce, N. F., *J. Exp. Med. 137*:1009 (1973).
35. Zenser, T. V., and Metzger, J. F., *Infect. Immun. 10*:503 (1974).
36. Cuatrecasas, P., *Biochemistry 12*:3547 (1973).
37. Cuatrecasas, P., *Biochemistry 12*:3558 (1973).
38. van Heyningen, W. E., and Mellanby, J., *Naunyn-Schmiedeberg's Arch. Pharmacol. 276*:297 (1973).
39. King, C. A., and van Heyningen, W. E., *J. Infect. Dis. 127*:639 (1973).

40. Cuatrecasas, P., Parikh, I., and Hollenberg, M. D. *Biochemistry* 12:4253 (1973).
41. van Heyningen, S. *Science (Washington, D. C.) 183*:656 (1974).
42. Fishman, P. H., Moss, J., and Osborne, J. C., Jr., *Biochemistry 17*:711 (1978).
43. Mullin, B. R., Aloj, S. M., Fishman, P. H., Lee, G., Kohn, L. D., and Brady, R. O., *Proc. Natl. Acad. Sci. U. S. A. 73*:1679 (1976).
44. Moss, J., Osborne, J. C., Jr., Fishman, P. H., Brewer, H. B., Jr., Vaughan, M., and Brady, R. O., *Proc. Natl. Acad. Sci. U. S. A. 74*:74 (1977).
45. van Heyningen, W. E., *Naunyn-Schmiedeberg's Arch. Pharmacol. 276*:289 (1973).
46. Haksar, A., Maudsley, D. V., and Peron, F. G., *Nature (London) 251*:514 (1974).
47. Revesz, T., Greaves, M. F., Capellaro, D., and Murray, R. K., *Br. J. Haematol. 34*:623 (1976).
48. Hansson, H.-A., Holmgren, J., and Svennerholm, L., *Proc. Natl. Acad. Sci. U. S. A. 74*:3782 (1977).
49. O'Keefe, E., and Cuatrecasas, P., *J. Membrane Biol. 42*: 61 (1978).
50. Holmgren, J., Lönnroth, I., Månsson, J.-E., and Svennerholm, L., *Proc. Natl. Acad. Sci. U. S. A. 72*: 2520 (1975).
51. King, C. A., van Heyningen, W. E., and Gascoyne, N. *J. Infect. Dis. 133 (Suppl)*:S75 (1976).
52. Moss, J., Fishman, P. H., Manganiello, V. C., Vaughan, M., and Brady, R. O., *Proc. Natl. Acad. Sci. U. S. A. 73*:1034 (1976).
53. Fishman, P. H., Moss, J., and Vaughan, M., *J. Biol. Chem. 251*:4490 (1976).
54. Moss, J., Manganiello, V. C., and Fishman, P. H., *Biochemistry 16*:1876 (1977).
55. Gill, D. M., *Proc. Natl. Acad. Sci. U. S. A. 72*:2064, (1975).
56. Gill, D. M., *J. Infect. Dis. 133 (Suppl)*:S55 (1976).
57. Bennett, V., and Cuatrecasas, P., *J. Membrane Biol. 22*: 1 (1975).
58. Bennett, V., Mong, L., and Cuatrecasas, P., *J. Membrane Biol. 24*:107 (1975).
59. Bennett, V., Craig, S., Hollenberg, M. D., O'Keefe, E., Sahyoun, N., and Cuatrecasas, P., *J. Supramol. Struct. 4*:99 (1976).
60. Johnson, G. L., and Bourne, H. R., *Biochem. Biophys. Res. Commun. 78*:792 (1977).
61. Moss, J., and Vaughan, M., *Proc. Natl. Acad. Sci. U. S. A. 74*:4396 (1977).

62. Lin, M. C., Welton, A. F., and Berman, M. F., *J. Cyclic Nucl. Res. 4*:159 (1978).
63. Enomoto, K., and Gill, D. M., *J. Supramol. Struct. 10*: 51 (1979).
64. Malbon, C. C., and Gill, D. M., *Biochim. Biophys. Acta 586*:518 (1979).
65. Doberska, C. A., Macpherson, A. J. S., and Martin, B. R., *Biochem. J. 186*:749 (1980).
66. Enomoto, K., and Gill, D. M., *J. Biol. Chem. 255*:1252, (1980).
67. Nakaya, S.,, Moss, J., and Vaughan, M., *Biochemistry 19*:4871 (1980).
68. Klee, C. B., Crouch, T. H., and Richman, P. G., *Annu. Rev. Biochem. 49*:489 (1980).
69. Brostrom, C. O., Huang, Y-C., Breckenridge, B. McL., and Wolff, D. J., *Proc. Natl. Acad. Sci. U. S. A. 72*: 64 (1975).
70. Brostrom, M. A., Brostrom, C. O., Breckenridge, B. M., and Wolff, D. J., *J. Biol. Chem. 251*:4744 (1976).
71. Lynch, T. J., Tallant, E. A., and Cheung, W. Y., *Biochem. Biophys. Res. Commun. 68*:616 (1976).
72. Lynch, T. J., Tallant, E. A., and Cheung, W. Y., *Arch. Biochem. Biophys. 182*:124 (1977).
73. Cheung, W. Y., Bradham, L. S., Lynch, T. J., Lin, Y. M., and Tallant, E. A., *Biochem. Biophys. Res. Commun. 66*:1055 (1978).
74. Cheung, W. Y., Lynch, T. J., and Wallace, R. W. *Adv. Cyclic Nucl. Res. 9*:233 (1978).
75. Le Vine, H., III, and Cuatrecasas, P., *Biochim. Biophys. Acta 672*:248 (1981).
76. Pinkett, M. O., and Anderson, W. B., *Biochim. Biophys. Acta 714*:337 (1982).
77. Schleifer, L. S., Kahn, R. A., Hanski, E., Northup, J. K., Sternweis, P. C., and Gilman, A. G., *J. Biol. Chem. 257*:20 (1982).
78. Cassel, D., and Pfeuffer, T., *Proc. Natl. Acad. Sci. U. S. A. 75*:2669 (1978).
79. Gill, D. M., and Meren, R., *Proc. Natl. Acad. Sci. U. S. A. 75*:3050 (1978).
80. Johnson, G. L., Kaslow, H. R., and Bourne, H. R., *J. Biol. Chem. 253*:7120 (1978).
81. Watkins, P. A., Moss, J., and Vaughan, M., *J. Biol. Chem. 256*:4895 (1981).
82. Hebdon, G. M., Le Vine, H., III, Sahyoun, N. E., Schmitges, C. J., and Cuatrecasas, P., *Life Sci. 26*: 1385 (1980).
83. Ross, E. M., and Gilman, A. G., *Annu. Rev. Biochem. 49*:533 (1980).

84. Rodbell, M., *Nature (London)* *284*:17 (1980).
85. Northup, J. K., Sternweis, P. C. Smigel, M. D., Schleifer, L. W., Ross, E. M., and Gilman, A. G., *Proc. Natl. Acad. Sci. U. S. A. 77*:6516 (1980).
86. Sternweis, P. C., Northup, J. K., Smigel, M. D., and Gilman, A. G., *J. Biol. Chem. 256*:11517 (1981).
87. Hanski, E., Sternweis, P. C., Northup, J. K., Dromerick, A. W., and Gilman, A. G., *J. Biol. Chem. 256*:12911 (1981).
88. Cassel, D., and Selinger, Z., *Proc. Natl. Acad. Sci. U. S. A. 74*:3307 (1977).
89. Burns, D. L., Moss, J., and Vaughan, M., *J. Biol. Chem. 257*:32 (1982).
90. Burns, D. L., Moss, J., and Vaughan, M., *J. Biol. Chem. 258*:1116 (1983).
91. Moss, J., and Vaughan, M., *Proc. Natl. Acad. Sci. U. S. A. 75*:3621 (1978).
92. Oppenheimer, N. J., *J. Biol. Chem. 253*:4907 (1978).
93. Moss, J., and Vaughan, M., *in* "Developments in Cell Biology, Vol. 6, Novel ADP-ribosylations of Regulatory Enzymes and Proteins" (M. E. Smulson, and T. Sugimura, eds.), p. 391. Elsevier/North Holland, New York, 1980.
94. Sack, R. B., *Annu. Rev. Microbiol. 29*:333 (1975).
95. Rašková, H., and Raška, K., *Biochem. Pharmacol. 26*: 1103 (1977).
96. Field, M., *Am. J. Clin. Nutr. 32*:189 (1979).
97. Holmgren, J., and Lönnroth, I., *in* "Cholera and Related Diarrheas" (O. Ouchterlony, and J. Holmgren, eds.), p. 88. Karger, Basel (1980).
98. Carpenter, C. C. J., *in* "Secretory Diarrhea" (M. Field, J. S. Fordtran, and S. G. Schultz, eds.), p. 67. American Physiological Society, Bethesda, Maryland (1980).
99. Moss, J., and Vaughan, M., *in* "ADP-Ribosylation Reactions" (O. Hayaishi, and K. Ueda, eds.), p. 623. Academic Press, New York (1982).
100. Holmgren, J., Fredman, P., Lindblad, M., Svennerholm, A-M., and Svennerholm, L., *Infect. Immun. 38*:424 (1982).
101. Moss, J., Garrison, S., Fishman, P. H., and Richardson, S. H., *J. Clin. Invest. 64*:381 (1979).
102. Moss, J., Osborne, J. C., Jr., Fishman, P. H., Nakaya, S., and Robertson, D. C., *J. Biol. Chem. 256*:12861 (1981).
103. Nalin, D. R., and McLaughlin, J. C., *J. Med. Microbiol. 11*:177 (1978).
104. Gill, D. M., and Richardson, S. H., *J. Infect. Dis. 141*:64 (1980).

105. Gill, D. M., Evans, D. J., Jr., and Evans, D. G., *J. Infect. Dis.* *133* Suppl:S103 (1976).
106. Tait, R. M., Booth, B. R., and Lambert, P. A., *Biochem. Biophys. Res. Commun.* *96*:1024 (1980).
107. Moss, J., and Richardson, S. H., *J. Clin. Invest.* *62*: 281 (1978).
108. Moss, J., Garrison, S., Oppenheimer, N. J., and Richardson, S. H., *in* "Proceedings of the 14th Joint Conference US–Japan Cooperative Medical Science Program, Cholera Panel, Symposium on Cholera, Karatsu, 1978" (K. Takeya, and Y. Zinnaka, eds.), p. 274. Fuji Printing Co., Ltd., Tokyo, 1979.
109. Moss, J., Garrison, S., Oppenheimer, N. J., and Richardson, S. H., *J. Biol. Chem.* *254*:6270 (1979).
110. Tamura, M., Nogimori, K., Murai, S., Yajima, M., Ito, K., Katada, T., Ui, M., and Ishii, S., *Biochemistry 21*: 5516 (1982).
111. Yajima, M., Hosoda, K., Kanbayashi, Y., Nakamura, T., Takahashi, I., and Ui, M., *J. Biochem.* *83*:305 (1978).
112. Katada, T., and Ui, M., *J. Biol. Chem.* *254*:469 (1979).
113. Katada, T., and Ui, M., *J. Biol. Chem.* *255*:9580 (1980).
114. Hazeki, O., and Ui, M., *J. Biol. Chem.* *256*:2856 (1981).
115. Katada, T., and Ui, M., *J. Biol. Biol. Chem.* *256*:8310 (1981).
116. Katada, T., Amano, T., and Ui, M., *J. Biol. Chem.* *257*: 3739 (1982).
117. Katada, T., and Ui, M., *Proc. Natl. Acad. Sci. U. S. A.* *79*:3129 (1982).
118. Katada, T., and Ui, M., *J. Biol. Chem.* *257*:7210 (1982).
119. Hildebrandt, J. D., Sekura, R. D., Codina, J., Iyengar, R., Manclark, C. R., and Birnbaumer, L., *Nature (London) 302*:706 (1983).
120. Burns, D. L., Hewlett, E. L., Moss, J., and Vaughan, M., *J. Biol. Chem.* *258*:1435 (1983).
121. Murayama, T., Katada, T., and Ui, M., *Arch. Biochem. Biophys.* *221*:381 (1983).
122. Bokoch, G. M., Katada, T., Northup, J. K., Hewlett, E. L., and Gilman, A. G., *J. Biol. Chem.* *258*:2072 (1983).
123. Kurose, H., Katada, T., Amano, T., and Ui, M., *J. Biol. Chem.* *258*:4870 (1983).
124. Murayama, T., and Ui, M., *J. Biol. Chem.* *258*:3319

BIOCHEMICAL MECHANISMS OF THE CYTOTOXIC ACTION
OF THE ANTITUMOR ELLIPTICINE DERIVATIVES

Claude Paoletti[1]
Christian Auclair

Laboratoire de Biochimie
Institut Gustave Roussy
Villejuif, France

Bernard Meunier[2]

Laboratoire de Pharmacologie et
Toxicologie Fondamentales CNRS
Toulouse, France

I. INTRODUCTION

Since ellipticine was first described as an antitumor compound by Dalton et al. (1) many studies have been carried out in these series; they led our group to propose a new drug (2, 3), 2-methyl-9-hydroxyellipticinium, as a therapeutic agent active against some human cancers, especially bone and skin metastatic forms of breast cancer (4, 5) (Fig. 1). This drug is under phase I and II clinical trials in several European and U.S. clinical centers (for general reviews, see 6, 7).

Ellipticine and many derivatives are cytotoxic; they probably owe their pharmacological action to this property which must be understood at the molecular level for improving a

[1] Part of these studies have been generously supported by SANOFI, France.
[2] Present address: Laboratoire de Chimie de Coordination CNRS, Toulouse, France.

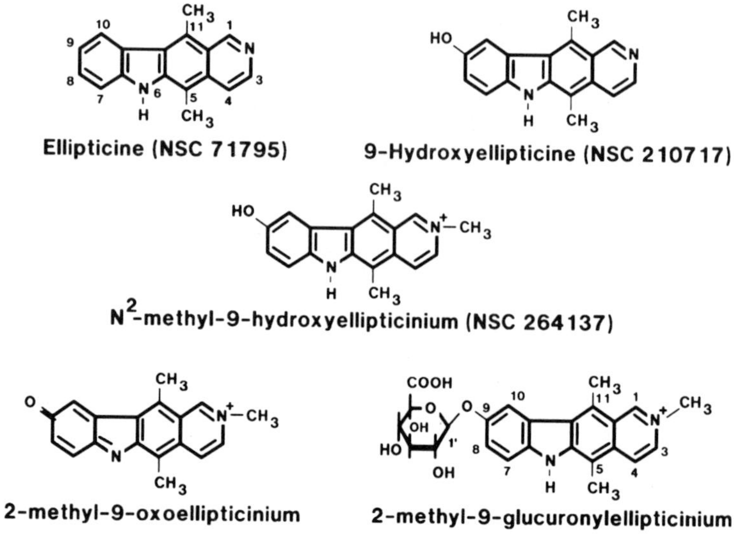

FIGURE 1.   Structure of ellipticine and main derivatives.

further biochemical screening of new active compounds in these
series. The in vitro search for any specific mode of interaction between these substances and some components of the
living systems might help in understanding their chemical
reactivity; it might, in addition, provide some clues –
although quite wooly – to the nature of the in vivo biochemical
interactions sustained by these drugs. For instance, it has
been established that ellipticine and most derivatives, owing
to their flat structure, bind to DNA into which they intercalate (K_{app} ~ $10^6 M^{-1}$ in usual conditions) (8, 9). However,
such an investigation must be extended to the identification
of the true pharmacological target, i.e., the one whose
hitting at is responsible for the cytotoxic effects. This
identification requires prerequisite steps, some of which are
described here:

(1)   Metabolites must be tracked down, isolated, characterized, and studied for their reactivity; such data may allow
an outlining of the true mechanisms of biochemical reactions.

(2)   Genetic evidence must be provided: known mutants
affecting characterized enzymatic pathways or biochemical con-
stituents, which are assumed to make up the pharmacological
target, should be responsive to the drugs, according to the
type of mutation.

(3) Biochemical data correlating the amount of drug or its metabolites bound in vivo to their supposed biochemical target and the pharmacological (or biological) responses must be looked for.

The main conclusions drawn from experiments worked out along these lines are presented here. Their implications to the understanding of the cytotoxic properties of the ellipticines will be briefly presented. All experimental details are published elsewhere.

II. METABOLISM OF ELLIPTICINE AND DERIVATIVES

A. Description

The metabolism and the biodisposition of ellipticine and its N^2-CH_3 derivative have been studied in rats and humans in our group (12, 25). Figure 2 summarizes the results.

1. After an iv or an ip administration, these compounds are first hydroxylated; minor 7OH-E and 9OH-E metabolites are detected; this oxidation process has been reconstituted in vitro with rat liver microsome preparations at a lower yield.

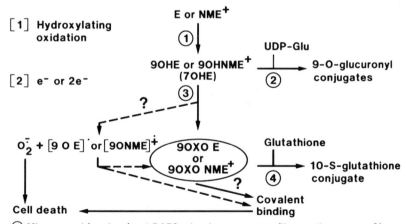

[1] Hydroxylating oxidation

[2] e⁻ or 2e⁻

① Microsomal (nuclear) cyt P450 mixed oxygenases (liver, other organs?)
② Glucuronyltransferases (liver).
③ Peroxydases, Prostaglandin endoperoxide synthetases?
④ Glutathione S-transferases (liver).

FIGURE 2. Metabolic pathways of ellipticine and N^2-CH_3 ellipticinium (NME⁺).

In vivo, most of the drug is oxidized along this pathway; the relative amounts of the two metabolites detected depends on the type of cytochrome P450 which has been induced by pre-treating the animals. These results might have some bearing on the pharmacological properties of the ellipticines since the 9OH derivatives are, as a general rule, more cytotoxic and more antitumoral than their non-hydroxylated counterparts, whereas the 7OH derivatives were by far less active (for instance, ID_{50} of in vitro grown L1210 cells after 48 hrs of exposure are respectively 0.015 μM and 5.4 μM). However, these hydroxylated derivatives are mostly eliminated as non-cytotoxic 9-0-glucuronide conjugates in the bile and the urine.

2.   A minor part of the N^2-methyl-9-hydroxylated metabolites is submitted to a second subsequent oxidation process which generates after abstraction of two hydrogen atoms a p-quinone imine ellipticinium derivative (9-oxo-ellipticinium). This component is a potent electrophile which binds covalently to nucleophilic glutathione to form a 10-S-glutathione adduct which has been recovered from the bile of rats (Fig. 3).

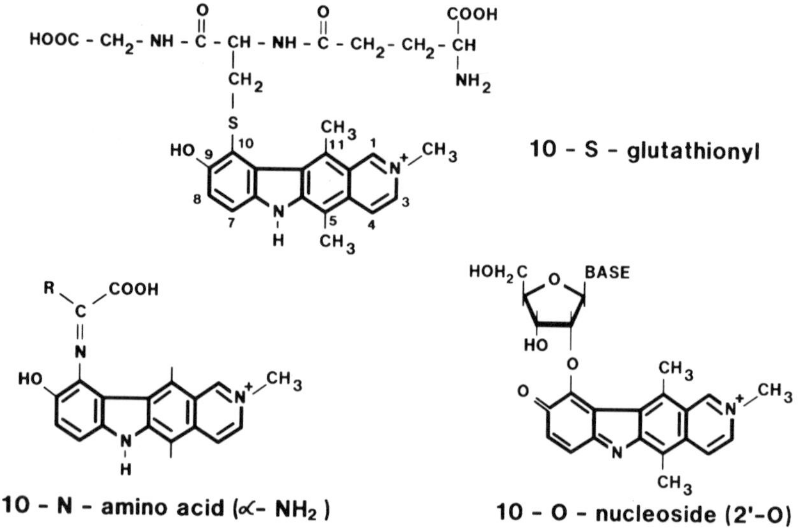

FIGURE 3.   Structure of the adducts formed either in vitro or in vivo (S-adducts) from 9-oxoellipticinium. Each structure reported here has been ascertained by NMR and mass spectrometry studies.

Urines of rats and humans iv treated by 2-methyl-9-hydroxy-
ellipticinium contain 10-S-adducts generated by a further
degradation of the glutathione adduct. The occurrence of such
adducts provides an indirect but compelling evidence for the
existence of the second oxidative pathway, subsequent to the
first one, along which electrophilic quinone imine metabolites
(oxoellipticines) are generated. The compounds might be
responsible in vivo for an oxidative alk(r)ylation process.
   3. In addition, we have been able to demonstrate in vitro
that 9-OH-ellipticine (nium) oxidation might proceed through a
stepwise removal of the two electrons; the first univalent
step generates transient radical species.
   In the following sections, we comment on the biooxidative
alkylation process and on the production of radical species.

B.   Chemical Studies on the Oxoellipticinium Derivatives

   The oxoellipticines, the occurrence of which was disclosed
by the metabolic studies, are difficult to handle, owing to
their high reactivity. They are, however, likely to occur
frequently because most animal cells contain peroxidases
and/or oxidases endowed with peroxidase activity, or prosta-
glandin-synthetase complexes which might be peroxidative prone
systems (14).   They are potent electrophiles able to spontaneously bind to many biological nucleophiles. Binding to
vital targets might induce cell death. Along this line, our
work has been focused (a) on the preparation of the oxoellipticine derivatives and (b) on the chemical reactivity of these
new products, especially on their electrophilic capabilities.

   1. Formation of oxoellipticine derivatives. These derivatives are easily obtained in vitro through oxidation of 9-OH-
ellipticines by horseradish or myelo-peroxidases in the presence of H_2O_2. This oxidation might also arise spontaneously
at a slower rate in the presence of atmospheric oxygen as the
electron acceptor. Their structure and physicochemical characteristics have been thoroughly documented (15). The oxo-
ellipticiniums are more reactive than the oxoellipticines and
must be extemporaneously manipulated.

   2. Chemical reactivity of oxoellipticinium derivatives.
In the presence of a variety of nucleophilic molecules, N^2-
methyl-9-oxoellipticinium undergoes an attack from which in-
variably results the formation of a covalent bond at the 10
position on the ellipticine nucleus. This regioselectivity
might be due to the existence of a tautomeric structure
arising from an electronic rearrangement around the four conjugated cycles facilitated by the pyridine nitrogen (Fig. 4).

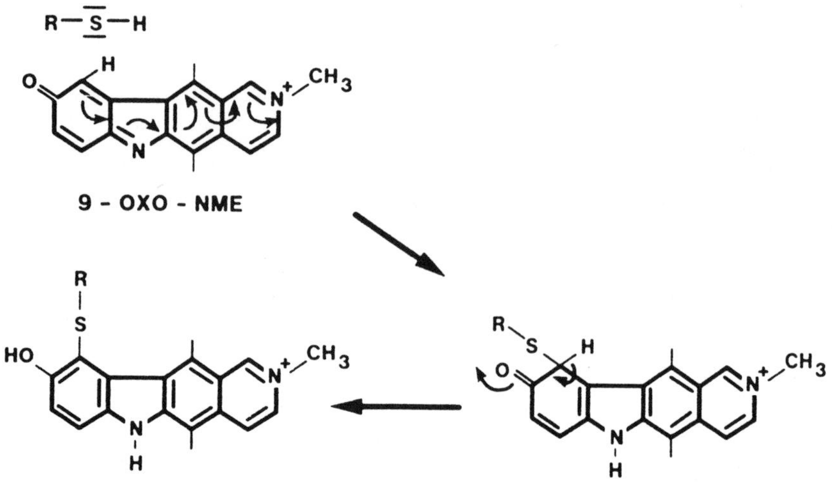

FIGURE 4. Mechanism of formation of 10-S-glutathione adduct.

H_2O (at acidic pH) and H_2O_2 at a neutral pH are capable of generating 9-10 orthoquinone derivatives which are side products of most alkylation reactions in these series.

Most amino acids can be bound by the α-NH_2 group to N^2-methyl-9-oxoellipticinium and form new stable adducts after a secondary oxidation process (Fig. 3). However, cysteine and glutathione form exclusively S-adducts (Fig. 4). The NH_2-adducts fluoresce; the quantum yield of fluorescence is increased by about 20-fold when these adducts intercalate into DNA. The new derivatives are very stable; surprisingly, they are not oxidizable in spite of the presence of a p-aminophenol structure.

An extensive study of the interactions of N^2methyl-9-oxo-ellipticinium and various other nucleosides, nucleotides, dinucleotides (NAD^+) and polynucleotides is under way.

Adducts are formed from ribonucleosides (Fig. 3); they result from an unexpected regioselective arylation at the 2'-0 position of the sugar which leaves untouched any other nucleophilic atom of the nucleoside. Neither bases alone nor ribose nor 2'-deoxyribonucleoside nor arabinofuranoside are able to react in the same conditions. The reason for this regioselectivity is still unknown; it might be the consequence of a preliminary stacking of the nucleoside base with the pyridocarbazole part of the ellipticinium as suggested by the better yield of these reactions when purine nucleosides are used.

This phenomenon might have significant bearings on under-standing some topological constraints which characterize the intercalative binding of several drugs into DNA. The ribonu-cleotides react also with N^2-CH_3-9-oxoellipticinium; however, the presence of a 5'-phosphoryl group entails the loss of the regioselectivity. The structure of the ribonucleotide adducts is not yet known with certainty. The deoxyribonucleotide adducts are fluorescent; consequently they provide convenient markers for the detection and the characterization of the adducts formed after binding of ellipticine derivatives or metabolites on DNA either _in vivo_ or _in vitro_.

The _in vitro_ covalent binding of N^2-methyl-9-oxoellipti-cinium on RNA and DNA can be followed directly by fluores-cence. Acid hydrolysis of DNA previously exposed to N^2-CH_3-9-oxoellipticinium yields fluorescent products which can be iso-lated by HPLC. Adenine might be a site of binding _in vitro_.

C. Generation of Radical Species. The formation of 9-oxoellipticine and N^2-CH_3-9-oxoellipticinium involves the univalent removal of one electron only as its first step and generates intermediate radical species, among which the super-oxide anion, O_2,$^-$ and some free radical form of the drug itself have been identified _in vitro_ by enzymatic studies and RPE determinations carried out in alkaline solutions or at a physiological pH with the spin trap DMPO. Both radical species dismutate and yield H_2O_2 or the oxoellipticine deriva-tives.

The standard potential of oxido-reduction of the univalent transfer of the first electron has been measured by electro-chemical techniques; it lies around +0,600 volt, slightly depending on the type of ellipticine derivatives and on the pH. The value shows that the intermediate free radical 9-OH species is a potent reducing agent able to abstract electrons from neighbor molecules and to propagate new radical species which might subsequently form covalent bonds. However, its formation is difficult to explain on simple thermodynamic grounds if O_2 is the only electron acceptor since the standard potential of the $O_2 \rightleftharpoons O_2^-$ redox couple is around -0,300 volt.

III.   IS DNA THE TARGET OF ELLIPTICINE DERIVATIVES?

A.   Mutagenesis by Ellipticine Compounds

Most ellipticine derivatives are potent mutagens in bacteria (16), in yeast (17), and in mammalian cells (18). This property suggests that DNA interacts directly with these compounds or some of their metabolites in vivo. This conclusion has been reinforced by experiments establishing that the mutagenic ability of ellipticine derivatives depend on the bases sequences information which is encoded in DNA or on the DNA repair capabilities of the cells (18). Experiments have been carried out on Salmonella strains provided by Ames. Ellipticine and 9-OH-ellipticine were able to reverse mutations of the histidine operon to prototrophic phenotypes. (a) Such reversions were observed only on frameshift mutants. The ellipticine derivatives are totally unable to reverse the base pair substitution mutants. (b) The frequency of the reversion mutant varied according to the type of frameshift mutations. (c) The strains which carried uvrB mutants were more sensitive to the mutagenic actions of the ellipticines than their wild-type counterparts. The uvrB enzyme is specific for removing thymine dimers or bulky groups on DNA.
  Such results do not establish that the cytotoxicity elicited by some ellipticines is due to the same biochemical determinants which control the mutagenicity. Nevertheless, they prove that DNA is the specific target of these drugs responsible for one of their biological effects.
  Many ellipticine derivatives can inhibit the growth of some bacterial strains according to defined dose effect curves. The establishment of such curves according to the genetic environment of the Salmonella strains shows, for instance, that the valine-ellipticinium adduct (see IIB2 above) is twenty-fold more bacteriostatic on uvrB strains than on wild type.

B.   Biochemical Evidence for the Binding
of some Ellipticine Derivatives on DNA in vivo
and its Correlation to Cytotoxic Effects

Two different sets of data indicate that some ellipticine derivatives are able to bind to DNA either irreversibly and/or through a reversible intercalative process. In this last case, one result suggests that the importance of some biological effects caused by these drugs to bacteria is related to the number of bound molecules on inside nucleic acids.

1. N^2-methyl-9-hydroxyellipticinium has been added to in vitro grown L1210 cells at a concentration of 10 µM for 2 hours. After mechanical disruption, isolation of a membrane and a nuclei enriched fraction and treatment by TritonX100, hydrolysis in HCl 0.1 N for 12 hours at 70°C and HPLC separation, a fluorescent adduct was recovered at the same retention time that the marker guanylate-ellipticinium adduct (see IIB2 above). Identification of these adducts is in progress.

Besides the covalent binding of the drugs to DNA in vivo, it has been shown that ellipticine itself can induce breaks on DNA inside mammalian cells (19).

2. In an attempt to simplify the study of any quantitative relationship between the amount of ellipticine derivatives bound to DNA and the biological effects resulting from this binding, we selected in these series compounds whose binding to DNA must proceed in simplified and easily quantifiable ways. We therefore took advantage of several peculiar properties of a class of ellipticinium adducts prepared from four aliphatic amino acids.

(a) They constitute a congener series which can be ranked according to their hydrophobicity; the more hydrophobic the drug, the more accessible nucleic acids inside bacterial cells exposed to it.

(b) They bind in vitro to DNA ($K_{app} \sim 10^5 M^{-1}$) into which they intercalate; they do not generate oxo-ellipticinium derivatives in the usual conditions applied to 9-hydroxylated ellipticines; consequently, they are unable to produce free radicals or electrophilic species; in any case, the 10-C position is already occupied. They can be considered mere DNA intercalators.

(c) Their quantum yield of fluorescence is markedly enhanced when they bind on double-stranded polynucleotides (about 20-fold at $\lambda exc = 320$ nm with DNA). This property provides a convenient tool to follow the binding of these compounds on DNA and RNA after their penetration inside cells, since control experiments on disrupted bacteria have revealed that no other cell components but DNA and RNA are able to form fluorescing complexes with them.

(d) They inhibit the growth of Ames S. typhimurium, their ED_{50}, ranging from 1.6 µM to 100 µM.

The interesting observation here is that these ED_{50} which express the magnitude of the pharmacological effect are roughly correlated with the amount of compound internally bound to nucleid acids at saturation.

IV. DISCUSSION AND SUMMARY

Most ellipticine derivatives are antitumoral compounds which, in addition to their DNA intercalating ability which has long been known (8), are also capable of generating free radical species and electrophilic alkylative species after a process of metabolic oxidation. Both species are very reactive and might be the ultimate metabolites responsible for the cytotoxic effects of these drugs, probably by interacting with DNA. The formation of the electrophilic species has been shown to occur in rats and in humans. The nitroaromatics radiosensitizers and other antitumoral substances, among which are bleomycin , procarbazine, mitomycin C and the anthracyclines, daunomycin and adriamycin, share with the ellipticines the capability to generate free radicals (for general review, see 20). Common structural features, i.e., a p-quinone or a p-quinoneimine structure, characterize the anthracyclines, mitomycin C and the 9-oxoellipticine metabolites.   More specifically, "oxidative stress" has been put forward as a mechanism of toxicity which requires redox cycling of some of these compounds through radical intermediates that can reduce molecular oxygen to superoxide anion (21). An identical mechanism can be proposed for ellipticinium derivatives although it has not yet received any experimental support from in vivo studies.

The generation of electrophilic metabolites has also been described for the nitroaromatics and for several antitumor compounds: dacarbazine, 6-thiopurine, mitomycin C and m-AMSA (for general review, see 20). The main metabolite of m-AMSA has been shown to be a glutathione conjugate which must result from an oxidative bioactivation of m-AMSA to a quinoidal diimine (22), according to a metabolic pathway analogous to the one described here.

A bioreductive alkylation model has been proposed by Moore (23) to account for the cytotoxicity, mostly mitomycin C and the anthracyclines. Alternatively, a biooxidative alkylation model founded on the conjugate and consecutive metabolic action of cyt P-450 mixed oxygenases and peroxidases is presented here and discussed elsewhere (7, 13); it might provide some clues for understanding the molecular mechanisms of the cytotoxicity of many ellipticine derivatives as well as other antitumor drugs whose action seems to depend on an oxidative process generating electrophilic metabolites (procarbazine, dacarbazine, possibly 6-thiopurine and m-AMSA). This model might offer features similar to those proposed by Mitchell, Gillette, and co-workers from their classical studies on the biochemical toxicity of acetanilides almost a decade ago (24).

ACKNOWLEDGMENTS

A.M. Armbruster, H. Banoun, J. Bernadou, J. Chenu, S. Cros, A. Gouyette, P. Lesca, P. Lecointe, C. Malvy, G. Meunier, M. Maftouh, J. Moiroux and B. Monsarrat have been involved in several aspects of the work summarized in this presentation.

REFERENCES

1. Dalton, L.K., Demerac, S., Elmes, B.C., Loder, J.W., Swan, J.M., and Teitei, T., Aust. J. Chem. 20:2715 (1967).
2. LePecq, J.B., Dat Xuong, N., Gosse, C., and Paoletti, C., Proc. Natl. Acad. Sci. USA 71:5078 (1974).
3. Paoletti, C., LePecq, J.B., Dat Xuong, N., Lesca, P. and Lecointe, P., Curr. Chemother. 1195 (1978).
4. Juret, P., Tanguy, A., Le Talaer, J.Y., Abbatucci, J.S., Dat Xuong, N., Le Pecq, J.B., and Paoletti, C., Eur. J. Cancer 14:205 (1978).
5. Juret, P., Heron, J.F., Couette, J.E., Delozier, T., and Le Talaer, J.Y., Cancer Treatment Reports 66:1909 (1982).
6. Paoletti, C., Le Pecq, J.B., Dat Xuong, N., Juret, P., Garnier, H., Amiel, J.L., and Rouesse, J., in "Recent Results in Cancer Research" (G. Mathe and F.M. Muggia, eds.) 74:107, Springer-Verlag, Berlin (1980).
7. Meunier, B., Auclair, C., Bernadou, J., Meunier, G., Maftouh, M., Cros, S., Monsarrat, B., and Paoletti, C., in "Structure-Activity Relationships of Antitumor Agents" (D.N. Reinhoudt, T.A. Connors, H.M. Pinedo and K.W. van de Poll, eds.), p. 149, Martinjs Niuhoff, The Hague (1983).
8. Festy, B., Poisson, J., and Paoletti, C., FEBS Lett. 17:321 (1971).
9. Kohn, K.W., Waring, M.J., Glaubiger, D., and Friedman, C.A., Can. Res. 35:71 (1975).
10. Paoletti, C., Lesca, C., Cros, S., Malvy, C., and Auclair, C., Biochem. Pharmacol. 28:345 (1978).
11. Paoletti, C., Cros, S., Dat Xuong, N., Lecointe, P., and Moisand, A., Chem. Biol. Interact. 25:45 (1979).
12. Meunier, G., Meunier, B., Auclair, C., Bernadou, J., and Paoletti, C., Tetrahedron Letters 24:365 (1983).
13. Auclair, C., Hyland, K., and Paoletti, C., J. Med. Chem. (1983) in press.
14. Marnett, L.J., Life Sci. 24:531 (1981).
15. Auclair, C., and Paoletti, C., J. Med. Chem. 24:289 (1981).
16. Lecointe, P., Lesca, P., Cros, S., and Paoletti, C., Chem. Biol. Interact. 20:113 (1978).

17. Pinto, M., Guerineau, M., and Paoletti, C., Biochem. Pharmacol. 31:2161 (1982).
18. DeMarini, D., Cros, S., Paoletti, C., Lecointe, P., and Hsie, A., Cancer Res. 43:3544 (1983).
19. Zwelling, L.A., Michaels, S., Erickson, L.C., Ungerleiger, R.S., Nichols, M., and Kohn, K.W., Biochemistry 20:6563 (1981).
20. Trush, M.A., Mimnaugh, E.G., and Gram, T.E., Biochem. Pharmacol. 31:335 (1982).
21. Nelson, S.D., J.Med.Chem. 25:753 (1982).
22. Shoemaker, D.D., Cysyk, R.L., Padmanabhan, S., Bhat, H.B., and Malspeis, L., Drug. Metab. Dispos. 10:35 (1982).
23. Moore, H.W., Science 197:527 (1977).
24. Hinson, J.A., Monks, T.J., Hong, M., Highet, R.J., and Pohl, L.R., Drug Metab. Dispos. 10:47 (1982).
25. Maftouh, M., Monsarrat, B., Ras, R.C., Meunier, B. and Paoletti, C., Drug. Metab. Dispos. (1983) in press.

STUDIES ON BACTERIAL MERCURIC ION REDUCTASE

Barbara Fox and Christopher Walsh

Departments of Biology and Chemistry
Massachusetts Institute of Technology
Cambridge, Massachusetts 02139

Introduction

This laboratory has been involved during the last decade in examination of flavoenzyme-catalyzed reactions where the processing of substrates has pharmacological or toxicological significances. A particularly interesting and unusual case is provided by the microbial enzyme mercuric ion reductase which reduces Hg^{II} ions to elemental mercury, Hg^{o} at the stoichiometric expense of NADPH oxidation. This is a crucial step in microbial resistance to and detoxification of inorganic mercury salts (Silver & Kinscherf, 1983).

$$RS...Hg^{II}..SR + NADPH + H^+ \xrightarrow{E-FAD} Hg^{o} + 2RSH + NADP$$

In the global scheme, the oceans contain about 2×10^8 tons of mercury, some 10^6 tons of that contributed by industrial activity since 1900. Inorganic mercury salts and elemental mercury are leached from rock resevoirs, the Hg^{II} reduced to Hg^{o} and ultimately methylated to methyl mercury the potent mammalian neurotoxin. Mercury resistant bacteria are widespread, having been isolated from mercury contaminated soils (eg. around Minamata, Japan) but also in about 50% of drug-resistant clinical isolates.

Bacterial mercury resistance is plasmid encoded, frequently transposon encoded as in the enzyme to be discussed here; resistance is inducible with low levels of mercurials and widespread, particularly among enteric and

MECHANISM OF DRUG ACTION

antibiotic-resistant strains. Broad and narrow spectrum resistances have been defined, with narrow spectrum comprising inorganic Hg^{II} salts and broad spectrum also extending to include organomercurials; broad spectrum resistance is less than 10% the narrow resistance frequency. The genes for mercury resistance are grouped in an operon, the mer operon which codes for proteins specifying transport of organomercurial or mercuric ion into the cytoplasm, cleavage of the carbon-mercury bond to hydrocarbon and mercuric ion (in broad spectrum resistance), enzymic reduction to elemental Hg^{o}, and nonenzymic removal of the volatile Hg^{o} from the growth medium (See, Silver & Kinscherf, 1983; Summers and Silver, 1978).

We initiated study of the bacterial mercuric ion reductase for several reasons. First it provides the molecular basis for bacterial resistance to inorganic mercuric salts and as such is of clear toxicologic significance. Second this enzyme, the mer A gene product, is the only known enzyme able to reduce mercuric ions catalytically (at rates up to 1000/min) in stark contrast to other enzymes and proteins which may bind Hg^{II} in divalent sulfhydryl chelation and become inhibited. Third, a paper by Schottel in 1978 had identified the reductase from an E. coli strain as an FAD enzyme. This suggested Hg^{II} may function as a specific dihydroflavin reoxidant in this enzyme. We have chosen to study the mercuric ion reductase from Pseudomonas aeruginosa PA09501 (a gift from Dr. Simon Silver) in which the enzyme is encoded on plasmid pVS1. In turn, within this plasmid it was known by 1979 that the transposable element Tn501 was present and the mer operon genes were in the transposon. Tn501 was the object of DNA sequence analysis in the laboratory of Nigel Brown in Bristol, England, and we had the hope, now realized, that DNA sequencing might provide protein primary structure (Brown et al, 1983).

Enzyme Isolation and Characterization

We have reported recently (Fox & Walsh, 1982) that from the Tn501-encoded mer A gene on PVS1 in P. aeruginosa, induction with merbromin causes greater than 1000-fold selective production of mercuric ion reductase. We have developed a two-step (65° heat step, Orange A matrex affinity column) purification that provides homogeneous enzyme in 80% yield after 15-fold purification. Thus, the enzyme is 6% of the soluble protein and we estimate that 160 grams of cells should yield one gram of the enzyme. Because the enzyme eluted from the matrex A column with

NADPH was green rather than yellow, reflecting a nicotin-
amide-enzyme FAD charge transfer complex, we monitored the
optical spectrum of the enzyme-FAD complex carefully on
reductive titrations.

The mercuric ion reductase takes up four electrons per
FAD before a reduced $FADH_2$ spectrum appears, mandating the
presence of another redox component. Also the two electron reduced intermediate showed charge transfer bands
which were highly similar to those seen previously with
lipoamide dehydrogenase and glutathione reductase
(Williams, 1976). Since these two enzymes both contain an
active site cystine disulfide which is reduced by transfer
of electrons from $FADH_2$, providing a net four electron
storage capacity, we felt mercuric ion reductase might be
of this category. In fact, titration of the oxidized
enzyme and the two electron reduced enzyme with dithiobis-
nitrobenzoate readily revealed that two cysteine dithiols
become specifically accessible in the EH_2 form of mercuric
ion reductase.

	Titratable Thiols
Oxidized Enzyme(-NADPH)	2.2 ± 0.10
Reduced Enzyme(+NADPH)	4.3 ± 0.47
Difference	2.1

At this juncture we felt it quite likely this enzyme
was structurally a new entry in the small class of enzymes
with FAD and a redox active cystine disulfide (Table I).

Table I
Enzymes with FAD and Redox Active Cystine Disulfide

Enzyme	Source	Physiologic Function
1. Glutathione Reductase	Procaryotes, Eucaryotes	Glutathione Disulfide Reduction
2. Lipoamide Dehydrogenase	Procaryotes, Eucaryotes	Dehydrogenation of dithiol form of lipoamide· enzyme

3.	Thioredoxin Reductase	Procaryotes, Eucaryotes	Reduction of Oxidized-Thioredoxin
4.	Asparagusate Dehydrogenase	Asparagus	Reduction of oxidized asparagusate
5.	Mercuric Ion Reductase	Bacterial Plasmids	Reduction of Hg^{II} to Hg^{o} in Bacterial Resistance to Hg^{II}

All other members of this class show catalytic activity towards disulfide or dithiol substrates. We have tested glutathione reductase, lipoamide dehydrogenase, and thioredoxin reductase: they cannot reduce mercuric salts. Nor can mercuric ion reductase catalyze reaction with glutathione, lipoamide, or thioredoxin. However, we have documented (Fox & Walsh, 1982) molecular weight similarities (all are dimers), reduction potential similarities, and charge transfer similarities among those four enzymes.

Structural Investigations

We began structural studies in two ways. First we analyzed the amino terminal sequence of the purified mercuric ion reductase. This was complicated by in vivo proteolysis (we see subunits of two sizes (61 and 56K)) but we could provide, from Edman degradation, the sequence of the first dozen residues to Nigel Brown and his colleagues at Bristol (Fox & Walsh, 1983a). This permitted identification of the start of the mer A gene which they then sequenced in toto (Brown et al, 1983). The mer A gene on Tn501 encodes a protein of 561 amino acids with a predicted molecular weight of 59,000.

In parallel with the N-terminal sequencing, we turned to iodoacetamide as a potentially specific label for alkylation of the active site thiols in the EH_2 form of the enzyme. This approach was based on the work of Williams and his colleagues on lipoamide dehydrogenase and glutathione reductase who had observed specific incorporation of one mole of carboxymethyl residue into the EH_2 forms, inducing complete inactivation (Thorpe and

ALKYLATION STRATEGY FOR MERCURIC REDUCTASE

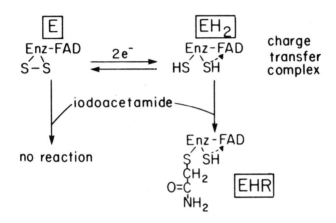

Williams, 1976; Arscott et al, 1981). With [^{14}C]-iodo-
acetamide, the inactivated enzymes were digested with
trypsin and a radioactive tryptic peptide isolated in each
case containing the active site cysteines. Sequence analysis of the peptide in each case revealed cysteines five
residues apart and preferential labeling of the amino
proximal cysteine of the pair. It was argued that the
carboxyl proximal cysteine was protected either by charge
transfer to the flavin in EH_2 or by inaccessibility. The
availability of a 2.0 A$^{\circ}$ map of human erythrocyte glutathione reductase has clearly revealed that the cysteine
that is not captured by iodoacetamide is closest to the
FAD in the oxidized form of the enzyme (Thieme et al,
1981).

   Our studies with iodoacetamide alkylation of mercuric
ion reductase have now dramatically proved out this structural similarity hypothesis (Fox & Walsh, 1983a). It is
again the EH$_2$ form that becomes specifically and stoichio-
metrically alkylated and we have isolated and sequenced
the major radiolabeled tryptic peptide. This active site
peptide has the two cysteine residues, with twelve of
thirteen residues identical to glutathione reductase,
including the invariant positioning and spacing of the
cys-val-asn-val-gly-cys sequence. Again it is the amino-
proximal cysteine of the pair that is specifically alkylated. The active site sequences of the three enzymes are
displayed below.

ACTIVE SITE SEQUENCE COMPARISON

		T7	T12	$[^{14}C]$-Iodoacetamide Labeling (T7/T12)
Mercuric Reductase	Gly	Thr Ile Gly Gly Thr Cys	Val Asn Val Gly Cys	val Pro Ser Lys	18 / 1
Glutathione Reductase[1]	His	Lys Leu Gly Gly Thr Cys	Val Asn Val Gly Cys	Val Pro Lys Lys	8 / 1
Lipoamide Dehydrogenase[2]	Asn	Thr Leu Gly Gly Val Cys	Leu Asn Val Gly Cys	Ile Pro Ser Lys	13 / 1

1. Arscott, Thorpe and Williams, 1981
2. Thorpe and Williams, 1976

The alignment of the active site tryptic peptide and the cystine bridge in the primary sequence of mercuric ion reductase could then be provided from the DNA sequence of Brown and his group (Brown et al, 1983). The active site cystine is located at residues 136 and 141 as noted in the

Location of Active Site in Amino Acid Sequence

	Location of Cys T7 and T12 (from NH_2-terminus)
Mercuric Reductase[1]	136,141
Glutathione Reductase[2]	58,63
Lipoamide Dehydrogenase[3]	45,50

– Cys - Val - Asn - Val - Gly - Cys –
T7   T12

Limited chymotryptic digestion of mercuric reductase cleanly removes 85 amino acids from the NH_2-terminus with no loss of catalytic activity.

1. Brown et al., 1983
2. Untucht-Grau et al., 1982
3. Williams, personal communication

table below. For comparison glutathione reductase and lipoamide dehydrogenase have the active site cystine bridge displaced some 100 residues closer to the amino terminus. This in turn suggested to us that mercuric ion reductase contained a long N-terminal extension which

might not be vital to catalysis. We have verified this by
limited exposure of mer reductase to chymotrypsin which
leads to a specific clipping at the amide bond after trp

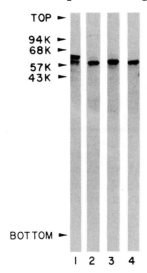

TOP ►
94K ►
68K ►
57K ►
43K ►

BOTTOM ►

1 2 3 4

Limited proteolytic digestion
of mercuric reductase
cleaves off ~85 a.a.,
indicating the presence of
a separate NH_2-terminal
domain. This brings the
active sites of mercuric
reductase and glutathione
reductase into register.

1. native mercuric reductase
2. enzyme + chymotrypsin,
   2 μg/ml
3. enzyme + trypsin, 5 μg/ml
4. enzyme + trypsin, 0.4 μg/ml

85 (determined by N-terminal sequencing of the 476 residue
long remaining enzyme). This shortened 476 residue enzyme
has no detectable loss in catalytic activity. The cysteine residues are now at positions 51 and 56 respectively
in much closer alignment with glutathione reductase and
lipoamide dehydrogenase (Fox and Walsh, 1983a). We have
prepared clipped mer reductase on a 10-20mg scale and
believe it a good candidate for crystallization and eventual high resolution analysis to compare with glutathione
reductase. That may eventually give some clues to how the
basic FAD, cystine redox domain has been subtly modified
to now reduce mercuric ions. Conversely mer reductase
will not reduce oxidized glutathione and this enzyme is
lacking the histidine equivalent to his467 of glutathione
reductase (Brown et al, 1983) which is argued to be a
crucial active site base/proton shuttle for that latter
enzyme's catalytic efficiency (Schulz et al, 1982).

Catalytic Studies:

    Studies on glutathione redutase and lipoamide dehy-
drogenase (summarized in Williams, 1976) have determined
the functional redox cycle is between oxidized enzyme(E)
and EH_2; EH_4 is a catalytically incompetent, kinetically
irrelevant species in turnover. We have not tested this
yet but anticipate that outcome for mercuric reductase.

It is likely that NADPH passes electrons to bound FAD via
hydride transfer in through flavin N5. Electron transfer
from dihydro FAD to active site cystine disulfide will
occur via covalent flavin 4a-thiol adduct with the amino
distal cysteine (cys 141). The overwhelmingly predominant
form of EH_2 on reductase titration is the E-FAD, cysteine
dithiol form. This EH_2 species has thiol ligands able to
chelate to incoming HgII, presented as a dithiol chelate.
It is likely that cys_{141} is in charge transfer complex to
FAD and cys_{136} is the thiol available for initial chelation to approaching $RS-Hg^{II}-SR$. Exchange of one thiol
ligand would yield initially the mixed E-cys-S..Hg..SR
species and what happens next may determine how this
enzyme survives. Does the cys_{141} then form a bidentate Hg
complex? Is that now a dead enzyme or still catalytically
competent? If a cys 136, 141-Hg bidentate complex is
active, how are electrons transferred uniquely in this
enzyme's microenvironment? If the enzyme stays monoden-
tate via cys_{136} how are electrons transferred there? Is
it a one or two electron process?

We have begun to accumulate some evidence which may
in the end be relevant from study of two species of
enzyme, the first the monoalkylated enzyme from iodoacetamide treatment (Fox & Walsh, 1983a), the second apo-
enzyme reconstituted with 5-deazaFAD (Fox & Walsh, 1983b).
Both are inactive for mercuric ion reduction but both have
actually increased Vmax rates for catalytic transhydrogenation to thio NADP, as noted in the table below. In

Enzyme Form	Turnover Number (min^{-1})	
	Hg^+ reduction	Transhydrogenation
Haloenzyme	220	40
Monoalkylated Enzyme	4	220
5deazaFAD Enzyme	0	135

the specifically monoalkylated enzyme, the FAD can still
be reduced by NADPH but electrons cannot flow on to HgII.
The $E-FADH_2$ accumulates and can transfer electrons back
out to thio NADP. By precedent with glutathione reductase
where the FAD coenzyme is sandwiched between bound NADPH
and the active site disulfide, alkylation of the active
site cysteine in mer reductase leaves the NADPH site
unaffected.

The second modification which blocks mercuric salt reduction but leads to an increase in Vmax of transhydrogenase activity is use of 5deazaFAD in place of FAD.

Flavin   5-carba-5-deazaflavin

We have previously used this flavin analog (naturally occurring in methanogenic bacteria) to study flavoenzyme mechanisms (Walsh, 1978; 1980). While $FADH_2$ reacts with disulfides by way of flavin C_{4a} adducts, the $5dFADH_2$ show no propensity to reduce disulfides. Chan and Bruice (1977) observed that 8-cyano-5-deazaflavins, which are highly electron deficient, will be attacked by thiols but at C_5, not at C_{4a}, to form an unproductive thiol-C_5deazaflavin adduct.

Our prediction that when apoprotein of mercuric reductase was reconstituted with 5-deazaFAD, the enzyme cannot reduce the active site disulfide and so not reduce HgII has been borne out (Fox & Walsh, 1983b). NADPH will reduce the bound 5dFAD in the enzyme but there is no overall reduction of HgII. When one examines 5dFAD-enzyme for transhydrogenation, the Vmax is three-fold elevated over native enzyme as shown in the above table. Again we interpret this increased rate to be due to steady state accumulation of the $5dFADH_2$ form of EH_2, reactive for transhydrogenation with thio NADP. The high catalytic competence of 5dFAD-mercuric reductase for nicotinamide transhydrogenation is dramatic and exceptional compared to other flavoenzymes where the lower reduction potential of 5dFAD (-310mv vs -210mv for FAD) and its inability to undergo facile one electron redox processes slow rates by 10^{-3} to 10^{-6} that of native FAD enzymes. Additional flavin analogs may be useful in mechanistic analysis of this unique enzymic reduction of mercuric ions.

REFERENCES

1.   Arscott, L. D., Thorpe, C., Williams, C. H. (1981)
      Biochemistry 20, 1513.

2.   Brown, N. L., Ford, S. J., Pridmore, R. D.,
      Pritzinger, D. C. (1983) Biochemistry 22, in press.

3.   Chan, R. L., Bruice, T. C. (1977) J. Amer. Chem. Soc.
      99, 6721.

4.   Fox, B. and Walsh, C. (1982) J. Biol. Chem. 257,
      2498.

5.   Fox, B. and Walsh, C. (1983a) Biochemistry 23, in
      press.

6.   Fox, B. and Walsh, C. (1983b) J. Biol. Chem. 258,
      submitted.

7.   Schottel J. (1978) J. Biol. Chem. 253, 4341.

8.   Schulz, G. E., Schirmer, R. H., Pai, E. F. (1982) J.
      Mol. Biol. 160, 287.

9.   Silver, S. and Kinscherf, T. (1983) in Biodegradation
      and Detoxification of Environmental Pollutants
      (Chakrabarty, A. M., ed) CRC Press, Boca Raton,
      Florida, in press.

10.   Summers, A. O., and Silver, S. (1978) Ann. Rev.
      Microbiol. 32, 637.

11.   Thieme, R., Pai, E., Schirmer, R. H., Schulz, G. J.
      Mol. Biol. 152, 763.

12.   Thorpe, C. and Williams C. H. (1976) J. Biol. Chem.
      751, 7726.

13.   Williams, C. H. (1976) in The Enzymes (Bayer, P. D.,
      ed) 3rd Ed. Vol. 13, p 89, Academic Press, N.Y.

14.   Walsh, C. (1978) Ann. Rev. Biochem. 47, 881.

15.   Walsh, C. (1980) Accts. Chem. Res. 13, 148.

CYTOCHROME P$_1$-450 INDUCTION BY TCDD: BIOCHEMICAL AND GENETIC ANALYSES IN MOUSE HEPATOMA CELLS[1]

James P. Whitlock, Jr.[2]
Donna Galeazzi
David Israel[3]
Arthur G. Miller[4]

Department of Pharmacology
Stanford University School of Medicine
Stanford, California

I. INTRODUCTION

Microsomal, cytochrome P-450-containing monooxygenases catalyze the initial reaction in the cellular metabolism of many lipophilic substrates. In some instances, this represents a step in a detoxificaion pathway; in other cases, the oxygenated metabolite is a chemically reactive, electrophilic species which can produce toxicity and/or neoplasia. Thus, the metabolism of a hydrophobic compound may be either beneficial or harmful to the cell; the net effect results from the balance between detoxification pathways and activation pathways and the relative activities of the enzyme systems involved (1,2).

[1]Supported by Research Grants CA24580 and GM17367 and Training Grant GM07149 from the NIH and Research Grant BC418 from the American Cancer Society.
[2]Recipient of a Faculty Research Award from the American Cancer Society.
[3]Recipient of an Advanced Predoctoral Fellowship in Pharmacology/Toxicology from the Pharmaceutical Manufacturers Association Foundation.
[4]Present address: The Salk Institute, San Diego, CA.

A number of compounds induce microsomal monooxygenase
activity. For example, the environmental contaminant
2,3,7,8,-tetrachlorodibenzo-p-dioxin (TCDD) is a potent
inducer of an isozyme (cytochrome P_1-450) associated with
aryl hydrocarbon (benzo(a)pyrene) hydroxylase (AHH) activity.
Induction involves the binding of TCDD to an intracellular
receptor protein and the accumulation of the TCDD-receptor
complex in the nucleus of the cell, followed by an increase
in enzyme-specific mRNA. Thus, AHH induction provides an
interesting system for studying eukaryotic gene expression
(3,4).

We are studying the mechanism of AHH induction using
mouse hepatoma (Hepa 1c1c7) cells in culture. We have
examined the induction process in parental (wild-type) cells,
in variant cells containing altered induction mechanisms,
and in hybrid cells constructed using cell fusion.

II. STUDIES OF WILD-TYPE CELLS: THE ROLE OF mRNA IN ENZYME INDUCTION

We have used a cDNA probe specific for a portion of the
cytochrome P_1-450 gene (5) to analyze the accumulation of
P_1-450-specific RNA in wild-type cells exposed to TCDD. We
isolated total and poly(A)-containing RNA from induced (1 nM
TCDD, 24 hr) cells and fractionated glyoxal-denatured RNA by
electrophoresis in agarose gels. We transferred the RNA to
nitrocellulose paper, hybridized it to cDNA labeled with ^{32}P
by nick-translation, and analyzed it by autoradiography. The
results (Fig. 1) indicate that TCDD induces the accumulation
of a single species of polyadenylated P_1-450 RNA with an
approximate size of 2900 nucleotides.

We analyzed total RNA using dot hybridization, autoradiography, and densitometry to compare the induction of P_1-450
mRNA to the induction of AHH activity with respect to both
the sensitivity of induction to TCDD and the kinetics of
induction. Figure 2 shows that for both mRNA induction and
enzyme induction 1) the half-maximal increase occurs at
about 10 pM TCDD, 2) the maximal increase occurs at about
100 pM TCDD, and 3) there is a 25-to 50-fold difference
between uninduced and maximally-induced cells.

Figure 3 shows that the accumulation of mRNA precedes
enzyme induction by several hours. RNA accumulation is half-
maximal about 2 hr and is maximal 4-6 hr after exposure to
TCDD. AHH activity is half-maximal about 4 hr and is maximal
8-16 hr after exposure to TCDD. These experiments indicate
that the accumulation of P_1-450 mRNA quantitatively accounts
for the induction of AHH activity by TCDD in these cells.

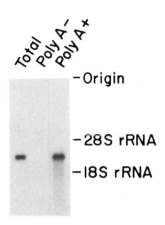

FIGURE 1. Analysis of RNA in TCDD-induced wild-type cells. Total RNA from induced (1 nM TCDD, 24 hr) cells was fractionated on oligo(dT)-cellulose, denatured with glyoxal, and electrophoresed in an agarose gel. Samples were transferred to nitrocellulose, hybridized to nick-translated P₁-450 cDNA, and analyzed by autoradiography. See Ref. 6 for details.

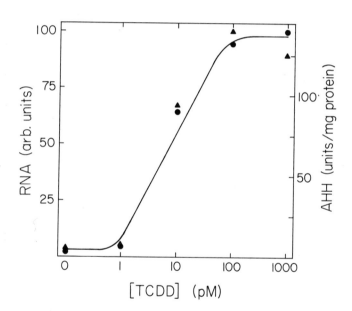

FIGURE 2. Induction of P₁-450 mRNA and AHH activity as a function of [TCDD]. Wild-type cells were exposed for 24 hr to TCDD; total RNA was analyzed by dot hybridization to P₁-450 cDNA, followed by autoradiography, and densitometry. AHH activity was measured using a spectrofluorometric assay which detects phenolic BP metabolites (7). See Ref. 6 for details. ▲, mRNA; ●, enzyme activity.

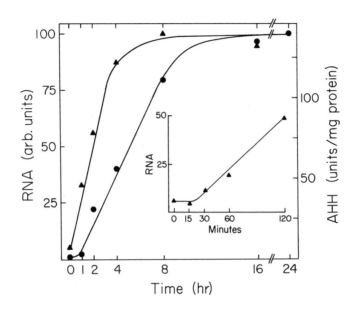

FIGURE 3.   Kinetics of induction of P_1-450 mRNA and AHH activity by TCDD (1 nM) in wild-type cells.   See legend to Fig. 2 and Ref. 6 for details.   ▲, mRNA; ●, enzyme activity.

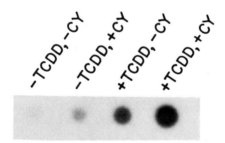

FIGURE 4.   Effect of cycloheximide on the induction of P_1-450 mRNA by TCDD in wild-type cells.   Cells were exposed for 4 hr to TCDD (1 nM) and/or cycloheximide (CY, 10 μg/ml). Total RNA was analyzed by dot hybridization to P_1-450 cDNA, followed by autoradiography.   See Ref. 6 for details.

The inset in Figure 3 indicates that we can detect an increase in P_1-450 mRNA 30 min after exposing cells to TCDD. Thus, the increase in P_1-450 mRNA is an early cellular response to TCDD.   In addition, TCDD induces an increase in P_1-450 mRNA in cells in which protein synthesis has been

inhibited 95-97% by cycloheximide (Fig. 4). The rapidity of
mRNA accumulation and its insensitivity to cycloheximide
both suggest that the induction of P_1-450 mRNA is a primary
response to TCDD. Additional experiments (not shown) suggest
that the accumulation of P_1-450 mRNA is not due to a decrease
in its rate of degradation. Therefore, we infer that TCDD
increases the rate of synthesis of P_1-450 mRNA, leading to
a higher steady-state level of the message.

Thus, our studies in wild-type cells indicate that the
mechanism of induction of AHH activity by TCDD involves the
accumulation of P_1-450 mRNA. This represents a primary
response to TCDD, and probably reflects an increased rate
of transcription of the P_1-450 structural gene.

III. ISOLATION OF VARIANT CELLS

We used the fluorescence-activated cell sorter (FACS) to
measure the metabolism of benzo(a)pyrene (BP) in single,
viable cells. We showed that the loss of BP fluorescence
from cells reflects the metabolism of the compound and that
we could use the FACS to isolate variant cells with either
enhanced or diminished BP-metabolizing enzyme activity. For
example, we sorted from a population of induced cells a subpopulation which lost BP fluorescence very slowly. We grew
this subpopulation, resorted it, and repeated this sequence
again. FACS analysis of these cells yields a fluorescence
histogram indicating a marked enrichment for cells which
metabolize BP much less rapidly than wild-type cells (Fig. 5).
These cells also grow well in high concentrations of BP,
due to their inability to metabolically activate the compound.
Thus, we designate these variants "BP^r" (BP-resistant).

We subcloned these cells, and we analyzed several representative subclones, to identify the defects responsible for
their diminished ability to metabolize BP.

IV. STUDIES OF BP^r VARIANT CELLS: THE ROLE OF A TCDD RECEPTOR PROTEIN IN ENZYME INDUCTION

Table I shows that several representative BP^r variants
contain less than 10% of wild-type basal and TCDD-inducible
AHH activity and that the variants comprise two classes:
those with low, but detectable, AHH activity (exemplified by
BP^rc4 and $TAOc1BP^rc1$) and those with no AHH activity (exemplified by BP^rc1 and BP^rc3).

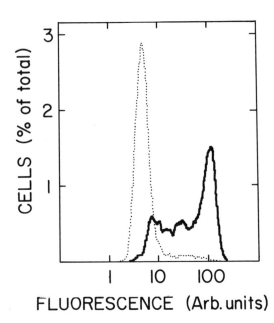

FIGURE 5.   FACS analysis of variants with decreased BP-
metabolizing enzyme activity.   Cells with high fluorescence
were sequentially selected three times from populations of
induced cells.   These cells (solid line) and wild-type cells
(dotted line) were incubated at 37°C for 20 min with 25 nM
BP and analyzed on the FACS.   See Ref. 8 for details.

We chose TAOc1BP^{r}c1 and BP^{r}c3 as representatives of the
two classes for further study.

TABLE I.   AHH Activity in Wild-Type and Variant Cells

Cell	Basal AHH[a]	Induced[b] AHH
Wild-type	1.0	127
BP^{r}c1	<0.1	<0.1
BP^{r}c3	<0.1	<0.1
BP^{r}c4	<0.1	4.3
TAOc1BP^{r}c1	0.1	5.3

[a]Units/mg protein
[b]TCDD (1 nM, 24 hr)
See Ref. 9 for details.

Fig. 6 shows that, as shown previously (Fig. 2), the
ED50 for AHH induction in wild-type cells is about 10 pm
TCDD. In contrast, in TAOc1BP^{r}c1 the ED50 for induction is
about 10-fold higher; again, BP^{r}c3 contains no AHH activity.

The decreased sensitivity of the induction response to
TCDD in TAOc1BP^{r}c1 suggested that the cells might contain
a lesion in a gene which regulates the induction mechanism,
rather than a lesion in a structural (enzyme) gene. Therefore, we analyzed the cells for their content of an intracellular receptor protein for TCDD. The results (Fig. 7)
indicate that TAOc1BP^{r}c1 cells contain about 10-fold less of
an 8S TCDD-binding protein than do wild-type cells, but in a
nuclear/cytoplasmic ratio similar to wild-type. Thus, these
variants contain a receptor which is reduced either in amount
or in affinity for TCDD, but they retain their ability to
accumulate the TCDD-receptor complex in the nucleus. In
contrast, BP^{r}c3 cells bind the same amount of TCDD as do
wild-type cells, but in an abnormal nuclear/cytoplasmic
proportion. Thus, these variants contain normal amounts of
receptor (with normal affinity for TCDD - not shown) but
are unable to accumulate the inducer-receptor complex in
the nucleus. Thus, these two classes of variant cells
contain different lesions, which can account for the altered
induction responses in the variant cells.

We used cell fusion to study the expression of the two
variant phenotypes and to determine whether the defects were
located on different genes. We selected cells resistant to

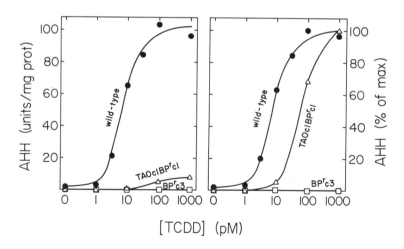

FIGURE 6. Induction of AHH activity in wild-type and
variant cells as a function of [TCDD]. Cells were exposed
to TCDD for 24 hr. See Ref. 9 for details.

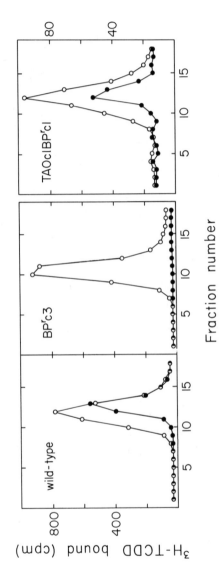

FIGURE 7. TCDD receptors in wild-type and variant cells. Cells were incubated at 37° for 1 hr with 1 nM ^{3}H-TCDD. See Ref. 9 for details. O, cytosolic; ●, nuclear.

6-thioguanine and 8-azaguanine and to ouabain (designated "TAO"), fused them to cells containing no drug markers, and selected hybrids in medium containing HAT and ouabain.

Fusion of variants with wild-type cells yields hybrids with wild-type enzyme activity (Table II), indicating that both variant phenotypes are recessive, and implying that the variants contain defective enzyme induction mechanisms rather than an intracellular inhibitor of enzyme activity.

We next performed a complementation analysis by fusing variant cells with each other. The results (Table III) indicate that the inter-class hybrids contain wild-type AHH activity, while the intra-class hybrids contain the expected low (or no) enzyme activity. The findings indicate that the two classes of variant are in different complementation groups and that the lesions in the two classes are on different genes. Further analyses of the interclass hybrids reveal 1) that the sensitivity of their induction mechanism to TCDD is identical to that of wild-type cells (Fig. 8), 2) that they contain wild-type amounts of TCDD receptor with a wild-type nuclear/cytoplasmic ratio (Fig. 9), and 3) that, in response to TCDD, they accumulate P_1-450 mRNA identical to that of wild-type in both amount and size (Fig. 10). Thus, by all these criteria, complementation has occurred.

The data in Fig. 10 reveal that the receptor-deficient variant cells (TAOc1BP^{r}c1) accumulate about 10-fold less TCDD-inducible mRNA than do wild-type cells; furthermore, the variant (BP^{r}c3) which fails to accumulate TCDD-receptor complex in the nucleus also fails to accumulate detectable mRNA in response to TCDD. These observations agree with the

TABLE II. AHH Activity in Wild-Type and
Wild-Type x Variant Hybrid Cells

Cell	Basal AHH[a]	Induced[b] AHH
Wild-type (wt)	0.8	126
wt TAO[c] x BP^{r}c1	2.0	190
wt TAO x BP^{r}c3	1.5	168
wt TAO x BP^{r}c4	0.6	137
wt x TAOc1BP^{r}c1	0.8	132

[a]Units/mg protein
[b]TCDD (1 nM, 24 hr)
[c]"TAO" indicates cells contain drug markers. See text and Ref. 9 for details.

TABLE III. AHH Activity in Variant x
Variant Hybrid Cells

Cells	Basal AHH[a]	Induced[b] AHH
Inter-class hybrids:		
BP^{r}c1 x TAOc1BP^{r}c1	1.5	161
BP^{r}c3 x TAOc1BP^{r}c1	1.5	138
BP^{r}c1TAO x BP^{r}c4	0.6	139
Intra-class hybrids:		
BP^{r}c1TAO x BP^{r}c3	<0.1	<0.1
BP^{r}c4 x TAOc1BP^{r}c1	0.2	13.7

[a]Units/mg protein
[b]TCDD (1 nM, 24 hr)
See Ref. 9 for details

AHH activity of these cells (Table I) and imply that transcription of the P_1-450 structural gene requires the accumulation of TCDD-receptor complex within the nucleus of the
cell.

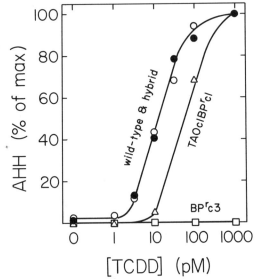

FIGURE 8. Induction of AHH activity in wild-type,
variant, and hybrid cells as a function of [TCDD]. Cells
were exposed to TCDD for 24 hr. See Ref. 9 for details.
●, wild-type; O, BP^{r}c3 x TAOc1BP^{r}c1; ☐ , BP^{r}c3; Δ,
TAOc1BP^{r}c1.

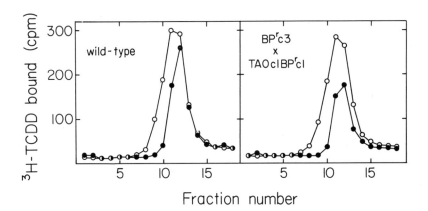

FIGURE 9. TCDD receptors in wild-type and hybrid cells. See legend to Fig. 7 and Ref. 9 for details. O, cytosolic; ●, nuclear.

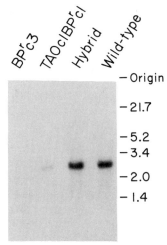

FIGURE 10. Analysis of P$_1$-450 mRNA in wild-type, variant, and hybrid cells. See legend to Fig. 1 and Ref. 9 for details.

V. SUMMARY

TCDD induces a marked increase in AHH activity in wild-type mouse hepatoma cells. A corresponding increase in cytochrome P$_1$-450-specific mRNA precedes the rise in enzyme activity; the accumulation of P$_1$-450 mRNA does not require protein synthesis. Variant cells with fewer receptors for

TCDD accumulate a lesser amount of P_1-450 mRNA in response
to TCDD. Variant cells which fail to accumulate inducer-
receptor complex in the nucleus do not contain detectable
P_1-450 mRNA. The lesions in the variant cells are on different genes, since the response to TCDD in variant x variant
hybrid cells is normal. We conclude that TCDD induces the
synthesis of P_1-450 mRNA, and that this requires the accumulation of the TCDD-receptor complex in the nucleus.

ACKNOWLEDGMENTS

We thank Dr. D.W. Nebert and Dr. M. Negishi for the
mouse cytochrome P_1-450 clone, Dr. O. Hankinson for our
original stock of mouse hepatoma cells, and Dr. A. Poland
for tritiated TCDD.

REFERENCES

1.   Sato, R. and Omura, T. (eds.) (1978). "Cytochrome P-450".
     Academic Press, New York.
2.   Estabrook, R.W. and Lindenlaub, E. (eds.) (1979). "The
     Induction of Drug Metabolism". F.K. Schattauer Verlag,
     Stuttgart.
3.   Nebert, D.W., Eisen, H.J., Negishi, M., Lang, M.A., and
     Hjelmeland, L.M. (1981). Annu. Rev. Pharmacol. Toxicol.
     21:431.
4.   Poland, A. and Knutson, J.C. (1982). Annu. Rev. Pharma-
     col. Toxicol. 22:517.
5.   Negishi, M., Swan, D.C., Enquist, L.W. and Nebert, D.W.
     (1981). Proc. Natl. Acad. Sci. USA 78:800.
6.   Israel, D.I. and Whitlock, J.P., Jr. (1983). J. Biol.
     Chem., in press.
7.   Nebert, D.W. and Gelboin, H.V. (1968). J. Biol. Chem.
     243:6242.
8.   Miller, A.G. and Whitlock, J.P., Jr. (1981). J. Biol.
     Chem. 256:2433.
9.   Miller, A.G., Israel, D., and Whitlock, J.P., Jr. (1983).
     J. Biol. Chem. 258:3523.

VI   CNS-DIRECTED AGENTS

COUPLING THE OPIATE RECEPTOR TO ADENYLATE CYCLASE

Arthur J. Blume

Department of Physiological Chemistry and Pharmacology
Roche Institute of Molecular Biology
Roche Research Center
Nutley, New Jersey 07110

Since the initial recognition by Sharma, Klee and Nirenberg (1) that opiates reduce accumulation of cAMP in certain
mouse x glia hybrid tissue cultured cells, a lot of additional
information about the "δ" opiate receptor and its effects on
cAMP synthesis have been reported (2-6). Most of the work has
been done on NG108-15 cells and thus far has uncovered three
functions for the "δ" opiate receptor; (i) bind opiates and
opioid peptides, (ii) stimulate hydrolysis of GTP and, (iii)
inhibit the ability of adenylate cyclase catalytic units to
make cAMP. In addition, we now know that sodium, magnesium
and guanine nucleotides regulate the binding of agonist to
these receptors and are required for the other two receptor
activities. A general outline of our current concept of how
these receptors are coupled to adenylate cyclase in NG108-15
is given in Fig. 1. Our ultimate goal is to understand the
mechanism(s) involved in the activation and interaction of
all of the membrane components responsible for opiate inhibition of cAMP synthesis. This article is intended as an
overview of recent studies[1],[2] carried out in my laboratory
which shed additional light on the coupling process. In
particular, we have uncovered a fourth activity of the δ -
receptor (i.e., regulation of guanine nucleotide binding) and
found that, at least in vitro, the relationship among the
various receptor activities is not fixed but actually can be

---

[1]Kilian, P. L., Mullikin-Kilpatrick, D. and Blume, A. J. (1983)
Submitted for publication.

[2]Mullikin-Kilpatrick, D., Sadler, K. L. and Blume, A. J. (1983)
Submitted for publication.

MECHANISM OF DRUG ACTION

altered by ions and nucleotides.

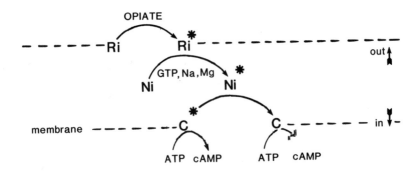

FIGURE 1. Hypothesized pathway of cascading reactions by which opiates direct a decrease in the synthesis of cAMP in NG108-15. Ri = "δ" receptor; Ni = guanine nucleotide regulatory component specific for mediating inhibition of C; C = catalytic unit of adenylate cyclase. *active state.

Central to the scheme outlined in Fig. 1, is the formation of a complex between the δ-opiate receptor (R) and a regulatory unit which is capable of interacting with guanine nucleotides (Ni). Although such a complex has not yet been isolated, two lines of evidence indirectly indicate that it exists. The first arises from studies done on the binding of [^{3}H]ligands (O) to R as outlined in rxn 1. By definition opiates (O), or opioid peptides, bind to R and guanine nucleotides (G) bind to Ni. Therefore, for nucleotides to

$$[^3\text{H}]\text{O}+\text{R}+\text{Ni} \rightarrow \rightarrow [^3\text{H}]\text{O}\cdot\text{R}\cdot\text{Ni}+\text{G} \longrightarrow$$
$$[\,[^3\text{H}]\text{O}\cdot\text{R}\cdot\text{Ni}\cdot\text{G}] \longrightarrow (\text{R}\cdot\text{Ni}\cdot\text{G}) + [^3\text{H}]\text{O} \qquad \text{rxn 1}$$

effect opiate binding, there would have to be an interaction of Ni and R (i.e., formation of the postulated R Ni complex). These studies have shown clearly that the addition of G (GTP, GppNHp or GTPγS) after the formation of the '[^{3}H]O·R' complex induces the opiate to dissociate from R. Such effects of G imply that the O·R·Ni·G complex was formed as an unstable intermediate in the process. The required specificity of Ni for guanine nucleotides is confirmed as ATP, UTP and CTP cannot replace GTP in these studies. In addition, guanine nucleotides also have been shown to decrease the potency of opiate agonists (or opioid peptides) to compete with [^{3}H]-antagonists for binding to R (7). Until recently, this effect was of a small magnitude (i.e., $\leq$ two-fold increases in agonist k_i.   However, in newer experiments performed with Mg^{++}, Na^+ and DTT present and utilizing highly washed membranes (see section on nucleotide release), the addition of G now decreases the potency of DAMA to compete [³H]naloxone binding up to 1000-fold (Table I). The magnitude depends on the guanine nucleotide used. No such changes in the affinity of R for the antagonist naloxone accompany any of these additions. The specific reasons for the recent increase in effectiveness of G to alter the affinity of R for O is not known. Nevertheless, these experiments add strong additional support that O·R·N·G complexes are formed transiently in NG108-15 membranes. The ability of G to so drastically alter agonist affinity yet not alter antagonist affinity for R parallels similar observations that had been made with the β-adrenergic receptor(βAR) and its associated guanine nucleotide regulatory component (N_s) (8-11). With the βAR, nucleotides specifically decrease only agonist affinity because the βAR and N_s are separate entities which can complex only after the agonist occupies (and activates) R. Subsequently, when G binds to the ternary complex (Agonist βAR· N_s) one gets an unstable quaternary complex from which A dissociates due to the fact that it has much lower affinity for βAR·Ns·G than for the βAR·Ns. It appears that a similar phenomenon may operate for the NG108-15 δ opiate receptor. Opiates certainly have much lower affinity for R·Ni·G than R·Ni. Yet, as outlined below, much remains to be understood about forming complexes

TABLE I. Nucleotides Control Agonist Affinity

Membranes	State of Components	Agonist Affinity K_d DAMA (nM)	
1. "N"-unfilled	R + N	8.5 ± 5	(100%)
2. "N"-filled with G_1	R + N_{G_1}	14 ± 8	(100%)
3. "N"-filled with G_1 and G_2 present as well	RN_{G_1} G_2		
	When G_2 = GTP	62 ± 26	(100%)
	G_2 = GppNHp	52 ± 46	(20%)
		9300 ± 4800	(80%)

G_1 = [³H]GppNHp. Data taken from Mullikin-Kilpatrick, Sadler and Blume².

between opiate receptors and Ni.

A second line of support for the occurrence of an R·Ni complex comes from studies on [^{3}H]G binding and its modification by opiates. As proposed by rxn 2, after first tightly

$$R + Ni \xrightarrow{[^3H]G; \text{ wash}} Ni \cdot [^3H]G \xrightarrow{+O} \longrightarrow_3$$
$$[O \cdot R \cdot Ni \cdot [^3H]G] \longrightarrow (O \cdot R \cdot Ni) + [^3H]G \qquad \text{rxn 2}$$

binding [^{3}H]GppNHp to NG108-15 membranes and removing all free [^{3}H]GppNHp, the bound [^{3}H]G dissociates from these membranes when they are suspended with opiates under appropriation conditions (i.e., with DTT, Mg^{++}, Na$^+$ and G; see Table II). This effect of opiates (and opioid peptides as well) is blocked by the pure opiate antagonist naloxone which, on its own, induces no [^{3}H]G release. Assuming again that opiates bind only to R and [^{3}H]G only to Ni, the effectiveness of O dissociate [^{3}H]G implies that a O·R·N·[^{3}H]G complex must have been formed as an intermediate in this process. Although the data are meager, they are sufficient to indicate that, in the R·Ni complex, opiates and guanine nucleotides have reciprocal activities; each inducing the dissociation of the other. However, the process of formation and dissociation of the actual intermediate is, itself, complex. The degree of complexity is evident based on the fact that Na$^+$ (at mM concentration) and G nucleotides (at µM concentrations) are required for dissociation of the complex (Table II). Sodium clearly depresses release in the absence but not the presence of opiates. This action is an exact reproduction of the

TABLE II. Effect of GTP and Na on Dissociation of G·Ni Complex.

		% Control[*] [^{3}H]GppNHp Released	
	Conditions	----	Opiate
1.	Basic system (buffer, Mg^{++}, DTT, GppNHp·Ni)	100[*]	100
2.	Basic system plus GTP (.1mM)	165	165
3.	Basic system plus Na (100mM)	107	165

[*]100% = 2.41 pmol/mg protein, opiate is 10uM DAMA

action Na^+ has on the GTP hydrolysis that is carried out by the high affinity GTPase activity present in NG108-15 membranes (4,5). In addition, specificity exists for which monovalent cation will suffice here ($Na^+ \geq Li > K >$ Choline). We believe that both opiate stimulation of GTP hydrolysis and G release may be the outcome of a single opiate action on R which removes the generally inhibitory influence that Na^+ has on the spontaneous activities of Ni. The actual relationship between G release and GTP hydrolysis has yet to be worked out.

What is equally intriguing about the dissociation process is the affinity of the R for agonists in $[^3H]GppNHp$ filled membranes devoid of other nucleotides. It must be noted here that, even with all else present including 100mM Na^+, opiates do not induce release in the absence of a second nucleotide. As expected, there is specificity for which nucleotides are active here and GTP or ITP work but ATP and AppNHp do not. Indeed, we find that the opiate receptor has the same high affinity for DAMA (i.e., k_d = 14nM) in GppNHp - filled and washed membranes suspended without G as seen in control "unfilled" membranes (i.e., k_d 8nM). Adding G to the "filled" membranes is what actually decreases the receptor's affinity for DAMA; approximately 8-fold when G is GTP and ~1000-fold when G is GppNHp. As depicted in rxn 3, we interpret these results as indicating that the original $[^3H]GppNHp$ is bound to a site on Ni (i.e., N_{1i}) from which it cannot be washed out but which is under the control of yet another guanine nucleotide specific site (i.e., N_{2i}). This

$$O \cdot R + [^3H]G \cdot N_{1i}^n \xrightarrow{\ G, N_{2i}\ } [O \cdot R \cdot [^3H]G \cdot (Ni)_n \cdot G] \longrightarrow \quad \text{rxn 3}$$
$$O + R \cdot (Ni)_n^1 \cdot G + [^3H]G$$

second site could be on the original Ni or on a second Ni component. When the N_{2i} site is filled with G, the agonist-receptor complex ($O \cdot R$) now couples to the first Ni site and induces the release of $[^3H]G$. Whereas the site binding $[^3H]G$ tightly does not appear to regulate the R affinity for agonists, the second nucleotide site apparently does. Whether there is one or two N components involved in these reactions, we feel that the components are Ni and not N_s. A formal distinction between Ni and N_s in NG108-15 seems to be indicated based on recent data on pertussis toxin effects in cells (12,13) and the following. Acetylcholine and epinephrine, but not PGE_1, also induce release of $[^3H]GppNHp$ from NG108-15 membranes and the former two neurotransmitters, along with opiates, inhibit NG108-15 adenylate cyclase while PGE_1 activates it. More support for the distinction between Ni and N_s is given below.

Having obtained evidence for the existence of a Ri•Ni complex, we wanted to know if it played an essential role in all three of the known "δ" opiate receptor activities: (i) G release, (ii) GTPase stimulation and, (iii) adenylate cyclase inhibition. Clearly, it controls the release of G from Ni. A possible way of testing its involvement in the other two events was suggested by finding that the receptor can be modified by either NEM or diamide in such a way that it loses its sensitivity to regulation by nucleotides but retains its high affinity for agonists at 4°C[1]. We believe this indicates that the proper complex of R and Ni cannot be formed after alkylation of certain sulfhydryls (by NEM) or formation of disulfides (by diamide) on either Ri or Ni. The positions of these reactive groups has not yet been identified. With this limitation in mind, we tested NEM and diamide treatments for cyclase and GTPase. About 10% of control adenylate cyclase remains and it is still stimulated to normal extents by PGE_1, but it is no longer inhibited by opiates. There is about 40% of the control GTPase activity but it, too, is no longer sensitive to opiates. Therefore, an Ri•Ni complex does seem to be required for all three receptor activities. Furthermore, we think that it is the same O•Ri•Ni complex for each of the activities as a rank ordering of maximal efficacy for a variety of opiates and opioid peptides is the same for G release, GTPase stimulation or adenylate cyclase inhibition. A comparison of the ordering for G release done in vitro with inhibition of cAMP accumulation done in intact cells (6) is given in Fig. 2.

Finally, we have tried to investigate how the three receptor activities are interrelated. As depicted in Fig. 1, they are sequential processes: activation of R triggers an activation of Ni, which in turn inactivates C. In support of the action of an activated Ni being inhibitory, there is the recent observation that in cells devoid of N_s but presumed to have an Ni, NaF and GppNHp (both of which activate N_s) produce an inhibition of adenylate cyclase activity (14).[s] We have tried to get information concerning the coupling by determining the dose of a single agonist (i.e., DAMA) that is required to be one-half maximally active for each of the three receptor activities when assayed under identical conditions. The affinity constants thus obtained, k_d, k_a and k_i for binding, release and cyclase inhibition, respectively, can then be directly compared. Where the relationship between any two processes is direct and simple, the k ratio would be 1:1; where it is complex (or, in other words, cascading), the k ratio would, therefore, be $>$ 1. For these studies, the membranes were all first "filled" with GppNHp, then washed and suspended under the regular conditions used either for

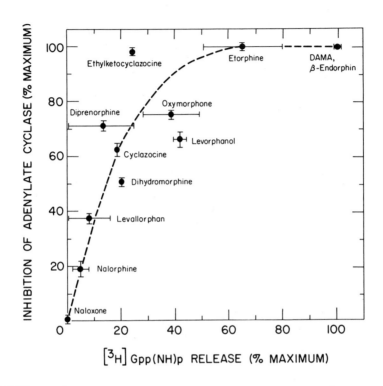

FIGURE 2. Comparison of the maximum efficacies for G release
and inhibition of adenylate cyclase as reported by (6).

the G release or adenylate cyclase. Binding affinity for
DAMA was assessed based on competition for [³H]naloxone.
Some of the results are summarized in Table III.

One thing readily visible is the fact that the ratio of
one receptor activity to another is variable. In 10mM Na⁺,
the k_a and k_d for DAMA are 11 and 14nM, respectively, a
ratio of one. However, under conditions used to assay
adenylate cyclase where the k_d is now 600-700nM, the k_a/k_d
ratio changes from 1:3 to 1:12 when Na⁺ is lowered from 100mM
to 10mM. Others have reported that the k_a for both
excitatory (16) and inhibitory (6) adenylate cyclase
signals decreases when Na⁺ is lowered. Under cyclase assay
conditions and low Na⁺, a cascade of effectiveness occurs
such that 1% receptor occupation translates into 12% G
release which, in turn, translates into 70% of maximal
adenylate cyclase inhibition. Often, with in vivo systems,
such relationships have been used to classify the system as

TABLE III. Relationships Among Receptor Activities[a]

Type of Coupling	Conditions	Activities	Coupling Ratios*
I. Direct			
	Low Na$^+$	Bi:Re	1:1
II. Cascade			
Partial	High Na$^+$ + AC**	Bi:Re:Inh	1:3:4
Full	Low Na$^+$ + AC	Bi:Re:Inh	1:12:70
III.	in vivo	Bi:Inh	1:7

*   Ratio of % maximal activities that would be seen
       with DAMA at 1/50th of its k_d dose.

**   AC = Nucleotide triphosphate regenerating system,
       ATP, cAMP, Ro20-1724.

       Low Na$^+$ = 10mM; high Na$^+$ = 100mM; all have 0.1mM
       GTP, 10mM Mg Cl$_2$.

[a]Data on in vivo taken from Fantozzi and Blume (15).

Bi = Binding; Re = Release; Inh = Inhibition.

having spare receptors. In fact, our studies with intact
NG108-15 cells suspended in physiological medium   indicated that DAMA k was 23nM, which was ~7 times its k_i for
inhibiting PGE$_1$-stimulated cAMP accumulation (15). It,
therefore, appears that in vivo the coupling of " δ " opiate
receptors to adenylate cyclase is of the 'cascade' type and
such coupling can be expressed in vitro. At present, we do
not know if coupling is a variable parameter under physiological conditions. Much work is clearly needed here to
identify the mechanisms responsible for the variable
coupling.
        In summary, we have definitely made headway in our
quest to understand the biochemical basis of regulation of

adenylate cyclase activity by opiates but we really still remain in a state of infancy in the matter. We may know about the existence of the basic units involved; a receptor, a coupler and adenylate cyclase catalytic units, but almost nothing is known about the molecular architecture of any of those components. There is some promising new data suggesting Ni is a heterodimer containing one unit in common with N_s and to dissociate like N_s when given GTP analogues (17,18). Yet, we do not know what is the normal stoichiometry among the basic units or even if the relationship is a fixed and not a variable one. Another unresolved area pertains to unraveling the relationship between GppNHp release, GTP hydrolysis and inhibition of catalytic units. Clearly, hormones which stimulate the catalytic activity of adenylate cyclase in a guanine nucleotide dependent manner also can induce release of guanine nucleotides from N_s and stimulate hydrolysis of GTP. How, then, could the same qualitative events be responsible for opiate-directed inhibition of the same catalytic units? One possibility is that the different Ni and N_s subunits generated by dissociation of the two different couplers could account for the differences observed between 'inhibitory' and 'excitatory' hormonal signals. Resolution of these questions and many others awaits better biochemical characterization of the units and reactions involved.

REFERENCES

1.   Sharma, S. K., Nirenberg, M. and Klee, W. A. (1972) Proc. Natl. Acad. Sci. USA 72, 590.
2.   Blume, A. J. (1978) Life Sci. 22, 1843.
3.   Blume, A. J., Lichtshtein, D. and Boone, G. (1979) Proc. Natl. Acad. Sci. USA 76, 5626.
4.   Koski, G. and Klee, W. A. (1981) Proc. Natl. Acad. Sci. USA 78, 4185.
5.   Koski, G., Streaty, R. A. and Klee, W. A. (1982) J. Biol. Chem. 257, 14035.
6.   Law, P. Y., Koehler, J. E. and Loh, H. H. (1982) Mol. Pharmacol. 21, 483.
7.   Blume, A. J., Boone, G. and Lichtshtein, D. (1979) In "Modulators, Mediators and Specifiers in Brain Function" (Y. H. Erhlich, J. Volavka, L. G. Davis and E. G. Brunngraber, eds.) Plenum Press, N. Y. pg. 163.
8.   Ross, E. M. and Gilman, A. G. (1980) Annl. Rev. Biochem. 49, 533.
9.   Rodbell, M. (1980) Nature, 284, 17.
10.   Limbird, L. E. (1981) Biochem. J. 195, 1.

11.   Stadel, J. M., DeLean, A. and Lefkowitz, R. J. (1982)
      Adv. Enzymol. 53, 1.
12.   Katada, T. and Ui, M. (1981) J. Biol. Chem. 256, 8310.
13.   Katada, T. and Ui, M. (1982) J. Biol. Chem. 257, 7210.
14.   Hildebrandt, J. D., Hanoune, J. and Birnbaumer, L.
      (1982) J. Biol. Chem. 257, 14723.
15.   Fantozzi, R., Mullikin-Kilpatrick, D. and Blume, A.
      J. (1981) Mol. Pharmacol. 20, 8.
16.   Howlett, A. C. (1981) J. of Cyclic Nucleotide Res. 8, 91.
17.   Burns, D. L., Hewlett, E. L., Moss, I. and Vaughan,
      M. (1982) J. Biol. Chem. 258, 1435.
18.   Katada, T., Bokoch, G. M., Northup, J. K. and Gilman,
      A. G. (1983) Fed. Proc. 42, 1850.

RECEPTOR-MEDIATED CONTROL OF CYCLIC NUCLEOTIDE
FORMATION IN THE CENTRAL NERVOUS SYSTEM

John W. Daly

Laboratory of Bioorganic Chemistry
National Institute of Arthritis, Diabetes, and
Digestive and Kidney Diseases
National Institutes of Health
Bethesda, Maryland

I. INTRODUCTION

Seminal discoveries concerning the possible importance of cyclic AMP and cyclic GMP to the function of the central nervous system were made in the sixties. At the time, the clear demonstration that putative neurotransmitters or neuro-modulators such as norepinephrine, serotonin, histamine, and adenosine could elicit accumulations of cyclic AMP in brain tissue (1,2) focused research onto receptor-mediated events. The seventies were then a decade of optimism and activity with literally thousands of published papers concerned with biochemical, physiological and behavioral aspects of cyclic nucleotides in the nervous system (see ref. 3-6). Receptor-mediated generation of cyclic nucleotides was proposed to be involved in both short term and long term modulation of synaptic transmission and/or neuronal excitability. The close relationship of calcium to both cyclic AMP and cyclic GMP systems was realized. It has, however, proven difficult to establish clear roles for cyclic nucleotide-generating systems in specific physiological or behavioral functions of the nervous system and the eighties appear destined to be a time for focal efforts to correlate biochemical events with physiological phenomenon. The present brief review attempts only to provide lead references to the literature. A comprehensive two volume treatise on cyclic nucleotides has recently appeared (7).

MECHANISM OF DRUG ACTION

The classical sequence for cyclic nucleotides as second messengers invokes i) a hormone-receptor-mediated activation of adenylate cyclase, ii) cyclic AMP-mediated activation of cyclic AMP-dependent protein kinases, iii) phosphorylation of specific proteins, thereby altering their properties, iv) a resultant physiological response, v) termination of the response by phosphodiesterase-catalyzed hydrolysis of cyclic AMP and by protein phosphatase-catalyzed hydrolysis of phosphorylated proteins. In the case of cyclic GMP, it would appear that hormone-receptor-mediated activation of calcium channels initiates a calcium activation of guanylate cyclase, followed by cyclic GMP-mediated activation of cyclic GMP-dependent kinases, phosphorylation of specific proteins and a physiological response. Correlations of the biochemical events, namely hormone-receptor binding, cyclic nucleotide elevation, protein kinase activation, and specific protein phosphorylation with physiological events has proven difficult, even in simpler neuronal systems such as peripheral sympathetic ganglia of vertebrate (8) or sensory ganglia of invertebrates (9,10) let alone in an organ as complex as brain.

Cyclic AMP-generating systems are present in perhaps all eukaryotic cells. For brain tissue this means neurons, glia and the endothelial cells of the capillary bed. Thus, measurements of brain levels of cyclic AMP either in situ or in vitro with membranes or slices may or may not reflect the compartment relevant to a particular physiological response. Furthermore, even if a hormone-receptor interaction gives rise to an accumulation of cyclic AMP, it always remains possible that the physiological response involves another pathway in the same cell or another cell not involving adenylate cyclase.

Specific activators or inhibitors of adenylate cyclase or guanylate cyclase would be useful tools. A diterpene, forskolin, has proven to be a specific activator of most adenylate cyclases and to potentiate receptor-mediated activation of the enzyme (11). A variety of oxidants have been found to be selective activators of guanylate cyclase (see ref. 7). An adenosine analog, 2',5'-dideoxyadenosine is a general inhibitor of brain and other adenylate cyclases (see ref. 7). Phosphodiesterase inhibitors should selectively potentiate receptor-mediated responses only if generation of a cyclic nucleotide is involved. However, such inhibitors have proven far from selective agents (12) and efforts to develop and define specific selective inhibitors of cyclic AMP or cyclic GMP hydrolysis must continue. Cyclic nucleotide analogs, relatively stable to hydrolysis and incapable to conversion to an active adenosine analog, provide useful tools for direct activation of cyclic AMP- and cyclic GMP-dependent protein kinases (see ref. 7). One major consideration in the use of such agents which bypass the hormone-receptor stage is that in a system as complex as the nervous system general activation or inhibition of cyclic nucleotide mechanisms most certainly will involve many interrelated compartments and cells. The resultant alteration in physiology or behavior may or may not be interpretable in terms of one receptor-controlled compartment.

II. ADENYLATE CYCLASE

The control of activity of the adenylate cyclase system has proven very complex (13): Two sets of hormone-receptor-mediated inputs pertain. One is stimulatory and involves a so-called stimulatory guanyl nucleotide-binding subunit (N_s). It is at this subunit, that cholera toxin catalyzes activation via an ADP-ribosylation. After ribosylation, the subunit is no longer capable of hydrolysing GTP to GDP and thus remains in the GTP-activated form. GTP analogs, such as GppNHp, which are stable to hydrolysis by the N_s-subunit, can also stabilize the system in an active form. Cholera toxin has proven of limited usefulness in probing the role of activation of cyclic AMP-mechanisms in the central nervous system, in part due to a relatively slow onset of action and irreversibility. Stable GTP analogs might prove useful in situations where intracellular injection is possible (see ref. 14). The other receptor-mediated input to adenylate cyclase is inhibitory and involves a so-called inhibitory guanyl nucleotide-binding subunit (N_i). It is at this subunit that a <u>Bordetella</u> <u>pertussis</u> toxin catalyzes an ADP-ribosylation (15,16). After ribosylation the N_i subunit appears no longer capable of inhibiting adenylate cyclase (15,17). Pertussis toxin should prove useful in probing the role inhibitory inputs to cyclic AMP-generating systems in the nervous system but like cholera toxin its usefulness may be limited by a relatively slow onset of action and irreversibility. The N_i-input, like the N_s-input to adenylate cyclase, requires GTP, but a stable analog such as GppNHp can also function (18). Both guanyl nucleotide binding subunits catalyze the hydrolysis of GTP.

There are a large number of putative neurotransmitters or neuromodulators which have been shown to affect adenylate cyclase <u>via</u> such N_s- or N_i-pathways (Table I). In addition, certain amines can potentiate adenosine (A_2)-receptor mediated activation of N_s-input in brain slices (<u>vide infra</u>). Such potentiation involves calcium ions. It should be noted

TABLE I. Putative Neurotransmitters or Neuromodulators which
are Inhibitory or Stimulatory to Adenylate Cyclase of the
Central Nervous System

Agent	Nature of Receptor Modulation of Adenylate Cyclase		
	Inhibitory (N_i)	Stimulatory (N_s)	Potentiation of N_s
Norepinephrine	α_2	β_1, β_2	α_1
Dopamine	D-2	D-1	—
Histamine	—	H_2	H_1
Serotonin	—	5-HT_1	5-HT
Adenosine	A-1	A-2	—
Prostaglandin	—	E_1, D_2	—
Vasoactive Intestinal Peptide	—	VIP	—
Acetylcholine	muscarinic	—	—
Enkephalins	μ,δ	—	—

that brain adenylate cyclase unlike many cyclases can be
activated by calmodulin (19). This activation appears independent of guanyl nucleotides but may depend on the state of
phosphorylation of membrane proteins (20).

An interplay between receptors and N_s- and N_i-subunits is
evident in a decrease in apparent affinity of agonists for
the receptor when the subunits are exposed to GppNHp or GTP
(21 and ref. therein). This might provide a means to assess
whether or not a particular receptor as assayed with ligand
binding is linked to adenylate cyclase or not. However, it
appears that guanyl nucleotides can affect binding of
agonists at receptors which are probably not linked to
cyclase, for example the D-3-dopamine receptor (22), the
glutamate receptor (23), the H_1-histamine receptor (24), and
the substance P receptor (25).

In addition to modulation by receptor-agonist input via
N_s and N_i-subunits, brain adenylate cyclase is subject to
activation by calcium-calmodulin, inhibition at a so-called
P-site by adenosine, inhibition at a divalent cation site by
calcium, activation at the same cation site by manganese, and
activation at a hitherto unsuspected site by the diterpene

forskolin. Forskolin activation has marked effects on other
inputs to the enzyme (11). In particular, forskolin potenti-
ates hormone-receptor mediated activation of the enzyme.
Thus, a "priming" low concentration of forskolin can markedly
augment the response of cyclic AMP-generating systems to
norepinephrine, histamine, vasoactive intestinal peptide and
prostaglandin E_1 in brain slices (26). Two effects of forskolin are seen, one an apparent increase in the potency of
the receptor agonist and the other an increase in the efficacy (maximal response) to the agonist. One or both of the
effects are seen depending on the tissue and/or the agonist.
Not only does forskolin potentiate effects of receptor
agonist on cyclic AMP-generating systems, but the converse is
true. Thus, a "priming" dose of an agonist can increase both
the potency and efficacy of forskolin as an activator of
cyclic AMP-generating systems (27). Forskolin-activated
cyclic AMP-generating systems can be inhibited by N_i-input
(11,18), but in intact cells, forskolin actually appears to
stabilize adenylate cyclase to inhibitory input (A. Siegl and
J.W. Daly, unpublished data). Forskolin should prove a very
useful tool for investigation of receptor-mediated activation
and inhibition of adenylate cyclase in brain. In peripheral
systems (platelets, adipocytes, etc.) forskolin elicits
physiological responses appropriate to cyclic AMP (11). As
yet forskolin has been used to probe the involvement of
cyclic AMP in only a limited number of physiological responses of neuronal system. In all cases, it has elicited a
response similar to that evoked by cyclic AMP analogs and/or
phosphodiesterase inhibitors. The systems were blockade of
accommodation of pyramidal cell discharge in hippocampus(28),
shifts in phase of circadian pacemaker in eye of the mollusc
Aplysia (29), decrease in gap-junction coupling in retina
(30), potentiation of after discharge in peptidergic neurons
of Aplysia (31) and reduction of potassium conductances in
neurons of the snail Helix (32). It should be noted that at
high concentrations, forskolin may become inhibitory to
physiological functions not because of activation of cyclic
AMP-systems, but due to partial energy deficit resulting from
shunting of large amounts of ATP into the cyclic AMP metabolic cycle (see ref. 33).

                III. RECEPTORS TO AMINES AND TO ADENOSINE

     Amine receptors coupled to adenylate cylase represent a
probable site of action of many centrally active drugs
including drugs with antidepressant, antipsychotic, anti-

hypertensive, neuroleptic, and sedative actions. Furthermore, prolonged treatment with drugs often results in homeostatic changes in the responsiveness of the cyclic AMP-
generating system, the direction of which depended on whether
or not the drug heightened or reduced interactions at the
receptor (see ref. 34).

In the first years of research on receptor-mediated
accumulations of cyclic AMP in brain slices, it was realized
that adenosine played a pivotal and ubiquitous role as an
activator. Adenosine caused accumulations of cyclic AMP in
tissue from all regions of brain. But in cerebral cortex and
hippocampus norepinephrine through a calcium-dependent α_1-
adrenergic receptor, histamine through a H_1-histaminergic
receptor, and serotonin through a serotonin receptor,
markedly potentiated the adenosine-response (35,36). In
addition, unknown factors released by depolarizing agents or
by glutamate markedly potentiated adenosine-elicited accumulations of cyclic AMP in brain slices (37). The profound
depressant effects of adenosine on neurons in all regions of
brain (38) and the potentiative depressant effects of adenosine and norepinephrine on cortical neurons (39) appeared to
provide physiological correlates of the biochemical effects.
However, it is now realized that adenosine interacts with two
major classes of receptors in brain (40). One is a so-called
"high affinity" A_1-adenosine receptor which interacts with
adenylate cyclase through the inhibitory N_i-subunit. The
other is a so-called "low affinity" A_2-adenosine receptor
which interacts with adenylate cyclase through the stimulatory N_s-subunit. Whether both such adenosine receptors occur
in one cell type is as yet unknown. The definition as "high
affinity" and "low affinity" is probably meaningless with
respect to the physiology of adenosine. It is not the biochemical half maximal inhibition of cyclic AMP-generation or
half maximal stimulation of cyclic AMP-generation which will
be important. Instead, for the inhibitory A_1-receptor it
will be the concentration of adenosine necessary to reduce
stimulated cyclic AMP levels below the threshold for maintaining protein kinase activation, thereby turning off the
physiological response initially triggered by stimulatory
(N_s) input to the cyclase. Conversely, for the stimulatory
A_2-receptor it will be the concentration of adenosine necessary to increase cyclic AMP levels to the threshold for
triggering protein kinase activation and the physiological
response. Although this threshold value for endogenous
cyclic AMP may vary from cell to cell, it appears that the
relevant concentration of adenosine for physiological control
of both A_1- and A_2-receptor-mediated input to adenylate
cyclase will be similar.

In addition to the ubiquitous A_2-receptor which increases cyclic AMP in brain slices and interacts synergistically with amines in cerebral cortical and hippocampal slices, there appears to be another higher affinity A_2-adenosine receptor which increases adenylate cyclase activity in striatal membranes, but not in membranes of other major brain regions (41). It would appear that this higher affinity A_2-receptor is associated with a relatively minor cyclic AMP-generating compartment and hence is not detected in slices of striatum, where the response to the ubiquitous lower affinity adenosine receptor is predominant.

The inhibitory A_1-adenosine receptor linked to adenylate cyclase was known only from adipocytes until its discovery in the late seventies in cultured cells from fetal mouse brain (42). Inhibitory effects of adenosine analogs on adenylate cyclase in both membranes (43) and in slices (44) from brain have now been documented. In the case of slices the presence of a low concentration forskolin and a phosphodiesterase inhibitor were required in order to manifest the inhibitory effects of the adenosine analog.

The development of a radioligand binding assay for the brain A_1-adenosine receptor (45) made possible detailed studies on structure-activity profiles and on localization and possible function in the central nervous system. A_1-adenosine receptors show a significantly different potency profile with respect to interaction with adenosine analogs than do A_2-adenosine receptors (see ref. 40). Such differences allow, with a select group of adenosine analogs, the investigation of the relevance of A_1- or A_2-adenosine receptors to a particular physiological or behavioral phenomenon. A_1-adenosine receptors appear to be localized in brain on presynaptic terminals associated with excitatory pathways (46). Such a localization is consonant with an apparent inhibitory physiological role for A_1-adenosine receptors for excitatory neurotransmission in hippocampus (47-49). Whether or not such inhibitory A_1-receptors are coupled to presynaptic adenylate cyclase has not been delineated. In other studies, it was concluded that an A_2-adenosine receptor was involved in adenosine-mediated depression of hippocampal pyramidal cells (50) and cerebral cortical neurons (51). Intrastriatal injection of adenosine analogs appeared to block dopamine responses resulting in rotation towards the injected side (52). The effect appeared to involve A_2-adenosine receptors. Attempts to relate behavioral effects of adenosine analogs and of adenosine antagonists with interaction at A_1-adenosine receptors have provided preliminary positive correlations (53). However, pharmacokinetic factors and the lack of satisfactory selective antagonists of A_1- and

A_2-adenosine receptors complicate any interpretation of these preliminary results. Theophylline and caffeine probably owe their behavioral effects to interactions at adenosine receptors. However, neither of these methylxanthines are selective towards either A_1- or A_2-receptors (41).

PROSPECTUS

Further studies on relationships of receptors and cyclic nucleotides in the nervous system must now focus more and more on well defined physiological functions. There are four steps to be considered:

I. The Interaction of the Neurotransmitter, Neuromodulator or Neurohormone with the Receptor and a Resultant Activation or Inhibition of Adenylate Cyclase. There is extensive knowledge of the receptors concerned with control of adenylate cyclase in brain membranes and slices and of their sensitivity to a variety of centrally active drugs. Further data are needed on the cellular localization of such systems and of guanylate cyclase systems. Selective toxins such as 6-hydroxydopamine, dihydroxytryptamines, and kainic acid have provided evidence concerning neuronal and glial localization of receptor sensitive adenylate cyclase systems (54-59, Table II) as have the use of mutant animal strains and neonatal x-irradiation in which certain neuronal cell types develop abnormally or not at all (3,46,60,61). Further studies aimed at specific localization are needed. A biochemical strategem for identifying receptors linked to adenylate cyclase is of prime importance. Delineation of selective phosphodiesterase inhibitors and of specific and potent inhibitors of adenylate cyclase are needed. The selective stimulatory effects of forskolin on basal activity of adenylate cyclase and the potentiative effects of forskolin on receptor-mediated activation need to be exploited.

II. Activation of Cyclic AMP-Dependent Protein Kinases and a Resultant Phosphorylation of Specific Protein Substrates. There is extensive knowledge of the effects of cyclic AMP on protein phosphorylation patterns in brain preparations (3,4,62) but again further studies are needed on the cellular and compartmental localization of such substrates.

III. The Relationship of Protein Phosphorylation to a Physiological Response. There is very little knowledge as to the functional significance of cyclic AMP-dependent phosphorylation of proteins in brain preparations. The increase in activity of tyrosine hydroxylase upon phosphorylation is

TABLE II. Effects of Kainic Acid on Receptor-Mediated
Activation of Cyclic AMP-Generating Systems in Brain:
↑ Increase, ↓ Decrease, (↑) Slight Increase

Agonist	Brain Region	Effect of Kainic Acid Lesion
Norepinephrine	Hippocampus	β_1 ↓; β_2 ↑
Adenosine	"	A_1 ↓
Histamine	"	↓
Isoproterenol	Striatum	β_1, β_2 ↑
Adenosine	"	A_2 (↑)
Dopamine	"	D-1 ↓
PGE_1	"	↑
VIP	"	↓

almost a unique case (see ref. 14). Indeed, most phosphorylated proteins of brain preparations are proteins in
search of function let alone an altered function upon phosphorylation. These include even the highly characterized
Synaptsin I, formerly known as Protein I (see ref. 14).
There are, however, a number of proteins which serve as
substrates for cyclic AMP-dependent proteins, for example
the nicotinic acetylcholine receptor (see ref. 14),
the voltage-dependent sodium channel (63), Na^+-K^+-ATPase
(64), and certain components of the cyclic nucleotide systems (see ref. 3,4,7,62). The physiological relevance of
such phosphorylations to function of neurons is unclear.
Correlations of physiological responses to biochemical
events have as yet mainly correlated the response to the
generation of cyclic AMP rather than to alterations in
phosphorylation of a functional protein. Such correlations of cyclic AMP levels with a physiological response
remain suspect since a receptor-mediated non-cyclic AMP
pathway may also pertain and may be responsible for the
physiological response with the cyclic AMP pathway
playing an independent or a modulatory role.

IV. Correlation of Cyclic AMP-Dependent Alterations
in Physiological Responses to Behavioral Changes in the
Intact Organism. For vertebrates, few answers have
been forthcoming, although cyclic nucleotides have been
considered to be involved in anxiety, aggression, depression,
epilepsy, psychosis, nociception, sleep, learning, and

memory. Receptor agonists and antagonists, forskolin, phosphodiesterase inhibitors and cyclic AMP analogs must be used in much more defined ways in inducing behavioral changes. Otherwise little is learned beyond the gross behavioral alterations resulting from a summation of increases or decreases in cyclic AMP at many sites throughout the brain. The successful analysis of behavioral roles of cyclic AMP in learning and habituation in invertebrates (9,10) does, however, provide the neuroscientist with some optimism concerning ultimate delineation of the role of receptor-mediated activation of adenylate cyclase and guanylate cyclase to the function of the vertebrate central nervous system.

REFERENCES

1. Kakiuchi, S., and Rall, T.W., Mol. Pharmacol. 4:379 (1968).
2. Sattin, A., and Rall, T.W., Mol. Pharmacol. 6:13 (1970).
3. Daly, J.W., "Cyclic Nucleotides in the Nervous System", Plenum Press, New York, 1977.
4. Greengard, P., "Cyclic Nucleotides, Phosphorylated Proteins and Neuronal Function", Raven Press, New York, 1978.
5. Bartfai, T., in "Current Topics in Cellular Regulation", Vol. 16 (B.L. Horecker and E.R. Stadtman, ed.), p. 226. Academic Press, New York, 1980.
6. Dunwiddie, T.V., and Hoffer, B.J., in "Handbook of Experimental Pharmacology", Vol. 58/II (J.W. Kebabian and J.A. Nathanson, ed.), p. 389. Springer-Verlag, New York, 1982.
7. Kebabian, J.W., and Nathanson, J.A. (eds.), "Handbook of Experimental Pharmacology", Vol. 58/I and 58/II, Springer-Verlag, New York, 1982.
8. Briggs, C.A., and McAfee, D.A., Trends Pharmacol. Sci. 3:241 (1982).
9. Kupfermann, I., Ann. Rev. Physiol. 42:629 (1980).
10. Kandel, E.R., and Schwartz, J.H., Science 218:433 (1982).
11. Seamon, K.B., and Daly, J.W., J. Cyclic Nucleotide Res. 7:201 (1981).
12. Stoclet, J.C., Trends Pharmacol. Sci. 1:98 (1979).
13. Ross, E.M., Pedersen, S.E., and Florio, V.A., Current Topics Membrane Res. 18:109 (1983).
14. Kennedy, M.B., Ann. Rev. Neuroscience 6:493 (1983).
15. Katada, T., and Ui, M., J. Biol. Chem. 257:7210 (1982).
16. Bokoch, G.M., Katada, T., Northrup, J.K., Hewlett, E.L., and Gilman, A.G., J. Biol. Chem. 258:2072 (1983).

17. Kurose, H., Katada, T., Amano, T., and Ui, M., J. Biol. Chem. 258:4870 (1983).
18. Seamon, K., and Daly, J.W., J. Biol. Chem. 257:1191 (1982).
19. Wolff, D.J., and Brostrom, C.O., Adv. Cyclic Nucleotide Res. 11:27 (1979).
20. Seamon, K.B., and Daly, J.W., Life Sci. 30:1457 (1982).
21. Burgisser, E., De Lean, A., and Lefkowtiz, R.J., Proc. Nat. Acad. Sci. USA 79:1732 (1982).
22. Freeman, S.B., Poat, J.A., and Woodruff, G.N., J. Neurochem. 37:608 (1981).
23. Sharif, N.A., and Roberts, P.J., Biochem. Pharmacol. 30:3019 (1981).
24. Chang, R.S.L., and Snyder, S.H., J. Neurochem. 34:916 (1980).
25. Cascieri, M.A., and Liang, T., J. Biol. Chem. 258:5158 (1983).
26. Daly, J.W., Padgett, W., and Seamon, K.B., J. Neurochem. 38:532 (1982).
27. Siegl, A.M., Daly, J.W., and Smith, J.B., Mol. Pharmacol. 21:680 (1982).
28. Madison, D.V., and Nicoll, R.A., Nature 299:636 (1982).
29. Eskin, A., and Takahashi, J.S., Science 220:82 (1983).
30. Gerschenfeld, H.M., Neyton, J., Piccolini, N., and Witkovsky, P., Biomed. Res. 3:21 (1982).
31. Strumwasser, F., Kaczmarek, L.K., and Jennings, K.R., Fed. Proc. 41:2933 (1973).
32. Deterre, P., Paupardin-Tritsch, D., Bockaert, J., and Gerschenfeld, H.M., Proc. Natl. Acad. Sci. USA 79:7934 (1982).
33. Ebstein, R.P., Seamon, K., Creveling, C.R., and Daly, J.W., Cell. Mol. Neurobiol. 2:179 (1982).
34. Sulser, F., Janowsky, A.J., Okada, F., Manier, D.H., and Mobley, P.L., Neuropharmacology 22:425 (1983).
35. Daly, J.W., Padgett, W., Nimitkitpaison, Y., Creveling, C.R., Cantacuzene, D., and Kirk, K.L., J. Pharmacol. Exp. Therap. 212:382 (1980).
36. Daly, J.W., Padgett, W., Creveling, C.R., Cantacuzene, D., and Kirk, K.L., J. Neuroscience 1:49 (1981).
37. Bruns, R.F., Pons, F., and Daly, J.W., Brain Res. 189:550 (1980).
38. Phillis, J.W., and Wu, P.H., Prog. Neurobiol. 16:187 (1981).
39. Stone, T.W., and Taylor, D.A., J. Physiol. 275:45P (1978).
40. Daly, J.W., J. Med. Chem. 25:197 (1982).
41. Daly, J.W., Butts-Lamb, P., and Padgett, W., Cell. Mol. Neurobiol., in press (1983).

42. Van Calker, D., Muller, M., and Hamprecht, B., Nature 276:839 (1978).
43. Cooper, D.M.F., Londos, C., and Rodbell, M., Mol. Pharmacol. 18:598 (1980).
44. Fredholm, B.B., Jonzon, B., and Linstrom, K., Acta Physiol. Scand. 117:461 (1983).
45. Bruns, R.F., Daly, J.W., and Snyder, S.H., Proc. Nat. Acad. Sci. USA 77:5547 (1980).
46. Goodman, R.R., Kuhar, M.J., Hester, L., and Snyder, S.H., Science 220:967 (1983).
47. Smellie, F.W., Daly, J.W., Dunwiddie, T.V., and Hoffer, B.J., Life Sci. 25:1739 (1979).
48. Reddington, M., Lee, K.S., and Schubert, P., Neurosci. Lett. 28:275 (1982).
49. Murray, T.F., Blaker, W.D., Cheney, D.L., and Costa, E., J. Pharmacol. Exp. Therap. 222:550 (1982).
50. Fredholm, B.B., Jonzon, B., Lindgren, E., and Lindstrom, K., J. Neurochem. 39:165 (1982).
51. Phillis, J.W., J. Pharm. Pharmacol. 34:453 (1982).
52. Green, R.D., Proudfit, H.K., and Yeung, S.-M.H., Science 218:58 (1982).
53. Snyder, S.H., Katims, J.J., Annau, Z., Bruns, R.F., and Daly, J.W., Proc. Natl. Acad. Sci. USA 78:3260 (1981).
54. Garbarg, M., Barbin, G., Palacios, J.M., and Schwartz, J.C., Brain Res. 150:638 (1978).
55. Minneman, K.P., Quik, M., and Emson, P.C., Brain Res. 151:507 (1978).
56. Quik, M., Emson, P.C., Fahrenkrug, J., and Iversen, L.L., Naunyn-Schmiedeberg's Arch. Pharmacol. 306:281 (1979).
57. Albano, J., Bhoola, K.D., Kerwin, R.W., Pay, S., Pycock, C.J., Brit. J. Pharmacol. 69:283 (1980).
58. Zahniser, N.R., Minneman, K.P., and Molinoff, P.B., Brain Res. 178:589 (1979).
59. Segal, M., Greenberger, V., and Hofstein, R., Brain Res. 213:351 (1981).
60. Murray, T.F., and Cheney, D.L., Neuropharmacology 21:575 (1982).
61. Ghetti, B., Truex, L., Sawyer, B., Strada, S., and Schmidt, M., J. Neurosci. Res. 6:789 (1981).
62. Rodnight, R., in "International Review of Biochemistry", Vol. 26 (K.F. Tipton, ed.), p. 1. University Park Press, Baltimore, 1979.
63. Costa, M.R.C., Casnellie, J.E., and Catterall, W.A., J. Biol. Chem. 257:7918 (1982).
64. Lingham, R.B., and Sen, A.K., Biochim. Biophys. Acta 688:475 (1982).

HOMOLOGOUS AND HETEROLOGOUS MECHANISMS
OF DESENSITIZATION OF ADENYLATE CYCLASE

Peter H. Fishman

Membrane Biochemistry Section, Developmental and Metabolic
Neurology Branch, National Institute of Neurological and
Communicative Disorders and Stroke, The National Institutes
of Health, Bethesda, Maryland

I. INTRODUCTION

    Current concepts envision the hormone-stimulated adenylate
cyclase as a plasma membrane complex consisting of at least
three identified components: a receptor (R), which recognizes
the hormone; a catalytic subunit (C), which converts ATP to
cyclic AMP; and a regulatory component (G/F), which binds
guanine nucleotides and "couples" R to C (1,2). The mechanism
for this coupling process, however, has not yet been elucidated. Continuous exposure of intact cells to a hormone often
results in an attenuation of the hormone response. This
phenomenon of desensitization or refractoriness may be
specific for the stimulating hormone (homologous) or general
(heterologous) and may or may not involve loss of the hormone
receptors (downregulation).
    Desensitization represents an important mechanism which
allows cells to regulate their responsiveness to physiological effectors. In this overview, I will summarize our current
knowledge about mechanisms of desensitization stressing the
role of the cyclase components. I will also consider the
role of protein synthesis and cyclic AMP in this phenomenon.

II. HOMOLOGOUS DESENSITIZATION BY β-AGONISTS

    Catecholamine-mediated desensitization has been extensive-
ly studied in a variety of tissues and cells, some of which

exhibit a more rapid loss of catecholamine-stimulated adenylate cyclase activity than of β-adrenergic receptors (3-6).
This pattern is observed in rat glioma C6 cells (Fig. 1). In
these experiments, intact cells were exposed to L-isoproteren-
ol (ISO) for different times (Fig. 1A) or at different concentrations (Fig. 1B), washed and assayed for β-receptors using
the β-antagonist L-iodopindolol or for cyclic AMP production
when rechallenged with ISO for 20 min in the presence of isobutylmethylxanthine (IBMX), a phosphodiesterase inhibitor.

Similar results were obtained when membranes were prepared
from the cells and assayed for receptors and adenylate cyclase
activity (5). Although ISO-stimulated cyclase activity was
reduced in membranes from ISO-treated C6 cells, there was no
loss in response to other effectors (Table I). These results
indicated that the desensitization process was homologous.

The ability of cholera toxin (CT) to activate adenylate
cyclase after ISO-mediated desensitization indicated that G/F,
which is ADP-ribosylated by the toxin, was still functional
(5,6). The functionality of G/F was shown directly by reconstituting adenylate cyclase activity in membranes of S49 cyc⁻
cells, which lack G/F, with detergent extracts containing G/F.
The G/F extracted from control and ISO-desensitized cells was

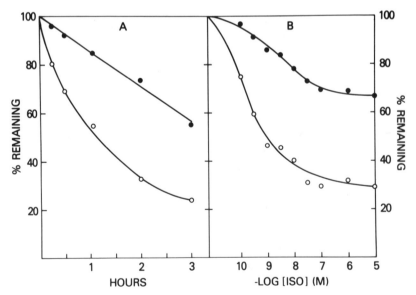

FIGURE 1. ISO-mediated desensitization and downregulation
in rat glioma C6 cells. Cells were incubated with 0.1 μM ISO
for the indicated times (A) or for 2 h with the indicated concentrations of ISO (B), washed and assayed for specific iodo-
pindolol binding (●) or for ISO-stimulated cyclic AMP (o).

TABLE I.   Effect of Catecholamine-Mediated Desensitization of Rat Glioma C6 Cells on Adenylate Cyclase Activities[a]

Effector	Adenylate Cyclase Activity (pmol/min/mg protein)		
	0 h	3 h	24 h
None	14.6	13.9	15.2
ISO	108	44.5	25.7
Gpp(NH)p	137	106	111
NaF	229	212	223
CT [b]	104	96.3	111
A_1 + NAD [c]	98.7	94.7	94.3

[a]Data from (5). Cells were incubated for the indicated times with 10 μM ISO, washed and assayed for adenylate cyclase activities. [b]Cells were incubated 1 h more with cholera toxin (CT). [c]Membranes were incubated with the A_1 subunit of CT and NAD. Gpp(NH)p, guanyl-5'-yl-imidodiphosphate.

equally effective in restoring ISO-stimulated activity to cyc⁻ membranes (6-9). Thus, desensitization did not induce any changes in G/F as it was able to couple R to C in the cyc⁻ membranes.

In some cells, catecholamine-mediated desensitization causes a reduction in the affinity of the agonist for the β-receptor (5,8-14). This can be detected either by a shift in the affinity of agonist to stimulate adenylate cyclase (Fig. 2A) or to compete with labeled antagonist for the receptors (Fig. 2B). It is well known that β-agonists exhibit a lower affinity for R in the presence of guanine nucleotides (see Fig. 2B, -----). The high affinity state is believed to represent an R·G/F complex which is dissociated by guanine nucleotides; the uncoupled R represents a low affinity state (14). The shift to lower affinity is consistent with an uncoupling of R from G/F. Desensitization, however, does not change the affinity of R for antagonists (3,5,10,11).

The uncoupling of R from G/F has been directly observed. Lysates of ISO-desensitized human astrocytoma cells, when sedimented on sucrose density gradients, exhibited an additional peak of β-receptors in a lighter membrane fraction that lacked ISO-stimulated cyclase activity (12). These receptors were in a low affinity state as measured by agonist affinity and absence of GTP modulation. Desensitization of frog erythrocytes led to a loss of β-receptors from the plasma membrane and their recovery in cytoplasmic vesicles (13). The vesicles were devoid of adenylate cyclase activity and G/F; the receptors in the vesicles were uncoupled and in a low af-

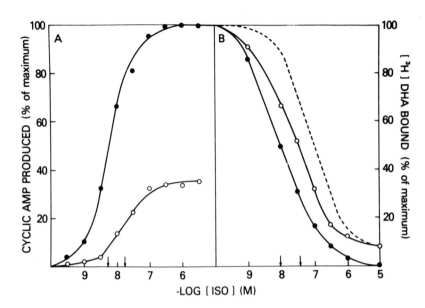

FIGURE 2. Reduction of Agonist Affinity in Desensitized
Rat Glioma C6 Cells. Cells were incubated with (o) and without (•) 0.1 μM ISO for 2 h and washed extensively. (A) Cells
were rechallenged with the indicated concentrations of ISO and
assayed for cyclic AMP production. (B) Membranes were prepared and assayed for [³H]dihydroalprenolol (DHA) binding in
the presence of the indicated concentrations of ISO. (-----),
binding in the presence of 0.1 mM GTP. Arrows indicate ISO
concentrations required for half-maximal effects.

finity state. It is not yet clear whether the sequestering of
R from other cyclase components is the cause or a consequence
of desensitization. Some cells such as human fibroblasts (6)
and S49 cyc⁻ cells (3,9,10) exhibited no loss in plasma
membrane β-receptors during agonist-mediated desensitization.
    The ability of S49 cyc⁻ cells to become desensitized (7,9)
clearly indicates that a functional G/F is not required for
desensitization to occur. It also suggests that the homologous desensitization mediated by catecholamines most likely
involves some change in the receptor. The functionality of
desensitized β-receptors was explored by using membrane/mem-
brane fusion techniques[1]. S49 cyc⁻ cells were used as the
donor of β-receptors; and Fc cells, which lack β-receptors but
have G/F and C as well as prostaglandin E₁ (PGE₁) receptors,
were used as the acceptor. Membranes from control and ISO-

[1]S. Kassis and P. H. Fishman, unpublished observations.

treated cyc⁻ cells were fused with membranes from Fc cells and the fusion products assayed for cyclase activity. β-receptors from ISO-treated cyc⁻ cells were less effective than control receptors in reconstituting ISO-stimulated activity in the hybrid membranes. These results indicate that homologous desensitization induced by β-agonists involves a change in the β-receptor that impairs its a ability to couple to G/F.

The nature of this change has not been determined. Turkey erthyrocytes were desensitized with ISO and their β-receptors covalently labeled with a β-antagonist photoaffinity probe (15). The labeled polypeptides from desensitized cells had a larger apparent size than those from control cells as determined by sodium dodecyl sulfate-polyacrylamide gel electrophoresis. ISO, however, causes a heterologous desensitization in turkey erythrocytes (16). When similar studies were done with frog erythrocytes, there was no change in the size of the desensitized β-receptor (13).

III. Heterologous Desensitization

When cultured human fibroblasts were exposed to PGE_1, the cells lost their ability to produce cyclic AMP when rechallenged with PGE_1 (6). The PGE_1-treated cells also became refractory to ISO and cholera toxin (6). This heterologous type of desensitization also was observed when membranes prepared from control and PGE_1-treated fibroblasts were assayed for adenylate cyclase activities (Table II). The reduction in

TABLE II. Heterologous Desensitization of Adenylate Cyclase in Human Fibroblasts Mediated by PGE_1[a]

Effector	Adenylate Cyclase Activity (pmol/min/mg protein)	
	Control Cells	PGE_1-treated Cells
GTP	49	33
GTP + ISO	89	66
GTP + PGE_1	403	299
Gpp(NH)p	215	179
NaF	443	360
CT	265	187
A_1 + NAD	170	118

[a]Data from (6). Membranes were prepared from cells incubated with and without 10 μM PGE_1 for 30 min. Cells or membranes were treated with CT or A_1 plus NAD as described in Table I.

all activities including cholera toxin suggested an effect on
G/F. Membranes were incubated with the A_1 subunit of cholera
toxin and $[^{32}P]NAD$ in order to label G/F subunits. As shown
in Fig. 3, the toxin substrates in human fibroblasts have Mr =
47,000 and 42,000. These same peptides were labeled in membranes from PGE_1-desensitized cells; there actually was more
^{32}P incorporated after desensitization.

In order to determine if there was a functional change in
G/F in the PGE_1-desensitized cells, G/F was extracted and used
to reconstitute adenylate cyclase activity in S49 cyc⁻ membranes (Fig. 4). G/F from PGE_1-treated cells was less effective than control G/F at all concentrations tested. In
addition, G/F from the desensitized cells was less efficient
in reconstituting adenylate cyclase activity in cyc⁻ membranes irrespective of the effector used to stimulate the
enzyme (Table III). Thus, the G/F extracted from human
fibroblast membranes exhibited the same impaired behaviour
when transfered to cyc⁻ membranes as it did in its original
membrane (compare Table II with Table III).

A soluble adenylate cyclase was prepared by extracting the
human fibroblast membranes with Triton N-101. The activity
was stimulated by GTP, Gpp(NH)p and NaF but not by ISO or PGE_1
(6). Thus, the soluble cyclase presumably represented a G/F·C
complex. When the soluble cyclase from control fibroblasts

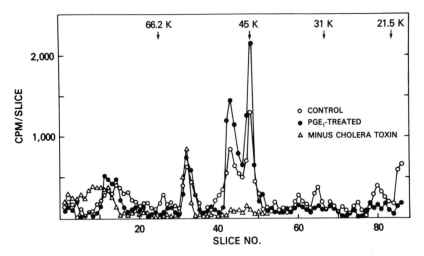

FIGURE 3. ADP-ribosylation of membranes from control and
PGE1-desensitized human fibroblasts. Membranes were prepared,
labeled with $[^{32}P]NAD$ in the presence and absence of the A_1
subunit of cholera toxin, and separated by sodium dodecyl
sulfate-polyacrylamide gel electrophoresis. From Kassis &
Fishman (6).

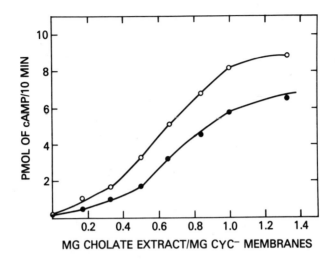

FIGURE 4.   Reconstitution of Adenylate Cyclase Activity in
S49 Cyc⁻ Membranes with Extracts from Human Fibroblasts.
Membranes were prepared from control (●) and PGE₁-treated (o)
cells and extracted with cholate; the extracts were used to
reconstitute adenylate cyclase in membranes of cyc⁻ cells.
From Kassis & Fishman (6).

was centrifuged on a linear sucrose gradient, it sedimented as
a single peak with an $S_{20,w}$ value of 6.2 (Fig. 5).   The enzyme
activity extracted from cells desensitized by PGE₁, however,
had an $S_{20,w}$ value of 5.0.   This shift in sedimentation value
could be due to a change in size of the cyclase complex (loss
of a subunit), a change in detergent binding or a change in
the interaction of G/F and C.   The observed sedimentation rate
of the complex depends not only on the sizes of G/F and C but

TABLE III.   Effect of PGE₁-Desensitization on G/F of Human
 Fibroblasts as Determined by Reconstitution of S49 Cyc⁻^{a}

Source of G/F	Adenylate Cyclase Activity (pmol/10'/mg protein)			
	GTP	GTP + ISO	Gpp(NH)p	NaF
Control	69	341	192	583
PGE₁-treated	60	190	109	299

^{a}Details are the same as in the legend to Fig. 4 except the
reconstituted cyc⁻ membranes were assayed for cyclase activity
with the indicated effectors.

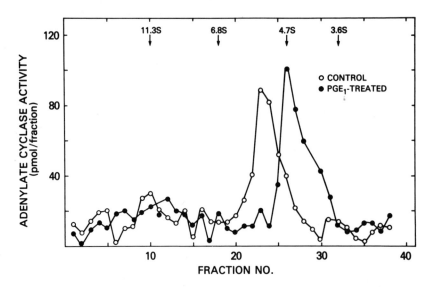

FIGURE 5. Sedimentation Behaviour of Soluble Adenylate
Cyclase from Human Fibroblasts. Membranes prepared from
control (o) and PGE1-treated (•) cells were extracted with 1%
Triton N-101; the extracts were centrifuged on linear sucrose
gradients and fractions collected and assayed for NaF-stimu-
lated adenylate cyclase activity. From Kassis & Fishman (6).

their affinity for each other. If the ability of G/F to interact with C is reduced in the PGE1-desensitized state, this
would be reflected in a shift in the equilibrium between them
and the complex would sediment at a slower rate.
   The above results clearly indicate that G/F is altered
during heterologous desensitization of human fibroblasts by
PGE1. Heterologous desensitization has also been observed in
rat adipocytes (17), turkey erythrocytes (16) and rat corpus
striatum (18). In the latter tissue, prolonged exposure to
dopamine led to a loss not only in dopamine-stimulated adenylate cyclase activity but also activity stimulated by NaF and
cholera toxin. These results are consistent with an an alteration in G/F. Thus, a modification of G/F may be a common
mechanism for heterologous desensitization. The nature of
this modification is not known. We have been able to hetero-
logously desensitize adenylate cyclase in a cell-free system[2].
Human fibroblast membranes were incubated with PGE$_1$ and GTP
and assayed for adenylate cyclase activity with various effectors. The loss in activity was both time and dose dependent

[2]S. Kassis and P. H. Fishman, unpublished observations.

and similar to that observed in intact cells. The desensitization was not observed in the absence of GTP. This cell-
free model may be usefully in understanding the biochemical
mechanism of heterologous desensitization.

IV. Role of Cyclic AMP and Protein Synthesis

It has been suggested that cyclic AMP may been involved in
the refractory state induced in rat glioma C6 cells by catecholamines as other agents such as dibutryl cyclic AMP, isobutylmethylxanthine and cholera toxin caused the cells to be
become less responsive to catecholamines (19-21). Our own
studies, however, indicated that C6 cells treated with these
agents retained their responsiveness to ISO (Table IV).
It also had been reported that prolonged exposure of C6
cells to either cholera toxin or dibutyryl cyclic AMP causes a
loss of β-receptors (22). We have confirmed (Table V) and extended these observations (23)[3]. The downregulation of β-receptors in cells exposed to cholera toxin, cyclic AMP derivatives or IBMX was much slower than that induced by ISO. The
loss began after a lag of 6 h and was ∿50% after 24 h when
ISO-treated cells had lost most of their receptors. Although
these agents induced downregulation of β-receptors, they did
not appear to cause desensitization. Thus, the concentration
of ISO required to half-maximally stimulate adenylate cyclase
or displace [^{3}H]DHA after C6 cells were incubated 24 h with
1 mM IBMX was not shifted to the right (compare with Fig. 2).
Also, there was little or no loss in ISO-stimulated adenylate
cyclase activity in membranes prepared from cells treated
with dibutyryl cyclic AMP and IBMX for 24 h.

TABLE IV. Responsiveness of Rat Glioma C6 Cells Treated
with Isoproterenol, Cholera Toxin or Isobutylmethylxanthine[a]

Pretreatment	Cyclic AMP Accumulation (pmol/mg protein)	
	- ISO	+ ISO
None	10.8	587
10 µM ISO, 3 h	10.9	51
1 mM IBMX, 3 h	22.2	529
10 nM CT, 2.5 h	450	922

[a]Data from (5). Cells were treated as indicated, washed and
incubated for 10 min with and without 10 µM ISO plus 1 mM IBMX

[3]P. H. Fishman and J. Hagmann, unpublished observations.

TABLE V. Downregulation of β-Receptors in Rat Glioma C6
Cells: Effects of Various Agents and Cycloheximide[a]

Agent	β-Receptors (% remaining)	
	− Cycloheximide	+ Cycloheximide
None	100	94
ISO (10 μM)	14	65
8-Bromo-cyclic AMP (1 mM)	55	115
IBMX (0.5 mM)	67	−[b]
CT (12 nM)	52	−

[a]Cells were incubated for 18 h with the indicated agents.
When present, 10 μg/ml of cycloheximide was added 2 h before.
[b]Not determined.

As indicated in Table V, inhibition of protein synthesis
blocked downregulation of β-receptors in C6 cells. Prior
exposure of the cells to cycloheximide, however, did not prevent ISO-mediated desensitization of adenylate cyclase. The
cycloheximide-treated cells, when incubated with ISO, rapidly
lost their ability to accumulate cyclic AMP upon rechallenge
with the agonist. Membranes prepared from these cells had
less ISO-stimulated adenylate cyclase activity than membranes
prepared from cells exposed only to cycloheximide. And finally, cycloheximide treatment did not prevent the shift in affinity of ISO as measured by competition for [^{3}H]DHA binding.
From these results, one can conclude that desensitization
of the β-adrenergic-stimulated adenylate cyclase system is
agonist specific, is not mediated by cyclic AMP and does not
depend on de novo protein synthesis. In contrast, downregulation of β-receptors can be induced both by agonist and cyclic
AMP and does require protein synthesis. As the time course
and extent of receptor loss is different, it is not clear that
both agonist and cyclic AMP utilize the same mechanism. A
similar phenomenon has been observed in murine Leydig tumor
cells that have receptors for human chorionic gonadotropin
(hCG) (24). When the cells were incubated with hCG, there
was a rapid loss of occupied receptors (half-life of 3 h)
followed by a loss of unoccupied ones 8 h after adding hCG.
The latter phase was mimicked by exposing the cells to cholera
toxin or dibutyryl cyclic AMP. Prior exposure of the cells to
cycloheximide inhibited the downregulation of receptors but
did not prevent hCG-mediated desensitization of adenylate cyclase. The ability of cyclic AMP to induce downregulation of
hormone receptors appears to be specific as there was no loss
of cholera toxin receptors in rat glioma C6 or murine Leydig
tumor cells exposed for 24 h to dibutyryl cyclic AMP or IBMX.

V. CONCLUSIONS

The mechanisms of homologous and heterologous desensitization of adenylate cyclase involve alterations in different components of the system. A decreased ability of R to couple to G/F is associate with the former whereas an impaired coupling between G/F and C is associated with the latter. An alteration in R and G/F, respectively, is implicated in these processes but the nature of the changes are unknown. It is tempting to speculate that a covalent modification is the underlining basis for desensitization. It has recently been demonstrated that receptors for insulin, epidermal growth factor and nerve growth factor have protein kinase activity associated with them and become phosphorylated when occupied by their ligands. Thus, there is some precedent for ligand-mediated phosphorylation of receptors. The requirement for nucleotide triphosphates, especially GTP, in cell-free desensitization is consistent with a phosphorylation process (25, 26,27)[2]. Phosphorylation of R could alter its ability to couple to G/F; similarly, phosphorylation of G/F could reduce its ability to couple to C. In addition, phosphorylation of R may provide a recognition marker for endocytosis and eventual degradation in lysosomes. Cyclic AMP-mediated downregulation may involve an induced protein kinase, which phosphorylates R at a separate site. Recent advances in covalently attaching hormones to their receptors by chemical crosslinking (28) and photoaffinity labeling (13,15) as well as receptor purification by affinity and immunoaffinity chromatography may provide the techniques for isolating and characterizing desensitizated receptors.

REFERENCES

1. Rodbell, M. (1980). Nature 284, 17.
2. Ross, E.M., and Gilman, A.G. (1980). Annu. Rev. Biochem. 49, 533.
3. Shear, M., Insel, P.A., Melmon, K.L., and Coffino, P. (1976). J. Biol. Chem. 251, 7572.
4. Su, Y.-F., Harden, T.K., and Perkins, J.P. (1979). J. Biol. Chem. 254, 38.
5. Fishman, P.H., Mallorga, P., and Tallman, J.F. (1981). Mol. Pharmacol. 20, 310.
6. Kassis, S., and Fishman, P.H. (1982). J. Biol. Chem. 257, 5312.
7. Green, D.A., and Clark, R.B. (1981). J. Biol. Chem. 256, 2105.

8. Iyengar, R., Bhat, M.K., Riser, M.E., and Birnbaumer, L. (1981). J. Biol. Chem. 256, 4810.

9. Green, D.A., Friedman, J., and Clark, R.B. (1981). J. Cyclic Nucleotide Res. 7, 161.

10. Su, Y.-F., Harden, T.K., and Perkins, J.P. (1981). J. Biol. Chem. 255, 7410.

11. Homburger, V., Lucas, M., Cantau, B., Barabe, J., Peni, J., and Bockaert, J. (1980). J. Biol. Chem. 255, 10436.

12. Harden, T.K., Cotton, C.U., Waldo, G.L., Lutton, J.K., and Perkins, J.P. (1980). Science 210, 441.

13. Stadel, J.M., Strulovici, B., Nambi, P., Lavin, T., Briggs, M.M., Caron, M.G., and Lefkowitz, R.J. (1983). J. Biol. Chem. 258, 3032.

14. Stadel, J.M., De Lean, A., and Lefkowitz, R.J. (1982). Adv. Enzymol. 53, 1.

15. Stadel, J.M., Nambi, P., Lavin, T.N., Heald, S.L., Caron, M.G., and Lefkowitz, R.J. (1982). J. Biol. Chem. 257, 9242.

16. Hoffman, B.B, Mullikin-Kilpatrick, D., and Lefkowitz, R.J. (1979). J. Cyclic Nucleotide Res. 5, 355.

17. Balkin, M., Melber, A., and Roginsky, M. (1982). Biochem. Biophys. Res. Commun. 106, 298.

18. Memo, M., Lovenberg, W., and Hanbauer, I. (1982). Proc. Natl. Acad. Sci. USA 79, 4456.

19. Terasaki, W.L., Brooker, G., de Vellis, J., Inglish, D., Hsu, C.-Y., and Moylan, R.D. (1978). Adv. Cyclic Nucleotide Res. 9, 33.

20. Nickols, G.A., and Brooker, G. (1979). J. Cyclic Nucleotide Res. 5, 435.

21. Koschel, K. (1980). Eur. J. Biochem. 108, 163.

22. Moylan, R.D., Barovsky, K., and Brooker, G. (1982). J. Biol. Chem. 257, 4947.

23. Zaremba, T., and Fishman, P.H. (1983). Fed. Proc. 42, 1852.

24. Rebois, R.V., and Fishman, P.H. (1983). Fed. Proc. 42, 1874.

25. Anderson, W.B., and Jaworski, C.J. (1979). J. Biol. Chem. 254, 4596.

26. Ezra, E., and Salomon, Y. (1980). J. Biol. Chem. 255, 653.

27. Iyengar, R., Mintz, P.W., Swartz, T.L., and Birnbaumer, L. (1980). J. Biol. Chem. 255, 11875.

28. Rebois, R.V., Omodeo-Sale, F., Brady, R.O., and Fishman, P.H. (1981). Proc. Natl. Acad. Sci. USA 78, 2086.

CHOLECYSTOKININ: ELECTROPHYSIOLOGIC AND RECEPTOR
AUTORADIOGRAPHIC STUDIES IN RODENT BRAIN

Robert B. Innis and George K. Aghajanian

Departments of Psychiatry and Pharmacology
Yale University School of Medicine
New Haven, Ct 06508

I. INTRODUCTION

Peptides are the most recent addition to the group of neurotransmitter candidates. During the past ten years the number of recognized peptide neurotransmitter possibilities has increased to about two dozen. Most of these are small, comprising 3-15 amino acids, though peptides up to 100 amino acids in length have been proposed as possible transmitters. Some are known to have definite electrophysiologic actions, either excitatory or inhibitory. However, many peptide neurotransmitter candidates do not display such clear-cut effects and have instead been proposed to act as neuromodulators, which modify responses of neurons to other neurotransmitters. Differentially labelling substances as neuromodulators or neurotransmitters may only be a semantic artifice to mask our ignorance of synaptic mechanisms. The numerous ways that a substance, localized in nerve endings and released upon depolarization, can affect other neurons may all "transmit" important information. For the purposes of simplicity, we consider substances that are highly localized to specific neuronal systems in the brain, released on depolarization, and produce changes in neuronal activity as "neurotransmitters."

For many years cholecystokinin (CCK), a 33 amino acid peptide, has been recognized as an intestinal hormone involved in the regulation of gallbladder and pancreatic

MECHANISM OF DRUG ACTION

375

function.   Recently, Dockray (1) and Rehfeld (2) reported
the existence of CCK-like immunoreactivity in the brain.
Shortly thereafter, CCK-like material was localized in
neurons by immunohistochemistry (Innis et al. (3), Larsson
and Rehfeld (4), and Loren et al.(5)). Receptor binding
sites for radiolabeled CCK have also been detected in the
brain   (Innis   and Snyder (6) and Saito et al. (7)).
Presently, a substantial body of evidence supports the
notion that CCK acts as a neurotransmitter in the CNS (see
Morley (8) for review). In this chapter, we will report on
the autoradiographic localization of CCK receptors in rodent
brain and on electrophysiologic studies of nociceptive
CCK-containing neurons in the midbrain central gray.

II. CCK RECEPTOR AUTORADIOGRAPHY

Receptor binding studies in tissue homogenates lack
sensitivity for localization of the receptors. A major
advance in the anatomic study of receptors has been   the in
vitro receptor autoradiographic technique developed by
Young and Kuhar (9). By this sensitive method, receptors
can be localized at the level of light microscopy in lightly
fixed tissue sections mounted on microscope slides. For
details of this technique, see Young and Kuhar (9) and
Unnerstall et al. (10).   Basically, tissue sections are
incubated in buffer containing the radioligand.   After
association of the ligand, non-specific binding is largely
washed away in solutions of excess buffer. Emulsion coated
coverslips are apposed to the dried tissue sections. After
adequate time for exposure of the radiographic grains, the
photographic emulsion is developed and the underlying tissue
histologically stained.
We have successfully labeled CCK receptors in rat and
guinea pig brain tissue sections (Innis et al. (11) and
Zarbin et al. (12)).   To label CCK receptors, 8 μm thick,
slide-mounted tissue sections of lightly fixed guinea pig
brain were incubated with ^{125}I-Bolton-Hunter labeled CCK
(^{125}I-CCK-33).   Nonspecific binding was determined by
incubating some tissue sections in the presence of excess
unlabeled displacer (0.1 μM cholecystokinin octapeptide).
This procedure gave specific to nonspecific binding ratios
of 2:1. The binding was saturable, reversible, of high
affinity, and was pharmacologically similar to that observed
in membrane homogenates. Autoradiograms were generated by
apposing emulsion-coated coverslips against the labeled
tissue sections. Exposure time was 2 months.
We found that CCK receptors were widely distributed
throughout the central nervous system with enrichment in

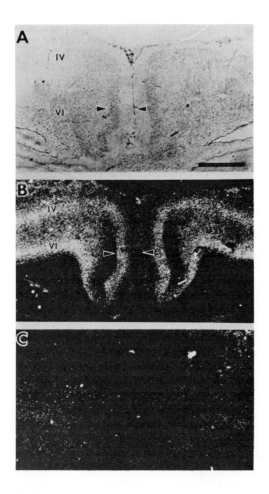

Figure 1.   Distribution of CCK binding sites in anterior
cingulate   cortex   of   guinea   pig.   A.   Bright field
photomicrograph of an autoradiogram of the guinea pig
cerebral   cortex.   At   this   magnification,   the
autoradiographic grains cannct be visualized. B. Darkfield
photogramicrograph of the autoradiogram shown in A.   In
darkfield illumination,   the autoradiographic grains appear
as white dots and the tissue is invisible.   Opposing
arrowheads mark the boundaries of lamina   IV (left) and
lamina I (right).   C.   Darkfield photomicrograph of an
autoradiogram generated by incubating a tissue section
consecutive to the one shown in A in the presence of 50 pM
^{125}I-CCK-33 and 100 mM CCK-8. The diffusely distributed, .
low density of grains in C represent non-specific binding.
Bar equals 2667 μm.

olfactory, visual, limbic, and cortical areas. In the olfactory system, CCK receptors are in the olfactory bulb, olfactory tract, and the superficial laminae of primary olfactory cortex. The presence of receptors on the fiber tract itself and in areas to which the tract projects suggests that these receptors are made in the neuronal cell bodies of the olfactory bulb and transported along the fiber tract to its projection areas. The axonal transport of CCK receptors has been demonstrated in the peripheral nervous system in the vagus nerve (13). These central CCK binding sites are situated in anatomic loci which would allow the modification of olfactory information at a very early point of entry into CNS circuits. CCK appears to play a crucial role in the control of food intake (see below). These olfactory CCK receptors may mediate eating behavior by modulating olfactory input through central feeding areas in the hypothalamus.

Within the visual system receptors are found on the primary sensory neuron of the eye (the retinal ganglion cell), the axon of this neuron (forming the optic tract), and in central projection areas of this neuron (the nucleus of the optic tract, the ventrolateral nucleus of the geniculate, and the superior colliculus). As with the olfactory system, some of these CCK receptors are probably located axonally and function to modulate at a presynaptic level the input of primary visual information. Consistent with this hypothesis, enucleation causes a drastic contralateral decrease in the density of CCK receptors along the optic tract and in central areas of projection (work in progress). This experiment suggests, therefore, that CCK receptors are made by neurons within the eye and are transported centrally.

In the limbic system, relatively high densities of receptors are found in the mammillary nuclei, in a laminar distribution in the hippocampal formation, and in the amygdala. Although the function of these receptors are unknown, one can speculate that they modulate emotions of the animal.

In the cerebral cortex, CCK receptors have a distinct laminar distribution, with highest concentrations in layers II-IV and VI, with a sparing of layers of I and V (Fig. 1). An interesting fact about CCK is that it is one of a small number of transmitters now known to be present in neurons intrinsic to the cerebral cortex (rather than just being in projection fibers to the cortex). Layers II and III contain cortical association neurons. Thus, the previous discovery of CCK containing neurons in layers II and III suggest that CCK plays a role in cortical-cortical information processing, including interhemispheric connections.

III.   CCK RECEPTORS FLOW IN THE RAT VAGUS NERVE

The most extensively studied behavioral effect of CCK is its modulation of food intake and apparent induction of satiety.   Schally et al. (14) demonstrated that "enterogasterone," an extract from the gut which is now known to be enriched in CCK, causes decreased food intake in the mouse. Gibbs et al.(15) later showed that exogenous CCK induces satiety in rat and monkey. Whether CCK induced satiety is mediated by the central nervous system or by peripheral mechanisms is uncertain (for review see Morley (8) and Smith and Gibbs (16)). In the rat, Smith et al.(17) have shown that abdominal vagotomy blocks the satiety effect of intraperitoneally injected CCK. We were unsuccessful in routine tissue homogenate binding studies to radiolabel a CCK receptor. The tough connective tissue surrounding the vagus nerve was difficult to homogenize and non-specific binding was very high. However, we were able to identify a CCK binding site in the rat vagus nerve with the in vitro receptor autoradiographic technique (19).

The vagus nerve was ligated approximately 1.5 cm distal to the nodose ganglion. Ligatures were allowed to remain in place for varying times between 0 and 24 hours. The nerves were then surgically removed, mounted for sectioning, and frozen in liquid nitrogen. Tissue sections were processed for routine CCK receptor autoradiography as described above.

Initial experiments were designed to detect the presence and transport of CCK receptors in the vagus nerve. An increased density of binding sites was detected proximal to the ligature (Fig. 2), suggesting that CCK receptor transport had occurred. To examine the time course of CCK receptor transport, rats were sacrificed after 6, 12 and 24 hours of ligation. After preparing autoradiographs, the grain densities, which reflect receptor densities, were measured and plotted as a function of distance from the ligature (Fig. 2). CCK binding sites accumulated proximal to the ligature in a time dependent manner, and the accumulation was approximately linear with time. Subsequent experiments demonstrated an appropriate pharmacologic profile for these binding sites, with sulfated CCK-8 much more potent that desulfated CCK-8 in displacing the radioligand. Also, the injection into the nerve trunk of colchicine (which is believed to disaggregate microtubules and to block fast axonal transport) blocks accumulation of CCK binding sites. This experiment suggests that microtubules are involved in the axonal flow of CCK receptors.

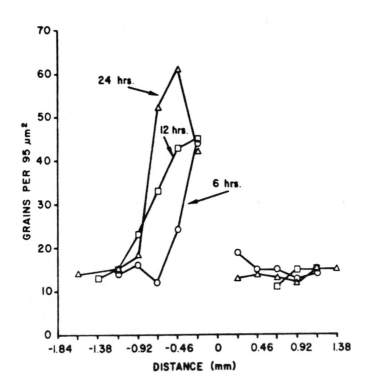

Figure 2. Time course of CCK binding site accumulation. Vagi were ligated for various times between 0 and 24 hours. The tissue was subsequently used to generate autoradiograms as described in the text. The x-coordinate 0 was assigned to the point at which the ligature was placed; negative x-values correspond to areas proximal to the ligature while positive x-values correspond to areas distal to the ligature. This experiment was repeated in nine animals (3 per time point) with essentially identical results. Data from a typical experiment are shown.

IV. ELECTROPHYSIOLOGIC STUDIES OF CCK CONTAINING NEURONS

A higher functional level to examine the role of CCK in the central nervous system is the physiologic study of electrical activity of CCK containing neurons. Besides the work described below, only one other group has successfully been able to record from CCK containing neurons.

Bunney and co-workers (18) recorded from mid-brain dopamine neurons which also contain CCK. The cell group which we chose to investigate is a dense cluster of CCK neurons located in the midline periaqueductal gray of rat anterior midbrain. This nucleus, which extends almost over the entire length of the aqueduct, is not notable with normal histologic stains, but corresponds in part with the nucleus linearis rostralis. The cellular cluster is only apparent with immunohistochemical staining and was first described by Innis et al.(2). The periaqueductal gray is a brain region involved in pain perception. Because of this, we speculated in that first report that CCK may be involved in pain perception. As will be explained below, this appears to have been serendipitously correct.

The technique used for this study was <u>in vivo</u> extracellular recording in chloral hydrate anesthetized rats. The strategy for locating these neurons took advantage of the fact that the CCK containing cluster of cells is located directly in the midline, the same depth from the surface of the brain as the serotonin containing dorsal raphe cells, and just anterior to these serotonin cells. Thus, the well-studied serotonin cells were first located and then the region just anterior to this was searched for neuronal firing patterns distinctive to the region known to contain CCK neurons. Such a firing pattern was found only in the region containing CCK neurons but not in adjacent regions. The neuron has a distinctive electrophysiologic characteristics. First, the spike is typically biphasic with an initial positive deflection followed by a smaller negative deflection. Second, the spontaneous firing rate is erratic. At times, the cell will fire in bursts and at other times fire fairly regularly (1-7 Hz) for up to an hour. Third, the cell responds to noxious stimuli such as toe pinch. Specifically, such painful stimuli cause an increase in firing rate, a decrease in amplitude, and an increase in the duration of pulse (Fig. 3). Continued painful stimuli will actually lead to a cessation of firing caused by depolarization blockade. That is, the increased firing rate is associated with a depolarization which ultimately causes an inhibition of firing presumably due to sodium-channel inactivation.

Several lines of evidence indicate that these cells are CCK containing neurons. First, dye spots deposited at the end of a recording session have always been histologically located in the narrow region of the CCK neuronal group. Second, co-localization experiments have shown the electrode tip (marked by a small area of tissue damage) surrounded by a dense cluster of immunohistochemically stained CCK

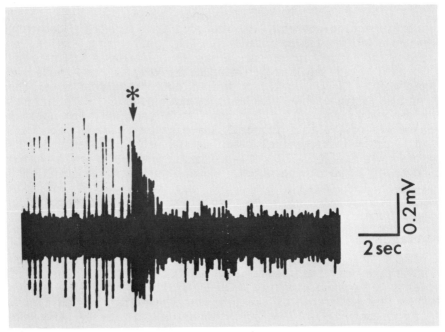

Figure 3. Single unit recording of a CCK neuron. This relatively slow sweep of the oscilloscope shown the firing of a single neuron. The first 5 sec of the recording shows a fairly regular firing of the neuron. Each "spike" consists of a positive and negative component (located respectively,, above and below the black band of background noise). At the time marked by the arrow, the hind paw was pinched. This noxious stimulus caused an increased firing rate (as indicated by the spikes moving so close together that they appear merged) and a decrease in amplitude of the positive and negative deflection. The cell goes into depolarization blockade, and firing is completely inhibited 1 sec after the toe pinch.

containing neurons. The definitive proof that we are recording from a CCK neuron would probably require in vivo intracellular recording and subsequent immunohistochemical demonstration that this individual neuron in fact contains CCK. Such an experiment is presently in progress. Without this definitive evidence, we should call these cells "putative CCK-containing neurons." For brevity, however, we will subsequently refer to these cells simply as "CCK neurons."

Recent reports show that CCK blocks the analgesic effect of opiates (19). Thus, the increased firing rate induced by toe pinch is consistent with this anti-analgesic action.

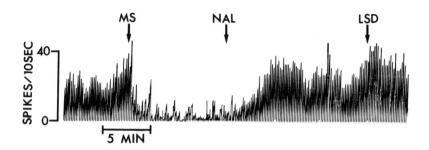

Figure 4. Cumulative rate histogram of a single CCK neuron in the periaqueductal gray. Athe the point labelled "MS," morphine sulfate (0.1 mg/kg) was injected via a single intravenous bolus. The cell's firing was markedly inhibited within one minute of this injection. At the point labelled "NAL," naloxone (10 µg/kg) was injected via a single intravenous bolus. The inhibition of firing induced by morphine is gradually reversed by naloxone and returned to slightly greater than control levels within 5 mins of injection of naloxone. LSD (10 µg//kg) was injected i.v. at point level "LSD," which appears to cause relatively small and transient increase in firing rate.

Furthermore, we found that intravenously administered morphine very potently inhibits the firing of these cells. As is shown in Fig. 4, doses of morphine as low as 0.1 mg/kg markedly and rapidly inhibit the firing of the cell. In addition, this morphine induced inhibition can be reversed by the specific opiate receptor antagonist, naloxone. Morphine can inhibit not only the spontaneous activity of a CCK cell but also block the toe pinch induced increase in firing.

The ability of morphine to inhibit the firing of CCK neurons could be mediated by opiate receptors located almost anywhere in the nervous system. If it is mediated by postsynaptic opiate receptors located on the CCK neurons, then the endogenous opiate peptide enkephalin should be located presynaptically adjacent to the CCK cells. In fact, we have recently been able to show with immunohistochemical staining a dense cluster of enkephalin containing terminal fibers in the neuropil of this neuronal cluster. However, it remains to be determined whether this enkephalin input is directly onto CCK cells or onto some interposed cell type.

V. CONCLUSION

The CCK receptor autoradiographic studies strongly indicate diverse roles for this nearly ubiquitous neuropeptide. CCK probably plays a significant role in the olfactory, visual, limbic, and cortical systems. Within the olfactory and visual systems, CCK receptors are probably located on axons, rather than their more traditional sites on dendrites and the neuronal cell bodies. These axonal receptors may act presynaptically to modify the input of sensory information. We have clearly shown that CCK receptors are located on the axons of the vagus nerve and flow distally towards the periphery.

In addition, we have very likely succeeded in recording the electrical activity of a dense cluster of CCK containing neurons in the periaqueductal gray. These cells have a distinctive firing pattern. Painful stimuli cause an increased rate of firing, and continued stimulation causes depolarization blockade. These neurons are exquisitely sensitive to morphine, which effect can itself be blocked by naloxone. Opiate induced analgesia is may be mediated in part by an inactivation of this neuronal cluster.

REFERENCES

1. Dockray, G.J. (1976). Nature. 264, 568.
2. Rehfeld, J.F. (1977). Acta Pharmacol. Toxicol. 24, 44.
3. Innis, R.B., Correa, F.M., Uhl, G.R., Schneider, B.S., and Snyder, S.H. (1979). Proc. Natl. Acad. Sci. 76, 521.
4. Larsson, L.I. and Rehfeld, J.F. (1979). Brain Res. 165, 201.
5. Loren, I., Alumets, J., Hakanson, R., and Sundler, F. (1979). Histochem. 59, 249.
6. Innis, R.B. and Snyder, S.H. (1980). Proc. Natl. Acad. Sci. 77, 6917.
7. Saito, A., Goldfine, I.D., and Williams, J.A. (1980). Science. 208, 1155.
8. Morley, J.E. (1982). Life Sci. 30, 479.
9. Young, W.S. and Kuhar, M.J. (1979). Brain Res. 179, 255.
10. Unnerstall, J.R., Kuhar, M.J., Niehoff, D.L., and Palacios, J.M. (1981). J. Pharmacol. Exp. Ther. 218, 7907.
11. Innis, R.B., Zarbin, M.A., Kuhar, M.J., and Snyder, S.H. (1983). In Methods in Neurobiology. Vol. 1, in press.

12. Zarbin, M.A., Innis, R.B., Wamsley, J.K., Snyder, S.H., and Kuhar, M.J. (1983). J. Neurosci. 3, 877.
13. Zarbin, M.A., Wamsley, J.K., Innis, R.B., and Kuhar, M.J. (1981). Life Sci. 29, 697.
14. Schally, A.V., Redding, T.W., Lucien, H.W., and Meyer, J. (1967). Science. 157, 210.
15. Gibbs, J., Young, R.C., and Smith, G.P. (1973). Nature. 245, 323.
16. Smith, G.P. and Gibbs, J. (1979). In Progress in Psychobiology and Physiological Psychology. Vol. 8, 179.
17. Smith, G.P., Jerome, C., Cushin, B.J., Eternu, R., and Simansky, K.J. (1981). Science. 213, 1036.
18. Skirboll, L.R., Grace, A.A., Hommer, D.W., Rehfeld, J., Goldstein, M., Hokfelt, T., and Bunney, B.S. (1981). Neuroscience. 6, 2111.
19. Itoh, S., Katsuura, G., and Maeda, Y. (1982). Eur. J. Pharmacol. 80, 421.

CHARACTERIZATION OF SOLUBLE
BENZODIAZEPINE RECEPTORS

John F. Tallman

Department of Psychiatry and Pharmacology
Connecticut Mental Health Center
Yale University School of Medicine
New Haven, Connecticut

I. INTRODUCTION

Since their introduction in 1960, the benzodiazepines have rapidly become one of the most widely used classes of drugs today. They are generally used as anxiolytics, anticonvulsants, sedative-hypnotics and muscle relaxants (1,2). A large body of evidence indicates that the pharmacological actions of the benzodiazepines are due in large part to their ability to interact with GABAergic neurons (3,4,5,6). The characterization of specific receptor binding sites for the benzodiazepines has permitted these interactions to be studied directly at the molecular level. Taken together, these studies provide evidence for a GABA receptor-benzodiazepine receptor-anionophore complex. While this complex explains in large part many of the actions of the benzodiazepines, it is not clear whether all the molecular actions of the benzodiazepines are mediated through this complex. To understand this, it will be imperative to study the molecular mechanisms of these interactions and these studies will require the solubilization, characterization, and isolation of each of the components of this complex. In this article, I will briefly describe some of the results for solubilization and characterization which have been obtained thus far.

MECHANISM OF DRUG ACTION

387

II.   SOLUBILIZATION

Since the benzodiazepine receptors are intrinsic membrane-bound proteins, it is necessary to remove them from the membrane by the use of detergents: high salt alone is generally ineffective (7). Unlike some receptors which have been solubilized and which require the use of a specific or particular detergent for solubilization, the benzodiazepine receptors have been solubilized by a wide number of detergents including Triton X-100 (8), Lubrol PX (9), Digitonin (10), and a number of synthetic and bile salt analog detergents (11).

In spite of the ability to solubilize benzodiazepine receptors in good yields, it has not yet been possible to solubilize all the benzodiazepine sites. At best about two-thirds of the sites are obtained in solubilized form. It is not clear whether this is a technical problem or whether it indicates heterogeneity of sites due to significant biological properties such as differences in attachment to cytoskeletal elements or in ability to interact hydrophobically with the membrane. Interestingly, the ability to differentially solubilize receptors by detergent and by detergent plus high salt has been useful in subdividing the receptor into two different species which have different pharmacological specificities. It has been suggested (12) that the drug CL-218,812 is a potent inhibitor of tritiated flunitrazepam binding in preparations solubilized by detergent alone, suggesting that this fraction is enriched in "type 2" sites while the pellet is enriched in "type 1" benzodiazepine receptors. This type of heterogeneity has been also studied by photolabeling and it has been suggested (13) that the higher molecular weight forms of the benzodiazepine receptors recognized more potently CL-218,812.

III.   AFFINITY CHANGES IN
SOLUBLE RECEPTORS

In general, the affinity of the benzodiazepine receptor is relatively unchanged by solubilization. A number of groups have looked fairly extensively at the ability of the benzodiazepine receptors to interact with other putative members of the complex such as GABA receptors. Initial reports on solubilized preparations were conflicting with some reports indicating that GABAergic agents affected benzodiazepine binding (10) while other reports indicated no affect on benzodiazepine bindings by GABA (9). Some of these initial differences were due to release of GABA upon solubilization. Apparently, membrane bound preparations can contain and even generate GABA which is released during solubilization. Dialysis of detergent extracts results in both soluble muscimol binding activity reappearing and at least partial restoration of GABAergic modulation of soluble benzodiazepine binding (14). In partly purified preparations it has been found that the benzodiazepine receptors and GABA receptors tend to co-purify (15). These results suggest that the both of the binding sites are contained within the same protein or complex of proteins which remains tightly associated following solubilization. However, since these preparations are not totally pure, additional purification may resolve these binding activities.

Other studies have suggested that the two activities may be resolved and depending on solubilization⁻ conditions it has been reported that GABA receptors alone, benzodiazepine receptors alone, or both can be solubilized together (16). Also autoradiographic studies have suggested the GABA sites and benzodiazepine sites have a different pattern of distribution in the brain (17) and ontogenic studies (18) suggest that benzodiazepine and GABA receptors develop at different rates. On the basis of this sort of evidence, therefore, it would appear unlikely that the GABA receptor and the benzodiazepine receptor are on the same protein. They may be part of a single complex or may represent the subunits of a more complex multimeric protein.

IV. PHYSICOCHEMICAL CHARACTERIZATION OF
BENZODIAZEPINE RECEPTORS

The molecular weight of solubilized benzodiazepine receptors has been investigated by a number of techniques including gel permeation chromatography, sucrose gradient centrification, polyacrylamide gel electrophoresis and, radiation inactivation. In general, the gel filtration studies have indicated an apparent molecular weight for the solubilized benzodiazepine receptor of about 200,000–250,000 daltons in non-ionic detergents (9,19). Considerably different values have been obtained using bile salt detergents where generally higher molecular weights are observed (20). The size of the solubilized benzodiazepine receptor has also been estimated by sucrose density gradient centrification. If the benzodiazepine receptor is assumed to be a globular protein and similar in shape and partial specific volume to the standards used, the corresponding apparent molecular weight is between 230,000-300,000 (7,9). Finally, size estimates for benzodiazepine receptors have been obtained using radiation inactivation. However, using this technique which measures the apparent in situ molecular weight of the receptor, the reported values have varied by nearly four-fold. Using a lyophilized bovine cerebral cortical preparation, a molecular weight of about 216,000 was reported (20). This value is very similar to the gel permeation chromatography. However, this may be a coincidental result. Using frozen rat brain preparation a value of approximately 57,000 has been obtained for tritiated benzodiazepine binding (21). This is similar to the values obtained by polyacrylamide gel electrophoresis for the photolabeled receptor on SDS gels. The third study using lyophilized rat brain membranes obtained an apparent molecular weight of about 90,000. This value was decreased to 63,000 if the membranes were treated with GABA before lyophilization (22). It is not clear why the various groups have obtained such varying molecular weights and size estimates using a similar technique.

The molecular weight of the photolabeled benzodiazepine receptor (23-26) has been determined using polyacrylamide gel electrophoresis and under the dissociating conditions. The subunit molecular weight various groups have indicated that the major photolabeled component has a molecular weight of 50,000. In addition, several groups have reported higher molecular weights species. Using unpurified hippocampal and rat striatial brain or mouse membranes, additional molecular weight species of 53,55, and 59,000 have been reported (13) and the pattern of these higher molecular weight species changes during development (27). Since the higher molecular weight bands are normally fainter bands, it is possible that they may represent synthetic precursors to the slightly lower molecular weight compounds.

V.   CHEMICAL MODIFICATION OF BENZODIAZEPINE RECEPTORS

A number of groups have attempted to study the amino acids present at the active site of the benzodiazepine receptor by chemical modification of functional groups in brain membranes.

By these techniques some implication of a histidine residue has been made (28); although the reagent used is fairly specific, it is possible that modification of other nucleophilic groups may contribute to the inactivation of binding by this reagent. Similarly, a number of acetylating agents which will acetylate phenolic groups have indicated that a tyrosine may be close to the active site (29). Finally, a number of groups have indicated that sulfhydryl reagents do not have major effects on benzodiazepine binding. These data would indicate that exposed cysteine residues are not intimately involved in the binding site (9). However, other studies have indicated that sulfhydryls may be involved in the secondary structure of the receptor itself (30). Decreases in binding due to sulfhydryl modification may actually have ultimate rather than specific effects at the binding site. Further work will be required to determine what the role of such functional groups at the receptor active site might be and to study the amino acids at the molecular site of action of the benzodiazepine receptor.

VI. PURIFICATION OF BENZODIAZEPINE RECEPTORS

A. Affinity Labeling

The number of groups have made use of affinity labeling to label the benzodiazepine receptor. These include photo affinity labeling described above and also a number of alkylating benzodiazepine derivatives have been prepared (31,32). These will inhibit benzodiazepine binding in vivo and in vitro in a non-competitive fashion, consistent with their ability to covalently modify the active site of the receptor.

B. Photo Affinity Labeling

A number of benzodiazepines containing a nitro group in position 7 appear capable of undergoing a photochemical reaction which results in their ability to covalently attach to the binding site (23-25). In particular, tritiated flunitrazepam will undergo this reaction and has provided a method of radioactively labeling the receptor. This type of technique has yielded valuable information concerning the molecular size, the localization (33), membrane configuration, and possible agonist-antagonist interaction at the benzodiazepine site (34-36).

C. Affinity Chromatography

Several different affinity gel resins have been prepared for purification of benzodiazepine receptors. Generally, these analogs of benzodiazepines contain a primary or secondary amine group. A flurazepam analog has been coupled to cyanogen bromide activated Sepharose through a seven carbon side arm (37,38). In early work using these resins, it was not possible to obtain affinity elution. Recently, however, the same compound has been coupled using an adipic acid dihydrazide spacer arm. An affinity elution has been obtained using high concentrations of chlorazepate (19,39). Using these columns, it has been possible to obtain over a 700-fold purification in one step. Hopefully in the near future, the use of affinity chromatography will result in rapid purification of the benzodiazepine receptors.

VII.   PROTEOLYTIC GENERATION OF PHOTOLABELED FRAGMENTS

Another approach based on the ability of limited proteolysis to release benzodiazepine receptor fragments of prelabeled receptors has been useful in generating small molecular weight fragments which are suitable for purification and for sequencing (Klotz, K., Neale, J. and Tallman, J., submitted). In general, proteolytic degradation of membrane bound benzodiazepine receptors results in the generation of smaller molecular weight fragments in the membrane and finally release of the material with approximately a molecular weight of 5,000 into the supernatant. It is possible to concentrate and purify these fragments using peptide methodology. In the not too distant future, we will obtain pure material in sufficient quantity for amino acid sequencing. Interestingly, the presence of an endogenous trypsin activity which is capable of degrading the benzodiazepine receptor in situ has also been demonstrated.

CONCLUSIONS

I am hopeful that these approaches which are complementary to each other will ultimately result in the very careful delineation of the molecular parameters of the benzodiazepine binding sites. Taken with possible purification of other members of the complex, we should have a very clear idea of the makeup of the benzodiazepine receptor, GABA receptor and anionophore complex. Understanding the function of this complex at a molecular level will allow us to develop better drugs for the treatment of anxiety.

REFERENCES

1. Sternbach, L. H., Randall, L. O., and Gustafson, S. R., in "Psychopharmacological Agents" (M. Gordon, Ed.), Vol. 1, p. 137. Academic Press, New York, 1964.
2. Randall, L. O., Schallek, W., Sternbach, L. H., Ning, R.Y., in "Psychopharmacological Agents" Vol. 3, pp. 175-281. Academic Press, New York, 1974.
3. Costa, E., and Guidotti, G., Ann. Rev. Pharmacol. Toxicol. 19:531-545 (1979).
4. Tallman, J. F., Paul, S. M., Skolnick, P., and Gallager, D. W., Science 207:274-281 (1980).
5. Haefely, W., Pieri, L., Polc, P., Schaffner, R., in "Handbook of Experimental Pharmacology" (Springer-Verlag), Vol.55/II, pp. 13-362, Berlin, Heidelberg, 1981.
6. Olsen, R. W., Ann. Rev. Pharmacol. Toxicol. 22:245-277 (1982).
7. Sherman-Gold, R., and Dudai, Y., Brain Res. 198:485-490 (1980).
8. Lang, B., Barnard, E. A., Chang, L. R., and Dolly, J. O., FEBS Lett. 104:149-153 (1979).
9. Yousufi, A. K. M., Thomas, J. W., and Tallman, J. F., Life Sci. 25:463-469 (1979).
10. Gavish, M., Chang, R. S., and Snyder, S. H., Life Sci. 25:783-789 (1979).
11. Stephenson, F. A., Watkins, A. E., and Olsen, R. W., Eur. J. Biochem. 123:291:298 (1982).
12. Lo, M. M. S., and Snyder, S. H., Soc. Neurosci. Abstr. 8:572 (1982).
13. Sieghart, W., Mayer, A., and Drexler, G., Eur. J. Pharm. 88:291-299 (1983).
14. Thomas, J. W., Characterization of mammalian benzodiazepine binding sites. Dissertation, George Washington University (1982).
15. Gavish, M. and Snyder, S. H., Proc. Natl. Acad. Sci. USA. 78:1939-1942 (1981).
16. Massotti, M., Guidotti, A., and Costa, E., J. Neurosci. 1:409-418 (1981).
17. Young, W. S., and Kuhar, M. J., Nature 280:393-395 (1979).
18. Palacios, J. M., Niehoff, D. L., and Kuhar, M. J., Brain Res. 179:390-395 (1979).
19. Martini, C., Lucacchini, A., Ronca, G., Hrelia, S., and Rossi, C. A., J. Neurochem. 38:15-19 (1982).
20. Chang, L. R., Barnard, E. A., Lo, M. M., and Dolly, J. O., FEBS Lett. 126:309-312 (1981).

21. Paul, S. M., Kempner, E. A., and Skolnick, P., Eur. J. Pharmacol. 76:465-466 (1981).
22. Doble, A., and Iversen, L. L., Nature 295:522-523 (1982).
23. Mohler, H., Battersby, M. K., and Richards, J. G., Proc. Natl. Acad. Sci. USA 77:1666-1670 (1980).
24. Thomas, J. W., and Tallman, J. F., J. Biol. Chem. 256:9838-9842 (1981).
25. Sieghart, W., and Karobath, M., Nature 286:285-287 (1980).
26. Sieghart, W., and Mohler, H., Europ. J. Pharmacol. 81:171-173 (1982).
27. Sieghart, W., and Mayer, A., Neurosci. Lett. 31:71-74 (1982).
28. Burch, T. P., and Ticku, M. K., Proc. Natl. Acad. Sci. 78:3945-3949 (1981).
29. Sherman-Gold, R. and Dudai, Y., FEBS Lett. 131:313-316 (1981).
30. Martini, C., and Lucacchini, A., J. Neurochem. 38:1768-1770 (1982).
31. Rice, K. C., Brossi, A., Tallman, J., Paul, S. M., Skolnick, P., Nature 278:854-855 (1979).
32. Williams, E. F., Rice, K. C., Mattson, M., Paul, S. M., and Skolnick, P., Pharmacol. Biochem. Behav. 14:487-491 (1981).
33. Battersby, M. K., Richards, J. G., Mohler, H., Europ. J. Pharmacol. 57:277-278 (1979).
34. Mohler, H., Europ. J. Pharmacol. 80:435-436 (1982).
35. Thomas, J. W., and Tallman, J. F., J. Neurosci. 3:433-440 (1983).
36. Kochman, R. L., and Hirsch, J. D., Mol. Pharmacol. 22:335-341 (1982).
37. Tallman, J. F., and Gallager, D. W., Pharmacol. Biochem. Behav. 10:809-813 (1979).
38. Gavish, M., and Snyder, S. H., Nature 287:651-652 (1980).
39. Sigel, E., Mamalaki, C., and Barnard, E. A., FEBS Lett. 147:45-48 (1982).

INDEX

A

AA oligomers, 17
AB oligomers, 17–18
N-Acetoxy acetoaminofluorene, 112
Acetylcholine
  gallamine and, 31
  positively cooperative interaction with, 32
Acetylcholine receptor, ligand occupation and
  response in, 9–24
Actinomycin D, 110
Adenosine deaminase, 109
Adenosine receptors, 355–358
Adenylate cyclase
  A_1-adenosine receptor and, 357
  activation by choleragen-catalyzed ADP
    ribosylation, 291–294
  activation by toxin-catalyzed ADP-
    ribosylation, 289–298
  choleragen and, 289
  cholera toxin activation of, 364
  desensitization of, 363–373
    heterologous, 367–371
    homologous, 363–367
    hormone-receptor-mediated activation of,
      352
    neurotransmitters or neuromodulators and,
      354, 358
    opiate receptor and, 341–349
    prostacyclin stimulation of, 210–211
    reconstitution of activity in S49 cyc⁻
      membranes, 369
    serotonin-activated, 200–202
    soluble, 368–370
Adenylate cyclase inhibitor, 229
Adenylate cyclase system, control of activity of,
  353–355
Adipose tissue LPL activity, endotoxin and, 177
ADP-ribosylation, requirements for, 291–292
ADP-ribocyltransferase activity, choleragen and,
  291, 296–297
Affinity, stereoselectivity and, 65–72

African trypanosomes, DFMO activity against,
  163–164, *see also* Trypanosomes
Agonist affinity control, nucleotides and, 343
Agonist-antagonist sites, irreversible inactivation
  of, 13–14
Agonist-elicited response, reversible antagonists
  and, 18–19
AHH [aryl hydrocarbon (benzo(a)pyrene)]
  hydrolase activity, 328–337
    TCDD and, 333
    in variant cell types, 331–336
Allopurinol metabolism, 148
Allopurinol ribonucleoside, HPP conversion to,
  150
Allopurinol ribonucleoside-5′-monophosphate,
  148
α-toxin association, as irreversible process, 13,
  see also Cobra α-toxin
Alprenolol, 39
Amines, receptors to, 355–358
Aminopyrazolopyrimidine-5′-monophosphate,
  148–150
Antagonist inhibition of ¹²⁵I-α-toxin binding,
  concentration dependence in, 21
Antiinflammatory drugs
  leukocyte infiltration and, 238
  in myocardial infarction, 236–237
Aquatic organisms, metal regulation, and
  toxicity in, 277–285
Aqueous media, metal speciation in, 278
Arachidonate, endothelium and, 246–247
Arachidonic acid
  exogenous, 233
  12-HETE and, 234
  lipoxygenase products and, 221
  leukotrenes and, 221–223
  prostacyclin and, 209
Arachidonic metabolism, vascular wall function
  and, 252–253
Aryl hydrocarbon (benzo(a)pyrene) hydroxylase,
  see AHH
Asparagine synthetase, 109